安徽省高等学校"十二五"规划教材

高等学校规划教材

药学系列

天然药物化学实验指导

TIANRAN YAOWU HUAXUE SHIYAN ZHIDAO

卫强 主编

北京师范大学出版集团
BEIJING NORMAL UNIVERSITY PUBLISHING GROUP
安徽大学出版社

图书在版编目(CIP)数据

天然药物化学实验指导/卫强主编. —合肥:安徽大学出版社,2014.12(2024.12重印)

高等学校规划教材.药学系列

ISBN 978-7-5664-0784-9

Ⅰ.①天… Ⅱ.①卫… Ⅲ.①生药学－药物化学－化学实验－高等学校－教材 Ⅳ.①R284-33

中国版本图书馆 CIP 数据核字(2014)第 134472 号

天然药物化学实验指导

卫 强 主编

出版发行:	北京师范大学出版集团
	安 徽 大 学 出 版 社
	(安徽省合肥市肥西路3号 邮编230039)
	www.bnupg.com
	www.ahupress.com.cn
印 刷:	安徽省人民印刷有限公司
经 销:	全国新华书店
开 本:	787 mm×1092 mm 1/16
印 张:	18.75
字 数:	456 千字
版 次:	2014 年 12 月第 1 版
印 次:	2024 年 12 月第 4 次印刷
定 价:	38.00 元

ISBN 978-7-5664-0784-9

策划编辑:李 梅 武溪溪	装帧设计:李 军
责任编辑:武溪溪 李 栎	美术编辑:李 军
责任印制:赵明炎	

版权所有 侵权必究

反盗版、侵权举报电话:0551—65106311
外埠邮购电话:0551—65107716
本书如有印装质量问题,请与印制管理部联系调换。
印制管理部电话:0551—65106311

《天然药物化学实验指导》编委会

主　编　卫　强

副主编　毛小明　包淑云　周国梁　汪涵涵

编　者（以姓氏笔画为序）

　　卫　强（安徽新华学院）

　　马世堂（安徽科技学院）

　　毛小明（安庆医药高等专科学校）

　　包淑云（皖南医学院）

　　刘金旗（安徽中医药大学）

　　汪涵涵（安徽新华学院）

　　张晓渊（安徽新华学院）

　　周国梁（安徽科技学院）

　　郭　庆（亳州中药科技学校）

　　尉成茵（安徽中医药大学）

　　熊有谊（安徽科技学院）

　　薛红梅（安庆医药高等专科学校）

前　言

实践和创新教育已成为21世纪高等教育的主流，是高校培养创新型人才的重要途径，也是我国高等教育改革和发展的重要方向。《天然药物化学实验指导》是"天然药物化学"理论教学的配套教材，本教材基于理论知识强化实验能力的锻炼和培养，深化和扩展理论知识，具有较强的实践性、应用性和探索性。

本教材以应用型人才培养为目标，以国际化人才培养为方向，让学生在实践中学习基本操作和实验技能的同时，夯实专业英语能力。教材实验指导部分摒弃理论性和学术性过强的内容，结合应用型人才培养实际，以提取、分离等实际操作技术为主要内容，具有一定的实用性。全书共选取20多个基本实验，涵盖了糖类、苯丙素类、醌类、黄酮类、萜类、三萜类、甾体类、挥发油类和生物碱类等内容。教材以中文为基础，配以相应的英文翻译，翻译力求符合英语语言习惯，同时配有英文词汇表，供初学者学习使用。为增加实验类教材的知识性和趣味性，教材中附有植物实物图、仪器图和化学结构图，并设有思考题和参考答案。实验部分包括验证性实验、设计性实验和综合性实验等3种，可满足人才培养和教师教学方式的多元化要求，有助于全面提升学生的应用能力。本教材适用于药学、制药工程、药物制剂、中药学等专业的双语教学，同时可以为相关专业研究生、科研工作者提供参考。

本教材第一章由卫强和周国梁编写；第二章和第三章由毛小明和薛红梅编写；第四章糖类、甾体类部分由薛红梅编写，苯丙素类部分由卫强编写，醌类部分由马世堂编写，黄酮类部分由熊有谊编写，萜类和挥发油部分由郭庆和卫强编写，三萜及其苷类部分由周国梁编写，生物碱类部分由毛小明、包淑云和卫强编写；第五章及附录三、附录四和附录五由卫强和刘金旗编写；附录一由包淑云、薛红梅、卫强编写；全书英文翻译及校译由卫强、汪涵涵、张晓渊、尉成茵、周国梁、熊自谊等完成。本教材在编写过程中得到相关兄弟院校专家和教授的指导，他们提出了许多建设性的意见和建议，在此表示衷心的感谢。同时特别感谢安徽中医药大学刘金旗副教授对本书所做的审核工作，感谢安徽新华学院08级药学专业的甘艳娇、杨淑芹同学以及09级药学专业的高燕玲、孙张章、周梅桂同学为本书的编写和翻译做出的大量工作。

由于双语教材的编写有一定难度，时间上比较仓促，加上编者水平有限，难免存在不足或错误之处，敬请读者予以指正。

编　者

2024年10月

目 录

天然药物化学实验守则 ··· 1
    一、实验要求 ··· 1
    二、实验安全 ··· 1
    三、伤害救护 ··· 2
    四、仪器洗涤 ··· 2
    五、仪器干燥 ··· 2
    六、实验报告 ··· 3

第一章 常用提取和分离技术 ·· 4
    一、溶剂提取法的原理 ··· 4
    二、影响提取效果的因素 ··· 4
    三、溶剂的选择 ··· 5
  第一节 常用提取技术 ·· 6
    一、浸渍法 ··· 6
    二、渗漉法 ··· 6
    三、煎煮法 ··· 7
    四、回流提取法 ··· 7
    五、连续提取法 ··· 8
    六、蒸馏法 ··· 8
    七、减压蒸馏法 ··· 9
    八、水蒸气蒸馏法 ··· 11
    九、超临界流体萃取技术 ··· 12
    十、超声波提取技术 ··· 13
    十一、微波提取技术 ··· 15
    十二、酶法提取和仿生提取技术 ····································· 16
  第二节 常用分离技术 ·· 16
    一、系统溶剂分离法 ··· 17
    二、两相溶剂萃取法 ··· 17
    三、沉淀法 ··· 19
    四、盐析法 ··· 20

五、透析法 ……………………………………………………………………… 20
　　六、分馏法 ……………………………………………………………………… 21
　　七、重结晶 ……………………………………………………………………… 21
　　八、液—液萃取、同时蒸馏/萃取、固相萃取和固相微萃取 ………………… 23

第二章　色谱分离技术 …………………………………………………………… 26
　　一、吸附色谱法 ………………………………………………………………… 27
　　二、分配色谱法 ………………………………………………………………… 29
　　三、离子交换色谱法 …………………………………………………………… 30
　　四、凝胶色谱法 ………………………………………………………………… 31
　　五、薄层色谱法 ………………………………………………………………… 32
　　六、纸色谱法 …………………………………………………………………… 33
　　七、气相色谱法 ………………………………………………………………… 34
　　八、高效液相色谱法 …………………………………………………………… 35
　　实验一　四季青中酚类化合物(原儿茶酸、原儿茶醛)的提取和分离 ……… 36
　　实验二　红辣椒中色素的分离 ………………………………………………… 38
　　实验三　绿叶中色素的提取和分离 …………………………………………… 43

第三章　结构鉴定技术 …………………………………………………………… 45
　　一、概述 ………………………………………………………………………… 45
　　二、结构鉴定方法 ……………………………………………………………… 48

第四章　各类成分的提取和分离实例 …………………………………………… 50
　　### 第一节　糖类 …………………………………………………………………… 50
　　　　实验一　香菇多糖的提取 ………………………………………………… 50
　　　　实验二　麻黄多糖的提取 ………………………………………………… 52
　　### 第二节　苯丙素类 ……………………………………………………………… 54
　　　　实验一　秦皮中七叶苷、七叶内酯的提取、分离和鉴定 ……………… 54
　　　　实验二　丹皮酚的提取、分离和鉴定 …………………………………… 56
　　### 第三节　醌类 …………………………………………………………………… 58
　　　　实验一　大黄中蒽醌类化合物的提取和分离 …………………………… 58
　　　　实验二　虎杖中大黄素的提取、分离和鉴定 …………………………… 62
　　### 第四节　黄酮类 ………………………………………………………………… 65
　　　　实验　芦丁的提取、分离和鉴定 ………………………………………… 65
　　### 第五节　萜类和挥发油 ………………………………………………………… 68
　　　　实验一　橙皮中柠檬烯的提取 …………………………………………… 68
　　　　实验二　穿心莲中穿心莲内酯的提取、分离和鉴定 …………………… 69
　　　　实验三　八角茴香挥发油的提取和鉴定 ………………………………… 73

  实验四 栀子中京尼平苷的提取、分离和纯化 ·················· 75
 第六节 三萜苷类 ···················· 77
  实验一 甘草酸的提取和鉴定 ···················· 77
  实验二 齐墩果酸的提取、分离和鉴定 ···················· 79
 第七节 甾体类 ···················· 82
  实验 薯蓣皂苷元的提取和鉴定 ···················· 82
 第八节 生物碱类 ···················· 84
  实验一 氧化苦参碱的提取、分离和鉴定 ···················· 84
  实验二 黄柏中小檗碱的提取、分离和鉴定 ···················· 88
  实验三 茶叶中咖啡因的提取及其红外光谱测定 ···················· 90
  实验四 延胡索生物碱的系统分离法 ···················· 94

第五章 各类成分预实验 ···················· 98

 第一节 天然药物化学成分系统预试验 ···················· 98
  一、实验目的 ···················· 98
  二、实验原理 ···················· 98
  三、实验步骤 ···················· 98
 第二节 天然物化学成分的鉴别方法 ···················· 101
  一、生物碱 ···················· 101
  二、酚类、鞣质 ···················· 101
  三、有机酸 ···················· 101
  四、氨基酸、蛋白质、肽 ···················· 102
  五、糖、多糖和苷 ···················· 102
  六、黄酮类 ···················· 104
  七、香豆素类 ···················· 104
  八、强心苷类 ···················· 105
  九、挥发油 ···················· 106
  实验 断血流化学成分预实验、提取和分离工艺设计 ···················· 106

附 录 ···················· 108

 附录一 实验思考题参考答案 ···················· 108
 附录二 常用溶剂性质及精制方法 ···················· 116
 附录三 常用干燥剂性能 ···················· 120
 附录四 常用试剂配制及显色方法 ···················· 124

参考文献 ···················· 131

Contents

Experimental Code for Chemistry of Natural Products ·········· 133

    1. Experimental Requirement ·········· 133
    2. Experimental Safety ·········· 133
    3. Injury Rescue ·········· 134
    4. How to Wash the Apparatus ·········· 135
    5. How to Dry the Apparatus ·········· 135
    6. Experimental Report ·········· 135

Chapter 1   Common Technology of Extraction and Separation ·········· 136

    1. Basic Principle of Solvent Extraction ·········· 136
    2. Factors of Influencing the Extraction Effect ·········· 136
    3. Selection of Solvents ·········· 137

    Section 1   Common Extraction Technology ·········· 138

        1. Impregnation ·········· 138
        2. Percolation ·········· 138
        3. Decoction ·········· 139
        4. Reflux ·········· 139
        5. Soxhlet Extraction ·········· 140
        6. Distillation ·········· 141
        7. Vacuum Distillation ·········· 142
        8. Steam Distillation ·········· 143
        9. Supercritical Fluid Extraction ·········· 145
        10. Ultrasonic Extraction ·········· 146
        11. Microwave Extraction ·········· 148
        12. Enzymatic Extraction and Bionic Extraction ·········· 149

    Section 2   Common Separation Technology ·········· 152

        1. Systematic Solvent Separation ·········· 152
        2. Two-Phase Solvent Extraction ·········· 153
        3. Precipitation ·········· 156
        4. Salt Fractionation ·········· 157

5. Dialysis ··· 157
　　6. Fractionation ··· 158
　　7. Recrystallization ·· 159
　　8. Liquid-Liquid Extraction, Coinstantaneous Distillation/Extraction, Solid-Phase Extraction and Solid-Phase Microextraction ················ 162

Chapter 2　Technology of Chromatographic Separation ············ 167

　　1. Adsorption Chromatography ·· 168
　　2. Distribution Column Chromatography ······························ 171
　　3. Ion Exchange Chromatography ·· 173
　　4. Gel Chromatography ··· 174
　　5. Thin Layer Chromatography ·· 175
　　6. Paper Chromatography ·· 177
　　7. Gas Chromatography ··· 178
　　8. High Performance Liquid Chromatography ······················· 180
　　Experiment 1　Extraction and Isolation of Phenolic compounds from *Ilex purpurea* Hassk ··· 182
　　Experiment 2　Isolation of Pigments from Red pepper ············· 186
　　Experiment 3　Extraction and Isolation of Chlorophyll in the Green Leaves ······ 192

Chapter 3　Technology of Structural Identification ···················· 195

　　1. Introduction ··· 195
　　2. Method of Structural Identification ·································· 200

Chapter 4　Extraction and Separation of Various Compositions ···· 203

Section 1　Saccharides ·· 203
　　Experiment 1　Extraction of Lentinan ····································· 203
　　Experiment 2　Extraction of Saccharide in Ephedra ················· 205

Section 2　Phenylpropanoids ··· 208
　　Experiment 1　Extraction, Isolation and Identification of Esculin and Esculetin in Ash Bark ·· 208
　　Experiment 2　Extraction, Isolation and Identification of Paeonol ······ 212

Section 3　Quinones ·· 215
　　Experiment 1　Extraction and Isolation of Anthraquinones from Chinese Rhubarb ······ 215
　　Experiment 2　Extraction, Isolation and Identification of Emodin from Polygonum Cuspidate ··· 220

Section 4　Flavonoids ·· 225
　　Experiment　Extraction, Isolation and Identification of Rutin ······ 225

Section 5　Terpenoids and Volatile Oil ············ 229
　Experiment 1　Extraction of Limonene from Orange Peel ············ 229
　Experiment 2　Extraction, Separation and Identification of Andrographolide from *Andrographis paniculata* ············ 232
　Experiment 3　Extraction and Identification of Volatile Oil from Star Anise ······ 237
　Experiment 4　Extraction, Isolation and Purification of Geniposide from Gardenia ······ 241
Section 6　Triterpenoids ············ 244
　Experiment 1　Extraction and Identification of Glycyrrhizic Acid ············ 244
　Experiment 2　Extraction, Isolation and Identification of Oleanolic Acid ············ 247
Section 7　Steroids ············ 250
　Experiment　Extraction and Identification of Diosgenin ············ 250
Section 8　Alkaloids ············ 254
　Experiment 1　Extraction, Isolation and Identification of Oxymatrine ············ 254
　Experiment 2　Extraction, Separation and Identification of Berberine from Phellodendron Bark ············ 259
　Experiment 3　Extraction and Infrared Analysis of Caffeine in Tea ············ 262
　Experiment 4　Systematic Separation of Corydalis's Alkaloids ············ 268

Chapter 5　Preliminary Test of Chemical Compositions ············ 273

Section 1　Systematic Preliminary Tests on Chemical Composition of Natural Medicine ············ 273
　1. Experimental Purpose ············ 273
　2. Experimental Principle ············ 273
　3. Experimental Procedure ············ 273
Section 2　Identification Method of the Chemical Composition of Natural Medicinal Chemistry ············ 276
　1. Alkaloid ············ 276
　2. Phenols and Tannin ············ 277
　3. Organic acid ············ 277
　4. Amino acid, Protein and Glycoside ············ 277
　5. Glycosides, Saccharides and Glucoside ············ 278
　6. Flavonoids ············ 280
　7. Coumarins ············ 281
　8. Cardiac glycosides ············ 282
　9. Volatile oil ············ 283
　Experiment　Preliminary Test, Extraction and Design of Separation process of Chemical Components from Herba Clinopodii ············ 283

天然药物化学实验守则

一、实验要求

(1)实验前应认真预习,做好预习笔记,明确实验目的,掌握实验原理,了解实验步骤。

(2)实验时要遵守实验制度,认真操作,正确使用各种仪器。观察到的实验现象和结果以及有关的重量、体积、温度或其他数据,应立即如实记录,养成及时记录的习惯。

(3)实验室内保持安静、整洁。不许大声喧哗,不许吸烟,上实验课不许迟到或随意离开。随时注意药品反应情况,及时做好下一步的准备工作。保持桌面、仪器、水槽、地面等清洁。废弃的固体和滤纸等须丢入废物缸内,绝不能丢入水槽或丢到窗外。

(4)实验后包好提取纯化的产品,贴上标签,交给老师。要认真分析实验现象,作出合理结论,写出实验报告。必要时还需查阅资料,进一步了解某些尚未理解的理论和知识。

(5)每次实验完毕,值日生负责整理公用仪器,将实验台和地面打扫干净,倒清废物缸,检查水电开关,关好门窗。

(6)使用仪器时要轻拿、轻放,未经老师允许不得擅自动用贵重仪器。一旦仪器损坏应及时报损、补领。

(7)公用试剂和药品不可调错瓶塞,以免试剂交叉污染。

二、实验安全

(1)在进行回流、蒸馏操作时,须检查冷凝水流动是否通畅,干燥管是否阻塞。在常压下进行蒸馏或回流操作时,仪器装置必须与大气相通,不能密闭。

(2)回流或蒸馏易燃溶剂(特别是低沸点易燃溶剂)时,不能使用明火加热,要根据溶剂的沸点选用水浴、油浴或电热套加热。溶液内要放几颗沸石,以防止溶剂过热冲瓶或发生暴沸。若在加热后发现未放入沸石,则应待溶剂冷却后再放入沸石。加热过程中也不得加入活性炭脱色,否则会发生暴沸。

(3)回流或蒸馏易燃、易挥发或有毒液体时,切勿使用漏气的仪器装置,冷凝管流出液应用弯接管导入接收瓶中,余气应用橡皮管通往室外或水槽。

(4)减压系统应装有安全瓶。加压色谱柱时,色谱柱及储液瓶的机械性能要高,连接要牢，注意控制压力的引入，以防净化管炸裂。

(5)使用易燃溶剂时，应在远离火源和通风处进行；启封易挥发溶剂时，脸部要避开瓶口，并慢慢开启，以防气体冲到脸上。

(6)有毒或有腐蚀性的药品应妥善保管，实验操作后立即洗手，避免药品沾到脸部及皮肤的伤口上。

(7)使用电器设备及各种分析仪器时，要事先了解电路情况及操作规程。使用时注意仪器和电线不要放在潮湿处，不要用湿手接触电源。

(8)欲将玻璃管插入橡皮塞时，可在塞孔处涂些水或甘油，用布包住玻璃管使其旋转而入，防止折断玻璃管。

(9)实验室一旦发生火灾事故，应保持镇静，并立即采取相应措施。应第一时间断绝火源，切断电源并移开附近的易燃物质。三角瓶内溶剂着火时可用石棉网或湿布盖熄。小火可用湿布或黄沙盖熄，火较大时应根据具体情况使用相应的灭火器材。

三、伤害救护

(1)创伤。伤口可用过氧化氢冲洗或涂抹红汞消毒。

(2)烫伤或烧伤。在伤口上涂抹烫伤药，或涂抹甘油、硼酸凡士林。

(3)酸碱腐伤。先用水冲洗伤口。若为酸腐伤，再用5%碳酸氢钠溶液或稀氨水冲洗；若为碱腐伤，再用1%乙酸溶液冲洗。最后均用水冲洗。若酸液或碱液溅入眼内，应立即用水冲洗。若为酸液，再用1%碳酸氢钠溶液冲洗；若为碱液，再用1%硼酸溶液冲洗。最后均用水冲洗。

(4)不慎误食有毒药品。应迅速取0.3～0.5 g硫酸铜溶于150～250 ml温水中，制成溶液内服，或用手指伸入咽喉部，促使中毒者呕吐以排出未消化的药品。

(5)上述各种伤害伤势较重者经急救后，应速送至医院检查和治疗。

四、仪器洗涤

常用的洗涤方法有以下几种。

(1)用水刷洗。用毛刷沾水刷洗，可使水溶性杂质、尘土和不溶物脱落下来，但不能洗去油污和有机物。

(2)用去污粉、合成洗涤剂洗。先把要洗的仪器用水湿润，用毛刷沾少许去污粉或洗涤剂擦洗瓶内外，再用水冲洗干净。

(3)用化学洗涤液洗。对于黏附在玻璃上的顽固斑迹或残渣，可用化学洗涤液来洗。最常用的洗涤液由等体积的浓硫酸和饱和的重铬酸钾溶液配制而成。

已洗净的仪器壁上不应附着不溶物或油污。如加水于仪器，将仪器倒转过来，水即顺着器壁流下，器壁上只留下一层既薄又均匀的水膜，而无水珠附着，则表示仪器已洗干净。

五、仪器干燥

(1)加热烘干。急用的仪器可放于烘箱内干燥(控制在105℃左右)，也可倒置在玻璃仪器烘干器上烘干。

(2)晒干和吹干。不急用的仪器可倒置于干燥处，使其自然晾干。带有刻度的计量器可加入少许易挥发的有机溶剂，再倾斜并转动仪器，倒出溶剂，低温烘干或晾干。

六、实验报告

实验报告要求字迹端正,条理清晰;实验报告的格式可以根据题目作适当调整。实验报告内容除包括专业、班级、实验组、姓名和实验时间外,还应包括以下几条。

(1)题目。

(2)目的和要求。

(3)基本原理。内容包括主要的提取、分离原理及鉴定原理。

(4)操作。以流程图表示操作流程,简明扼要,包括现象的记录。

(5)鉴定。记录化学反应的试剂、现象及结论,色谱鉴定条件,结果及结论。

(6)产品。记录产品的颜色、晶形、重量、熔点及得率。

(7)讨论。内容包括实验过程中的主要注意事项、关键步骤、实验成败的原因以及心得体会等。

(8)思考题。根据老师的要求,回答各实验中的思考题。

第一章 常用提取和分离技术

天然药物化学是研究天然药物中有效成分的学科。天然药物的化学成分非常复杂，往往含有大量无效成分或杂质。因此，必须将有效成分提取出来并进一步分离和精制，以得到纯的总成分或单体，才能为结构测定、药理作用等方面的研究奠定基础。提取就是用适当的溶剂或适当的方法将化学成分从药物中溶解出来的过程，是药品生产的前处理工作。

一、溶剂提取法的原理

溶剂提取法是根据天然药物中多种成分在溶剂中溶解性的不同，选用对活性成分溶解度大，对不需要溶出成分溶解度小的溶剂，将有效成分从药材组织中溶出的方法。当溶剂加到中草药原料（需适当粉碎）中时，由于扩散、渗透作用，溶剂逐渐通过细胞壁透入细胞内，溶解出可溶性物质，造成细胞内外浓度差，细胞内浓度较高的溶液不断向外扩散，溶剂不断进入药材组织细胞中。直至细胞内外溶液浓度达到动态平衡时，将饱和溶液滤出，继续多次加入新溶剂，就可以把所提成分近于完全溶出或大部分溶出。

二、影响提取效果的因素

溶剂提取法的关键在于选择合适的溶剂和方法，但是在提取过程中，药材的粉碎度、提取的温度和时间等都能影响药物成分的提取效率。

1. 粉碎度

溶剂提取过程包括渗透、溶解、扩散等过程。药材粉末越细，药粉颗粒表面积越大，提取效率就越高。但如果药材粉碎过细，药粉颗粒表面积太大，则吸附作用增强，反而影响扩散作用。另外，含蛋白质、多糖类成分较多的药材在用水提取有效成分时，如果药材粉碎过细，虽然有利于有效成分的提取，但蛋白质和多糖等杂质也溶出较多，使提取液黏稠，过滤困难，影响有效成分的提取和分离。因此，用水提取药物有效成分时，通常可将药材碾成粗粉或切成薄片。

2. 温度

因为随着温度升高，分子运动加快，溶解、扩散速度也加快，有利于有效成分的溶出，所以热提取效率常比冷提取效率高。但温度过高时，有些药物成分会遭到破坏，同时杂质的溶出量也增多，故一般加热温度不宜超过 60℃，最高不超过 100℃。

3. 时间

有效成分的溶出量随提取时间的延长而增加，直到药材细胞内外有效成分的浓度达到平衡为止。不必无限制地延长提取时间，一般用水加热提取以每次 0.5～1 h 为宜，用乙醇加热提取以每次1~2 h为宜。

三、溶剂的选择

溶剂提取法的关键是选择适当的溶剂。选择溶剂要注意以下三点：溶剂对有效成分的溶解度大，对杂质的溶解度小；溶剂不能与中药的成分发生化学反应；溶剂要具有经济、易得、使用安全等优点。

常见的提取溶剂可分为以下三类。

1. 水

水是一种强极性溶剂。优点：中草药中亲水性成分，如无机盐、低分子量的多糖类、鞣质、氨基酸、蛋白质、有机酸盐、生物碱盐及苷类等，都能被水溶出。为增加某些成分的溶解度，常采用酸水、碱水作为提取溶剂。酸水提取可使生物碱与酸生成盐类而溶出，碱水提取可使有机酸、黄酮、蒽醌、内酯、香豆素以及酚类成分溶出。缺点：用水提取时，易使苷类成分酶解和霉坏变质，某些含果胶、黏液质类成分的中草药，其水提取液常常很难过滤；沸水提取时，中草药中的淀粉可被糊化，从而增加过滤的难度。故中药传统用的汤剂多用中药饮片不经粉碎直接煎煮；用大量水煎煮会增加蒸发、浓缩的难度，溶出大量杂质，给成分的分离和提纯带来麻烦；中草药水提取液中含有皂苷及黏液质类成分，在减压浓缩时，还会产生大量泡沫，造成浓缩的困难。通常可在蒸馏器上装一个气一液分离防溅球加以克服，工业上则常用薄膜浓缩装置。

2. 亲水性溶剂

与水能混溶的有机溶剂，如乙醇、甲醇、丙酮等，称为亲水性溶剂，以乙醇最常用。

乙醇的优点：溶解性能比较好，对中草药细胞的穿透能力较强，亲水性的成分除蛋白质、黏液质、果胶、淀粉和部分多糖等外，大多能在乙醇中溶解，还可以根据被提取物的性质，采用不同浓度的乙醇进行提取；用乙醇提取比用水提取时溶剂用量少，提取时间短，溶解出的水溶性杂质也少；乙醇沸点低，毒性小，价格便宜，来源广，方便回收，提取液不易发霉变质。乙醇的缺点：燃点低，有一定危险性。

甲醇的性质和乙醇相似，沸点较低（64.5℃），但有视神经毒性，使用时应注意。

3. 亲脂性溶剂

与水不能混溶的有机溶剂，如石油醚、苯、氯仿、乙醚、乙酸乙酯、二氯乙烷等，称为亲脂性溶剂。优点：溶剂的选择性能强，不能或不容易提取出水溶性杂质。缺点：溶剂挥发性大，多易燃（氯仿除外），一般有毒，价格较高；透入植物组织细胞能力较弱，往往需要长时间反复提取才能将有效成分提取完全；如果药材中含有较多水分，用这类溶剂就很难浸出其有效成分。因此，在大量提取中草药原料时，直接应用这类溶剂提取有效成分有一定的局限性。

第一节 常用提取技术

一、浸渍法

1. 冷浸法

取药材粗粉,置适宜容器中,加入一定量的溶剂,如水、酸水、碱水或稀醇等,密闭,不断搅拌或振摇,在室温条件下浸渍 1~2 天,使有效成分浸出,过滤。向药渣中再加入适量溶剂,浸泡 2~3 次,使大部分有效成分浸出。然后将药渣充分压榨并过滤,合并滤液后,经浓缩即可得提取物。

2. 温浸法

具体操作与冷浸法基本相同,但温浸法的浸渍温度一般为 40~60℃,浸渍时间短,却能浸出较多的有效成分。由于温度较高,浸出液冷却后放置贮存时常析出沉淀,为保证提取液的质量,需滤去沉淀后再浓缩。

二、渗漉法

1. 渗漉装置

常用的渗漉装置见图 1-1。渗漉筒一般为圆柱形或圆锥形,筒的长度为筒直径的 2~4 倍。渗漉提取膨胀性不大的药材时用圆柱形渗漉筒,渗漉提取膨胀性较大的药材时则用圆锥形渗漉筒。

2. 操作方法

将药材粗粉放入有盖容器内,加体积为药材粗粉量 60%~70% 的浸出溶剂,均匀湿润后密闭保存,放置 15 min 至数小时,使药材粗粉充分膨胀后备用。另取脱脂棉一团,用浸出液润湿后,铺垫在渗漉筒的底部,然后将已湿润膨胀的药材粗粉分次装入渗漉筒

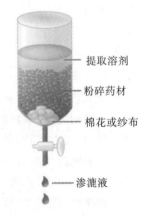

图 1-1 渗漉装置

中。每次装药后,均需摊匀、压平。松紧程度视药材质地及浸出溶剂性质而定,若为含水量较多的溶剂,宜压松些;若为含醇量多的溶剂,则可压紧些。药粉装完后,用滤纸或纱布覆盖在药材上面,并压上一些玻璃珠或碎瓷片等重物,以防加入溶剂时药粉被冲浮起来。然后向渗漉筒中缓缓加入溶剂,并注意先打开渗漉筒下方浸液出口处的活塞,以排除筒内空气,待溶液自下口流出时,关闭活塞。流出的溶剂应再倒回筒内,并继续添加溶剂至高出药粉表面数厘米,加盖放置 24~48 h,使溶剂充分渗透扩散。开始渗漉时,如以 1000 g 药粉计算,漉液流出速度以每分钟 1~5 ml 为宜。渗漉过程中需随时补充新溶剂,使药材中有效成分充分浸出。渗漉溶剂的用量一般为 1∶(4~8)(药材粉末∶渗漉溶剂)。

3. 注意事项

(1) 药材粉末不能太细,以免堵塞药粉颗粒间的孔隙,妨碍溶剂通过。一般大量渗漉时,将药材切成薄片或长 0.5 cm 左右的小段;少量渗漉时,将药材粉碎成粗粉。若粉碎时残留

的细粉较多,应待粗粉充分湿润后将其拌入一起装筒,这样可避免堵塞渗漉筒。

(2)药粉装筒前一定要先放入有盖容器中,用溶剂湿润,且须放置一段时间,使药粉充分湿润膨胀,以免药粉在渗漉筒中膨胀后造成堵塞,或药粉膨胀不均匀造成浸出不完全。

(3)装筒时,药粉的松紧及使用压力是否均匀对浸出效果影响很大。药粉装得过紧,会使出口堵塞,溶剂不易通过,无法进行渗漉;药粉装得过松,溶剂很快流过药粉,造成浸出不完全,消耗的溶剂量多。因此,装筒时要分次一层一层地装,每装一层,都要用木槌均匀压平,不能过松或过紧。

(4)渗漉筒中药粉量装得不宜过多,一般为渗漉筒容积的2/3,留有一定的空间以存放溶剂,可连续渗漉且便于操作。

(5)药粉填装好后,应先打开渗漉筒下口活塞,再添加溶剂,否则会因加溶剂造成的气泡冲动粉柱而影响浸出。渗漉过程中,溶剂必须保持高出药面,否则渗漉筒内药粉干涸开裂,再加入溶剂时则因溶剂从裂隙间流过而影响浸出。若采用连续渗漉装置(见图1-2),则可避免此现象发生。

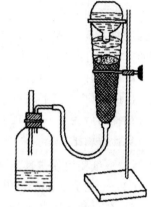

图1-2 连续渗漉装置

三、煎煮法

取药材饮片或粗粉,置于适当容器(勿用铁器)中,加水浸没药材。充分浸泡后,加热煎煮,待药液沸腾后,继续保持微沸,经一段时间后进行过滤,得到水煎液。药渣再加适量水,重复操作,至水煎液味道淡薄为止。最后合并水煎液并浓缩。

一般需煎煮2~3次,煎煮的时间可根据药材的量及质地而定。对少量、质松而轻薄的药材,第一次可煮沸20~30 min;药材量多或质地坚硬时,第一次煎煮1~2 h,第二次和第三次煎煮时间可酌减。

四、回流提取法

将药材粗粉装入圆底烧瓶内,倒入溶剂使其浸过药面1~2 cm,烧瓶内药材及溶剂的加入量为烧瓶容积的1/2~2/3。烧瓶上方接通冷凝管,置水浴中加热回流一段时间,滤出提取液,药渣再加新溶剂重新回流提取。一般需提取2~3次,最后合并提取液(见图1-3)。

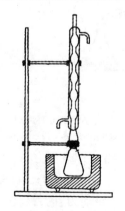

图1-3 回流提取装置

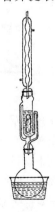

图1-4 索氏提取器

五、连续提取法

1. 装置

实验室中常用的索氏提取器一共分三部分,上部是冷凝管,中部是带有虹吸管的提取筒,下部为圆底烧瓶。三部分通过磨口严密连接(见图1-4)。

2. 操作

先将研细的药材粉末装入滤纸筒,然后放入提取筒,再将提取筒下端和盛有适量提取溶剂的烧瓶连接,上端接上冷凝管。安装完毕后,水浴加热,当溶剂沸腾时,蒸汽通过提取筒旁边的支管上升到冷凝管中,被冷凝成为液体后,滴入提取筒。当筒中液体的液面超过虹吸管的最高处时,由于虹吸作用,提取液自动全部流入烧瓶中,烧瓶内的溶液因受热气化而上升,而溶出的药材成分因不能气化而留在烧瓶中。如此循环提取,直至药材中的大部分可溶性成分被提出后为止,一般需要数小时才能完成。

3. 注意事项

(1)滤纸筒可用定性滤纸捆扎或者折叠而成。滤纸筒的高度以超过索氏提取器的虹吸管1~2 cm为宜。滤纸筒内径应小于索氏提取器的提取筒内径。

(2)药材粉末的装入量不宜过多,放入提取筒内后,药面应低于虹吸管端。应注意不要把药粉撒到滤纸筒外,以防堵塞虹吸管。

(3)加热前,应在烧瓶内加入沸石。

六、蒸馏法

1. 蒸馏装置及安装

最常用的常压蒸馏装置(见图1-5)由蒸馏瓶、蒸馏头、温度计、冷凝管、尾接管(牛角管)和锥形瓶组成。

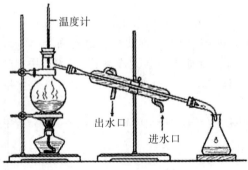

图1-5 蒸馏装置

选择大小合适的蒸馏瓶,调整温度计水银球下限和蒸馏瓶支管上限在同一水平线上。安装顺序一般是先从热源处开始,然后由下而上、从左到右依次安装。安装冷凝管时,铁夹应夹在冷凝管的重心部位,调整位置使之与蒸馏瓶支管在同一直线上,然后松开冷凝管铁夹,使冷凝管沿此直线移动并和蒸馏瓶相连,这样才不致折断蒸馏瓶支管。再装上尾接管和锥形瓶。各铁夹不应夹得太紧或太松,以夹住后稍用力尚能转动为宜。整套装置从正面或侧面观察,仪器各部件的中心线都应在一条直线上。

2. 蒸馏操作

(1) 加料。通过长颈漏斗加入待蒸馏的液体,必须防止液体从支管流出。加入数粒沸石,然后安装温度计,检查各仪器之间的连接是否紧密、有无漏气现象。

(2) 加热。先向冷凝管中缓缓通入冷水,然后开始加热。加热时当蒸汽的顶端到达温度计水银球部位时,温度计读数会急剧上升。这时应控制温度,调节蒸馏速度,通常以每秒钟蒸出 1~2 滴为宜。

(3) 收集蒸馏液。要准备多个接收器,因为在达到主要蒸馏液的沸点之前,可能有沸点较低的液体先蒸出。待此部分蒸完,温度趋于稳定后,蒸出的就是主要蒸馏液,此时应更换一个接收器。如果维持原来的加热温度不再有蒸馏液蒸出,而温度突然下降,这时就可停止蒸馏。应先停止加热,然后关闭水源,拆除仪器。

3. 注意事项

(1) 加入蒸馏液的体积不应超过蒸馏瓶体积的 2/3,一般不少于 1/3。

(2) 当蒸馏易挥发或易燃的液体时,不能用明火,一般以水浴为热源。

(3) 加热前必须加入沸石。若已经加热而未加入沸石,则补加时必须将蒸馏液冷却至沸点以下。切忌将沸石加入已近沸腾的蒸馏液中,否则蒸馏液可能突然放出大量蒸汽,而使大部分液体从蒸馏瓶口喷出,造成火灾及烫伤事故。如果因故中途停止蒸馏,那么再次加热前,应加入新的沸石。

七、减压蒸馏法

在常压下进行的蒸馏称常压蒸馏,也称普通蒸馏或简单蒸馏。常压蒸馏是分离和提纯液态有机化合物的常用方法。但是某些沸点较高的有机化合物在加热还未达沸点时往往发生分解或氧化,所以不能采用常压蒸馏,若使用减压蒸馏则可避免上述现象的发生。减压蒸馏是用真空泵与蒸馏装置相连接,将体系内部的压力减小,使有机物的沸点下降,从而使蒸馏操作在较低的温度下进行。减压蒸馏也称为真空蒸馏。

1. 减压蒸馏的装置

常用的减压蒸馏系统(见图 1-6)可分为蒸馏装置、抽气装置以及测压装置等三部分。

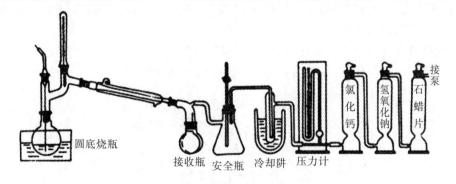

图 1-6　减压蒸馏装置

减压蒸馏装置由圆底烧瓶、克氏蒸馏头、直形冷凝管、真空接收管、接收瓶、安全瓶、压力计和真空泵(油泵或水循环式真空泵)组成(见图 1-7 至图 1-9)。减压蒸馏时,蒸馏瓶和接收瓶均不能使用不耐压的平底仪器(如锥形瓶、平底烧瓶等)、薄壁和破损仪器,以防由于装置内处于真空状态,外部压力过大而引起爆炸。减压蒸馏的关键是装置的密封性要好,因此,在安装仪器时,应在磨口接头处涂抹少量真空油脂,以起到保证装置密封和润滑接头的作用。

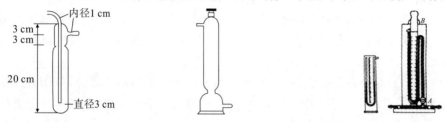

图 1-7　冷却阱　　　　图 1-8　吸收塔　　　图 1-9　压力计(左为开口式,右为封闭式)

在克氏蒸馏头的直口处插一根毛细管,直至蒸馏瓶底部,与底部距离越短越好,但要保证毛细管有一定的出气量。毛细管的作用是在抽真空时,将微量气体抽进反应体系中,起到搅拌和气化中心的作用,防止液体暴沸。因为在减压条件下,沸石已不能起气化中心的作用。在毛细管上端加一节乳胶管,再插入一根细铜丝,用螺旋夹夹住,可以调节进气量。

真空接收管上的支口与安全瓶连接,安全瓶不仅能防止压力下降或停泵时油或水倒流入接收瓶中,造成产品污染,而且可以防止物料进入减压系统。安全瓶连接着泵和压力计。

2. 减压蒸馏操作

减压蒸馏时,加入待蒸馏液体的量不能超过蒸馏瓶容积的1/2。待压力稳定后,蒸馏瓶内液体中有连续平稳的小气泡通过。如果气泡太大,已冲入克氏蒸馏头的支管,则可能有两种原因:一是进气量太大,二是真空度太低。此时,应调节毛细管上的螺旋夹,使其平稳进气。由于减压蒸馏时,一般液体在较低的温度下就可以蒸出,因此,加热不要太快。当馏头蒸完后转动真空接引管(一般用双股接引管,当要接收多组馏分时,可采用多股接引管),开始接收馏分,蒸馏速度控制在每秒1~2滴。在压力稳定或化合物较纯时,沸程应控制在1~2℃范围内。

3. 注意事项

蒸馏结束后将加热器撤走,打开毛细管上的螺旋夹。待稍冷却后,慢慢地打开安全瓶上的放空阀,使压力计(表)恢复到零的位置,再关泵。否则,系统中压力骤降,会发生油或水倒吸回安全瓶或冷却阱的现象。

随着现代仪器技术的不断发展,传统的减压蒸馏装置由于搭置困难、安全系数低,在提取液的浓缩环节已较少使用,逐渐被旋转蒸发仪所取代(见图 1-10)。

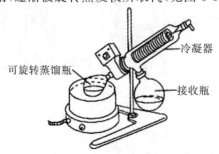

图 1-10　旋转蒸发仪

八、水蒸气蒸馏法

1. 水蒸气蒸馏装置

实验室常用水蒸气蒸馏的简单装置(见图1-11)由水蒸气发生器、蒸馏部分、冷凝部分和接收器四个部分组成。

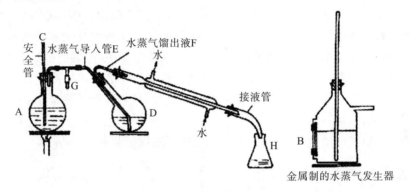

图1-11　水蒸气蒸馏装置

A是水蒸气发生器，一般用金属制成(也可用大的短颈圆底烧瓶代替)。玻管B为水位计，用来观察发生器内水面的高度。C为安全管(长1 m,内径约5 mm的玻璃管)，安全管应插到发生器A的近底部。当水蒸气发生器内的气压太大时，水可沿着安全管上升，以调节内压。如果蒸馏系统发生阻塞，水便会从安全管的上口喷出，此时应检查圆底烧瓶内的水蒸气导管下口是否已被堵塞。

蒸馏部分通常是用体积大于500 ml的长颈圆底烧瓶。为了防止瓶中液体受热后因跳溅而冲入冷凝管内，一般将烧瓶的位置向水蒸气发生器的方向倾斜45°。瓶内液体量不宜超过其容积的1/3。水蒸气导入管E的末端应弯曲，使之垂直于瓶底中央并伸到接近瓶底处。水蒸气导出管F(弯角约30°)的孔径应比管E略大一些，一端插入圆底烧瓶的双孔塞子中，露出约5 mm，另一端通过塞子和冷凝管相连接。蒸馏液通过接液管进入接收器H。必要时接收器外围可用冷水浴冷却。

水蒸气发生器与圆底烧瓶之间应装上一个T形管，T形管的支管连接橡皮管及螺旋夹G。T形管一方面用来除去水蒸气中冷凝下来的水，另一方面，当操作中发生不正常的情况时，可立即打开螺旋夹G，使水蒸气发生器与大气相通，以保证实验安全。

2. 水蒸气蒸馏操作

先将待蒸馏液(混合液或混有少量水的固体)置于D中，在水蒸气发生器中加入约占容器容积3/4的热水，并加入数片素烧瓷。待检查整个装置并发现不漏气后，旋开螺旋夹G，加热水蒸气发生器。当有大量水蒸气从T形管的支管冲出时，立即旋紧螺旋夹，水蒸气便进入圆底烧瓶内开始蒸馏。如果在蒸馏过程中，由于水蒸气的冷凝而使圆底烧瓶内液体量增加，以至超过圆底烧瓶容积的2/3，或水蒸气蒸馏速度不快，则可将圆底烧瓶隔石棉网直接加热。但应注意，防止圆底烧瓶内发生严重的蹦跳现象，以免发生意外。蒸馏速度应控制在2～3滴/秒。在蒸馏过程中，必须经常检查安全管中的水位是否正常，圆底烧瓶中有无严重的飞溅现象。一旦发生不正常现象，应立即旋开螺旋夹G，排出水蒸气，然后移去热源，拆下装置进行检查,排除堵塞后再继续进行蒸馏。当馏出液变得澄清、透明且无明显油珠时,便可停止蒸馏。然后旋开螺旋夹G,使之与大气相通,方可停止加热。否则,圆底烧瓶中的液体会倒吸入水蒸气发生器中。

3. 注意事项

(1)如果随水蒸气挥发的物质具有较高的熔点,在冷凝后易于析出固体,此时应将冷凝水的流速调小,使该物质在冷凝管中仍能保持液体状态,便于流出。假如冷凝管中已有固体析出,并且快要阻碍蒸馏液的流出时,可暂时关闭冷凝水,甚至可将冷凝水暂时放去,以使冷凝管的温度上升,蒸馏物熔融成液体状态后,随水流入接收器中。必须注意,在冷凝管夹套中重新注入冷却水时,要小心和缓慢,以免冷凝管因骤冷而破裂。如果冷凝管已被阻塞,应立即停止蒸馏,并设法疏通,如用玻棒将阻塞的晶体捅出,或在冷凝管夹套中灌入热水,使之熔融成液体而流出,然后再继续蒸馏。

(2)如果待蒸馏溶液的量较少,可用克氏蒸馏瓶代替圆底烧瓶。

九、超临界流体萃取技术

超临界流体萃取(Supercritical Fluid Extraction,SFE)是一项发展很快、应用很广的实用性新技术。传统的提取物质中有效成分的方法,如水蒸气蒸馏法、减压蒸馏法、溶剂萃取法等,工艺复杂,产品纯度不高,而且易残留有害物质。超临界流体萃取是利用流体在超临界状态时具有密度大、黏度小、扩散系数大等优良的传质特性而成功开发的技术,具有提取率高、产品纯度好、流程简单、能耗低等优点。

1. 超临界的概念

任何一种物质都存在三种相态——气相、液相和固相。三相呈平衡态共存的点称三相点。液、气两相呈平衡状态的点称临界点。处于临界点时的温度和压力称为临界温度和临界压力。不同的物质其临界点所要求的压力和温度各不相同。超临界流体(SCF)是指在临界温度(T_c)和临界压力(P_c)以上的流体(见表1-1)。高于临界温度和临界压力而接近临界点的状态称为超临界状态。

表1-1 超临界流体与气体、液体的物理性质比较

相	密度(g/ml)	扩散系数(cm^2/s)	黏度(g/cms)
气体(G)	10^{-3}	10^{-1}	10^{-4}
超临界流体(SCF)	0.3~0.9	10^{-4}~10^{-3}	10^{-4}~10^{-3}
液体(L)	1	10^{-5}	10^{-2}

2. 超临界萃取的原理

超临界流体萃取是利用超临界流体作为萃取剂,用于分离提取某一成分的过程。在超临界状态下,超临界流体具有很好的流动性和渗透性,将超临界流体与待分离的物质接触,使其有选择性地把成分按极性大小、沸点高低和相对分子质量大小依次萃取出来。当然,对应各压力范围所得到的萃取物不可能是单一的,但可以控制条件以得到最佳比例的混合成分,然后借助减压、升温的方法使超临界流体变成普通气体,被萃取物质则完全析出,从而达到分离和提纯的目的,所以超临界流体萃取过程是由萃取和分离组合而成的(见图1-12)。

影响超临界萃取的主要因素如下。

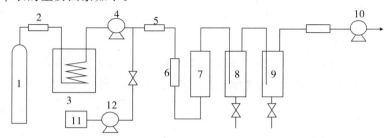

1. CO_2钢瓶　2.过滤器　3.冷冻机　4.高压计量泵　5.混合器　6.预热器
7.萃取器　8.分离器Ⅰ　9.分离器Ⅱ　10.累计流量计　11.夹带剂　12.离心泵

图1-12　超临界二氧化碳萃取装置

(1)密度。溶剂强度与SCF的密度有关。温度一定时,密度(压力)增加,可使溶剂强度增加,溶质的溶解度增加。

(2)夹带剂。适用于SFE的大多数流体极性小,这有利于选择性提取,但这也限制其对大极性化合物的应用。可在这些SCF中加入少量夹带剂(如乙醇等)以改变其极性,大幅度提高萃取的回收率。

(3)粒度。溶质在样品颗粒中的扩散,可用Fick第二定律加以描述。粒子的大小可影响萃取的回收率。一般来说,粒度小有利于$SFE-CO_2$的萃取。

(4)流体体积。提取物的溶解性与所需的SCF体积有关,增大流体的体积能提高萃取的回收率。

十、超声波提取技术

1. 简介

超声波提取(Ultrasonic Extraction,UE)是近年来应用到中药材有效成分提取和分离的一种最新的、较为成熟的技术。超声波是指频率为20~50 MHz的电磁波,它是一种机械波,需要能量载体——介质来进行传播。超声波在传递过程中存在着正负压强交变周期。在正相位时,对介质分子产生挤压,增加介质原来的密度;在负相位时,介质分子稀疏、离散,介质密度减小。也就是说,超声波并不能使样品内的分子产生极化,而是在溶剂和样品之间产生声波空化作用,导致溶液内气泡的形成、增长和爆破压缩,从而使固体样品分散,增大样品与萃取溶剂之间的接触面积,提高目标萃取物从固相转移到液相的传质速率。

超声波萃取的原理:超声波萃取中药材的优越性,主要基于超声波的特殊物理性质。超声波萃取主要通过压电换能器产生的快速机械振动波来减少目标萃取物与样品基体之间的作用力,从而实现固-液萃取分离。其基本过程包括:

(1)超声波能够加速介质质点的运动,将超声波能量作用于中药材药效成分质点上,使之获得巨大的加速度和动能,让中药材基体迅速逸出而游离于水中。

(2)超声波在液体介质中传播产生特殊的"空化效应",使中药材成分物质被"轰击"逸出,并使中药材基体被不断剥蚀,其中不属于植物结构的药效成分不断被分离出来,加速植物有效成分的浸出和提取。

(3)超声波的振动匀化,使整个样品萃取更有效。

综上所述,天然药物中的药效物质在超声波场作用下,不但作为介质质点获得巨大的加速度和动能,而且通过"空化效应"获得强大的外力冲击,因此能被高效而充分地分离出来。

2. 超声波萃取的特点

超声波萃取适用于中药材有效成分的萃取,是彻底改变中药材制药传统的水煮醇沉萃取方法的新方法、新工艺(见图1-13)。与水煮醇沉萃取方法相比,超声波萃取具有以下几个突出特点。

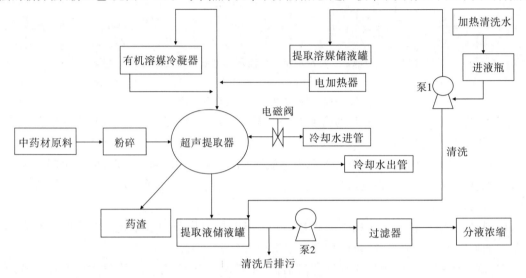

图1-13 工业生产超声波提取器示意图

(1)无需高温。在40～50℃水温下用超声波强化萃取,无水煮高温,不破坏中药材中某些对热不稳定、易水解或易氧化的药效成分。超声波能促使植物细胞破壁,提高中药材的疗效。

(2)常压萃取,安全性好,操作简单易行,维护保养方便。

(3)萃取效率高。超声波强化萃取20～40 min即可获得最佳提取率,萃取时间仅为水煮醇沉法的1/3或更少。萃取充分,萃取量是传统方法的2倍以上。据统计,超声波在65～70℃水温条件下工作效率非常高。而只要温度维持在65℃左右,中药材的有效成分基本就不会受到破坏。使用超声波后(在65℃条件下),中药材有效成分的提取时间约为40 min,而蒸煮法的蒸煮时间往往需要2～3 h,是超声波提取时间的3倍以上。每罐提取3次,基本上可提取出中药材90%以上的有效成分。

(4)具有广谱性。超声波萃取法适用性广,绝大多数中药材的各类成分均可使用超声波萃取。

(5)超声波萃取对溶剂和目标萃取物的性质(如极性)要求不高。因此,可供选择的萃取溶剂种类多,目标萃取物范围广泛。

(6)减少能耗。由于超声波萃取无需加热或加热温度低,萃取时间短,因此,大大降低了能耗。

(7)中药材原料处理量大,萃取效率成倍或数倍提高,且萃取液的杂质少,有效成分易于分离、纯化。

(8)萃取工艺成本低,综合经济效益显著提高。

(9)超声波具有一定的杀菌作用,萃取液不易变质。

十一、微波提取技术

1. 简介

微波提取(Microwave Extraction,ME)是一种常用的提取技术,一般是根据不同物质吸收微波能力的差异,使得基体物质的某些区域或萃取体系总的某些组分被选择性加热,使被萃取物质从基体或体系中分离,进入介电常数较小、微波吸收能力相对较差的萃取剂中,从而达到提取的目的。

微波提取的原理:微波是一种频率在300~300 000 MHz之间的电磁波。它具有波动性、高频性、热特性和非热特性四大基本特性。常用的微波频率为2450 MHz。微波加热是利用被加热物质的极性分子(如H_2O、CH_2Cl_2等)在微波电磁场中快速转向及定向排列,从而产生撕裂和相互摩擦而发热的一种方法。微波加热时能量直接作用于被加热物质,空气及容器对微波基本上不吸收、不反射,保证了能量的快速传递和充分利用。

2. 微波提取的特点

(1)微波具有选择性,能对极性分子选择性加热,从而使极性分子溶出。

(2)微波提取大大降低了提取时间,提高了提取速度。传统提取方法需要几小时至几十小时,超声波提取也需要半小时到1 h,微波提取只需要几秒到几分钟,提取速率提高了几十甚至几千倍。

(3)微波提取由于受溶剂亲和力的限制较小,可供选择的溶剂较多,同时还减少了溶剂的用量。

微波提取一般适合于热稳定性物质,对于热敏感性物质,微波加热易导致其变形或失活;微波提取要求物料有良好的吸水性,否则细胞难以吸收足够的微波能来将自身击破,产物也就难以释放出来;微波提取对组分的选择性差。随着现代技术的发展,连续微波提取已经进入工业化阶段(见图1-14)。

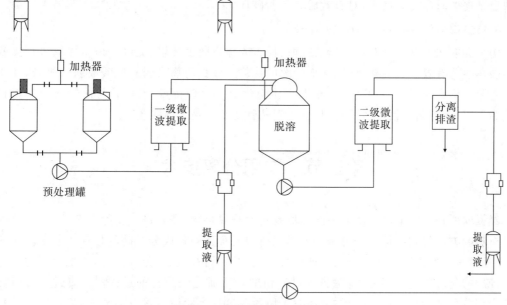

图1-14 连续提取工业微波系统

十二、酶法提取和仿生提取技术

1. 酶法提取

酶法提取是一项新技术。近年来,纤维素酶在各个领域的应用极为广泛,在中药材提取方面的工业化应用也已进入初开发阶段。大部分中药材的细胞壁是由纤维素构成的,植物的有效成分往往包裹在细胞壁内。纤维素是 β-D-葡萄糖以 1,4-β-葡糖苷键连接的,用纤维素酶可破坏 β-D-葡萄糖苷键,进而有利于中药材有效成分的提取。传统的提取方法如煎煮、回流提取等,提取时温度高、提取率低、浪费乙醇、成本高、不安全,而选用适当的酶,可以通过酶反应将植物组织温和地分解,加速有效成分的释放和提取。选用相应的酶可将影响液体制剂澄清度的杂质如淀粉、蛋白质、果胶等分解去除,也可促进某些极性低的脂溶性成分转化成糖苷类等易溶于水的成分而有利于提取。

酶法提取的影响因素有:

(1)药材预处理。为利于酶解,需要对药材进行预处理。如用球磨机作预处理,粉碎颗粒越细,越易悬浮在酶解液中,增加有效面积而易被酶水解,加快水解速度。

(2)pH、温度及酶解作用时间。由于所提取中药材的品种及所使用酶的种类不同,故酶解时的最适 pH 及最适温度也会有所不同,应根据实验结果来确定最佳值。

酶法在提取中有较大的应用潜力,但该技术也存在一定的局限性,表现在酶的寻找困难、提取过程比较复杂。

2. 半仿生提取法(Semi-Bionic Extraction,SBE)

半仿生提取法是一种将整体药物研究法与分子药物研究法相结合,从生物药剂学的角度,模拟口服给药及药物经胃肠道转运的原理,为经消化道给药的中药制剂设计的一种新的提取工艺。具体方法是将提取液的酸碱度加以生理模仿,分别用近似胃和肠道的酸碱水溶液煎煮 2~3 次。这样不仅充分发挥混合物的综合作用,又能利用单体成分控制制剂质量。其缺点是提取时需高温煎煮,对有效成分有所破坏。

3. 仿生提取法(Bionic Extraction,BE)

仿生提取法主要是针对口服给药提取,模拟人体胃肠道环境,克服半仿生提取法高温煎煮易破坏中药有效成分的缺点,又增加酶解的优势。多数药物是弱有机酸或弱有机碱,在体液中有分子型和离子型两种类型。根据人体消化道的生理特点,消化管与血管间的生物膜是类脂质膜,允许脂溶性物质通过,故分子型药物更容易被人体吸收。

第二节 常用分离技术

经提取所得的提取液和浓缩后的提取物仍然是混合物,需要进一步除去杂质,通过分离并进行精制方可得到单体。分离是根据提取所得混合物中各成分之间的物理或化学性质的差异,运用一定的方法使各成分之间彼此分开的过程。精制也是分离过程,是把得到的具有一定纯度的化合物进一步分离,除去少量残留的杂质而达到纯化的过程。分离过程可粗略地分为部分分离、组分分离和单体分离三个阶段。这三个阶段并没有明显界线,根据不同药材的化学成分的具体情况可以灵活取舍。常用的分离和精制方法有系统溶剂分离法、两相溶剂萃取法、沉淀法、盐析法、透析法、分馏法、重结晶、液—液萃取、同时蒸馏/萃取、固相萃取和固相微萃取等。

一、系统溶剂分离法

系统溶剂分离法是指将经提取得到的总提取物,用三四种不同极性的溶剂,由极性低到极性高分步依次进行提取,使总提取物中的各种成分依其在不同极性溶剂中溶解度的差异而分离,结合药理,确定有效部位,可为有效成分的分离提供方便。由于总提取物多为胶状物,难以均匀分散在低极性溶剂中,故常使提取难以完全。这时可拌入适量惰性填充剂,如硅酸土或纤维素粉等,低温干燥使之成为粉末状,再用溶剂依次提取,这样提取就比较完全。常用的溶剂有石油醚、乙醚、氯仿、乙酸乙酯、乙醇、水等。使用该方法时,如有成分化学性质不稳定,则需尽量避免或减少不利理化因素的影响,如过高温度、受热时间长、强酸或强碱等,防止有效成分发生分解、异构化等变化。

二、两相溶剂萃取法

1. 简单萃取法

简单萃取法是利用混合物中各成分在两种互不相溶的溶剂中分配系数的不同而达到分离的方法。萃取时,各成分在两相溶剂中的分配系数相差越大,则分离效率越高。如果在水提取液中的有效成分是亲脂性的物质,一般多用亲脂性有机溶剂进行两相萃取,如苯、氯仿或乙醚等。如果有效成分是亲水性的物质,就需要改用弱亲脂性的溶剂,如乙酸乙酯、丁醇等。还可以在氯仿、乙醚中加入适量乙醇或甲醇,以增大其亲水性。提取黄酮类成分时,多选用乙酸乙酯和水进行两相萃取;提取亲水性强的皂苷等,则多选用正丁醇、异戊醇和水进行两相萃取。

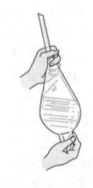

图 1-15 分液漏斗

(1)萃取装置。实验室最常使用的萃取仪器为分液漏斗(见图1-15)。

(2)萃取操作。操作时应选择容积比待分离液体体积大1倍以上的分液漏斗,把下端的活塞擦干,薄薄地涂上一层润滑脂,塞好后再把活塞旋转数圈,使润滑脂均匀分布,然后放在铁圈中。关好活塞,将待分离溶液和萃取溶剂(一般为待分离溶液体积的1/3)依次自上口倒入分液漏斗中,塞好塞子,上口的塞子不能涂润滑脂,但应注意旋紧,以免漏出液体。取下分液漏斗时,先用右手手掌顶住漏斗磨口玻璃塞子,手指可握住漏斗颈部或主体。左手握住漏斗下部的活塞部分,大拇指和食指按住活塞柄,中指垫在塞座下边,以防活塞脱出。振摇时将漏斗稍倾斜,漏斗的活塞部分向上,便于自活塞放气。开始时振摇要慢,每摇几次以后,将漏斗口朝向无人处开启活塞,放出因振摇而生成的气体,以便平衡漏斗内外压强。重复操作2~3次,然后再用力振摇一段时间,使两种不相溶的液体充分接触,提高萃取率。

将分液漏斗放回铁圈上静置,待溶液分成两层后,打开上面的塞子,再将活塞缓缓旋开,使下层液体自活塞放出。分液时一定要尽可能分离干净,有时在两相间可能出现的一些絮状物也应同时放去。然后将上层液体从分液漏斗的上口倒出,切不可也从活塞处放出,以免上层液体被残留在漏斗颈上的第一种液体所沾污。萃取次数取决于分配系数,一般为3~5次。

（3）注意事项。

①先用小试管猛烈振摇约1 min,观察萃取后两液层分层现象。如果容易产生乳化,大量提取时要避免猛烈振摇,可延长萃取时间。如碰到乳化现象,可将乳化层分出,再用新溶剂萃取;或放置较长时间并不时旋转,令其自然分层。乳化现象较严重时,可以采用两相溶剂逆流连续萃取装置。

②水提取液的比重最好为1.1~1.2,过稀则溶剂用量太大,影响操作。

③溶剂与水溶液应保持一定量的比例,第一次提取时,溶剂要多一些,一般为水提取液的1/3;以后的用量可以少一些,一般为水提取液的1/6~1/4。

④一般萃取3~4次即可。但当亲水性较大的成分不易转入有机溶剂层时,需要增加萃取次数,或改变萃取溶剂。

在工业生产中,大量萃取多在密闭萃取罐内进行,用搅拌机搅拌一定时间,使两液充分混合,再放置令其分层;有时将两相溶液喷雾混合,以增大萃取的接触面积,提高萃取效率,也可采用两相溶剂逆流连续萃取装置。

⑤当溶液呈碱性时,常常会产生乳化现象。

2. 逆流连续萃取法

逆流连续萃取法（CCE）是一种连续的两相溶剂萃取法。其装置包括数根萃取管。管内用小瓷圈或小不锈钢丝圈填充,以增加两相溶剂萃取时的接触面积。如可用氯仿从川楝树皮的水浸液中萃取川楝素（见图1-16）。将氯仿盛于萃取管内,而比重小于氯仿的水提取浓缩液储于高位容器内,开启活塞,则水浸液在高位压力作用下流入萃取管,撞击瓷圈而分散成细粒,使之与氯仿接触面积增大,萃取就比较完全。

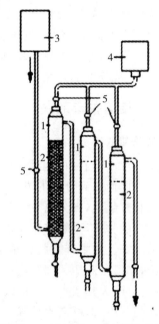

1.萃取管 2.填料层 3.水浸液高位容器
4.溶剂储液罐 5.控制阀

图1-16 逆流连续萃取法装置

如果一种中药材的水浸液需要用比水轻的苯、乙酸乙酯等进行萃取,则需将水提取浓缩液装在萃取管内,而将苯、乙酸乙酯装在高位容器内。可取样品用薄层色谱、纸色谱及显色反应或沉淀反应检查萃取是否完全。

3. 逆流分配法

逆流分配法（CCD）与两相溶剂逆流萃取法原理一致,但逆流分配法的加样量一定,并需在一定容量的两相溶剂中,经多次移位萃取分配而达到分离混合物的目的。本法所采用的逆流分布仪由若干只乃至数百只管子组成。若无此仪器,少量萃取时可用分液漏斗代替。预先选择对混合物分离效果较好,即分配系数差异大的两种不相混溶的溶剂,通过试验测知要经多少次的萃取移位才达到真正的分离。逆流分配法对于分离性质非常相似的混合物,往往可以取得良好的效果。但逆流分配法操作时间长,萃取管易因机械振荡而损坏,消耗溶剂亦多，应用上常受到一定限制。

4. 液滴逆流分配法

液滴逆流分配法（Droplet Countercurrent Chromatography，DCCC）又称液滴逆流色谱法，为近年来在逆流分配法基础上改进的两相溶剂萃取法。目前应用的仪器是：将内径为 2.4 mm、高为 60 cm 的分配萃取管每 25 管接连一板，共装 12 板，合计 300 管的连续分配萃取管。液滴逆流分配法对溶剂系统的选择基本同逆流分配法，但要求能在短时间内分离成两相，并可生成有效的液滴（见图 1-17 和图 1-18）。由于移动相形成液滴，在细的分配萃取管中与固定相有效地接触、摩擦，不断形成新的表面，促进溶质在两相溶剂中分配，故其分离效果往往比逆流分配法好，且不会产生乳化现象。用氮气压驱动移动相，被分离物质不会因遇大气中的氧气而被氧化。应用液滴逆流分配法能有效地分离多种微量成分，如柴胡皂苷、原小檗碱型季铵碱等。但是，此法必须选用能生成液滴的溶剂系统，且对高分子化合物的分离效果较差，处理样品量小（1 g 以下），并需要配备一定的设备。

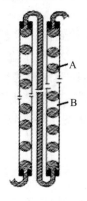

（A：流动相　B：固定相）

图 1-17　DCCC 法的移动相与固定相

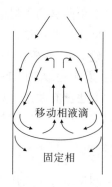

图 1-18　移动相液滴与固定相之间分配示意图

三、沉淀法

沉淀法是在中药材提取液中加入某些试剂使其产生沉淀，以去除杂质的方法。

1. 铅盐沉淀法

铅盐沉淀法是分离某些中药材成分的经典方法之一。乙酸铅及碱式乙酸铅在水及醇溶液中，能与多种中药材成分生成铅盐或络盐沉淀。此法常用于沉淀有机酸、氨基酸、蛋白质、黏液质、鞣质、树脂、酸性皂苷以及部分黄酮等。通常向中药材的水或醇提取液中先加入乙酸铅浓溶液，静置后滤出沉淀，再将沉淀洗液并入滤液，向滤液中加碱式乙酸铅饱和溶液至不发生沉淀为止，这样就可得到乙酸铅沉淀物、碱式乙酸铅沉淀物及母液三部分。将铅盐沉淀悬浮于新溶剂中，通常用硫化氢气体使其分解并转为不溶性硫化铅而沉淀。含铅盐的母液亦需先用上述方法进行脱铅处理，再浓缩精制。硫化氢脱铅比较彻底，但溶液中可能存有多余的硫化氢，必须先通入空气或二氧化碳，让气泡带出多余的硫化氢气体，以免在处理溶液时参与化学反应。新生的硫化铅多为胶体沉淀，能吸附药液中的有效成分，要注意用溶剂处理收回。

用硫酸、磷酸、硫酸钠、磷酸钠等也可除铅，但硫酸铅、磷酸铅在水中仍有一定的溶解度，除铅不彻底。用阳离子交换树脂脱铅快而彻底,但要注意药液中某些有效成分也可能被交换上去,同时脱铅树脂再生也较困难。还应注意脱铅后溶液酸度增加,有时需中和后再处理溶液,有时可用新制备的氢氧化铅、氢氧化铝、氢氧化铜、碳酸铅或明矾等代替乙酸铅、碱式乙酸铅。如在黄芩水煎液中加入明矾溶液,黄芩苷就与铝盐络合生成难溶于水的络合物而与杂质分离,这种络合物用水洗净就可直接供药用。

2. 试剂沉淀法

在生物碱盐的溶液中,加入某些生物碱沉淀试剂,则生物碱生成不溶性复盐而析出。水溶性生物碱难以用萃取法提取分离,常加入雷氏铵盐使之生成生物碱雷氏盐沉淀而析出。又如橙皮苷、芦丁、黄芩苷、甘草皂苷等,均易溶于碱性溶液,当加入酸后可使之沉淀析出。某些蛋白质溶液可以改变溶液的 pH,利用其在等电点时溶解度最小的性质而使之沉淀析出。此外,还可以用明胶、蛋白质溶液沉淀鞣质,用胆甾醇沉淀洋地黄皂苷等。

四、盐析法

盐析法是在中药材的水提液中加入无机盐至一定浓度,或达到饱和状态,可使某些成分在水中的溶解度降低并沉淀析出,从而与水溶性大的杂质分离。常用作盐析的无机盐有氯化钠、硫酸钠、硫酸镁、硫酸铵等。如三七的水提取液中加硫酸镁至饱和状态,三七皂苷即可沉淀析出,自黄藤中提取掌叶防己碱、自三颗针中提取小檗碱等,在生产上都是用氯化钠或硫酸铵盐析的方法。有些成分如原白头翁素、麻黄碱、苦参碱等的水溶性较大,在提取时,亦往往先在水提取液中加入一定量的食盐,再用有机溶剂萃取。

五、透析法

透析法是利用小分子物质在溶液中可通过半透膜,而大分子物质不能通过半透膜的性质,达到分离目的的方法。如分离和纯化皂苷、蛋白质、多肽、多糖等物质时,可用透析法除去无机盐、单糖、双糖等杂质。反之,也可将大分子的杂质留在半透膜内,而让小分子的物质通过半透膜进入膜外溶液中,而加以分离精制(见图1-19)。

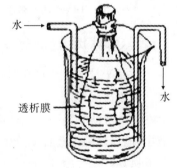

图 1-19 透析法示意图

小心加入需要透析的样品溶液,悬挂在清水容器中。经常更换清水,使透析膜内外溶液的浓度差加大,必要时适当加热,并加以搅拌,以利于增加透析速度。为了增加透析速度,还可应用电透析法,即在半透膜两旁纯溶剂中放置 2 个电极,接通电路,则透析膜中带有正电荷的成分如无机阳离子、生物碱等向阴极移动,而带负电荷的成分如无机阴离子、有机酸等向阳极移动,中性化合物及高分子化合物留在透析膜中。取透析膜内溶液进行定性检查,可得知透析是否完全。

透析是否成功与透析膜的规格关系极大。透析膜有动物性膜、火棉胶膜、羊皮纸膜(硫酸纸膜)、蛋白质胶膜、玻璃纸膜等。市售玻璃纸或动物性半透膜多扎成袋状,外面用尼龙网袋加以保护。一般透析膜可以自制。可采用动物半透膜,如猪、牛的膀胱膜,用水洗净,再用乙醚脱脂,即可供用;羊皮纸膜可浸入 50% 硫酸 15~60 min,取出铺在板上,用水冲洗制得,其膜孔大小与硫酸浓度、浸泡时间以及用水冲洗的速度有关；火棉胶膜是将火棉胶溶于乙醚及无水乙醇，涂在板上，阴干后放入水中即可供用，其膜孔大小与溶剂种类、溶剂挥发速度有关，溶剂中加入适量水可使膜孔增大，加入少量乙酸可使膜孔缩小；蛋白质胶（明胶）膜可用20%明胶涂于细布上，阴干后放入水中，再加甲醛使膜凝固，冲洗干净后即可供用。

六、分馏法

分馏法是用于分离液体混合物的一种方法，是利用液体混合物中各组分沸点的差别，经在分馏柱中多次反复蒸馏而达到分离目的。在天然药物化学研究中，分馏法常用于挥发油和一些液体生物碱的分离。

液体混合物中所含的每种成分都有各自固定的沸点，在一定的温度下，都有其一定的饱和蒸汽压。沸点越低，则该成分的蒸汽压越大，也就是说挥发性越大。当溶液受热汽化后，并呈气—液两相平衡时，沸点低的成分在蒸汽中的分压力高，因而在气相中的含量就较液相中大，即在气相中含较多的低沸点成分，而在液相中含有较多的高沸点成分。经过一次理想的蒸馏后，馏出液中沸点低的成分含量增加，而沸点高的成分含量降低。如果把馏出液再进行一次蒸馏，沸点低的成分含量会进一步增加，如此经过多次蒸馏，可将混合物中各成分分开。这种多次反复蒸馏而使混合物分离的过程称为分馏。

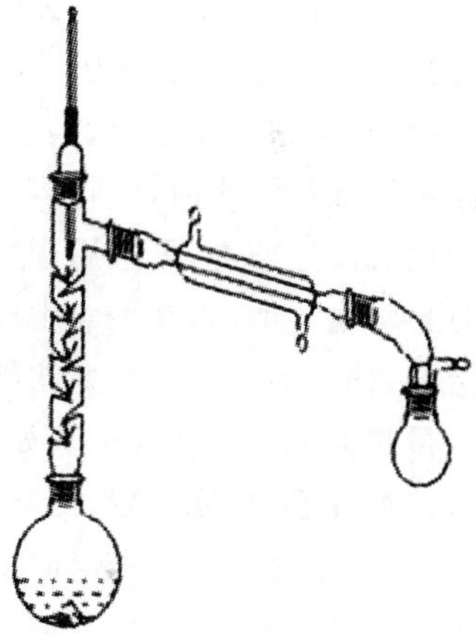

分馏的实际操作是在分馏柱中完成的（见图1-20）。在分

图 1-20 分馏法装置

馏柱内，由于柱外空气的冷却，进入分馏柱的部分蒸汽冷凝成液体，上行的蒸汽碰到下行的冷凝液，就产生了热交换而达到气—液两相平衡。如上行的蒸汽中包含几种成分，则沸点高的成分较易被冷凝，那么随着蒸汽在分馏柱上行升高，混合蒸汽中所含的高沸点成分越来越少，到了一定高度，即可获得某一沸点较低的纯组分。为增加气—液两相接触面，便于更快地达到平衡，常在蒸馏柱内放入填充物（如玻璃管、玻璃珠等）。

在分离液体混合物时，如液体混合物各成分沸点相差100℃以上，则可以不用分馏柱，如相差25℃以下，则需使用分馏柱，沸点相差越小，则需要的分馏装置越精细。若液体混合物能生成恒沸混合物，则达到恒沸点时，由于相互平衡的液体和蒸汽的成分一致，因此，不能继续用分馏法分离，必须用化学方法处理才能得到纯组分。

用分馏法分离挥发油时，由于挥发油中各成分沸点较高，并且有些成分在受热情况下易发生化学变化，因而常常需在减压情况下进行操作。由于挥发油成分较复杂，有些成分沸点相差小，故用分馏法很难得到单体成分，而常常得到成分较简单的组分，如果配合其他分离方法，如色谱法等，则容易得到单体化合物。

七、重结晶

1. 重结晶的操作

（1）溶剂的选择。重结晶对溶剂的基本要求是结晶物质在热溶剂中溶解度大，在冷溶剂中溶解度小。可以通过试验来选择合适的溶剂，其方法是：取0.1 g待重结晶的固体粉末于一小试管中，用滴管逐滴加入溶剂并不断振荡，待加入的溶剂约有 1 ml 时，小心加热至沸腾（严防溶剂着火），若此物质在 1 ml 冷的或沸腾的溶剂中全部溶解，则此溶剂不适用。若该物质不溶于 1 ml 沸腾溶剂中，分次再加入 0.5 ml 溶剂并加热至沸腾，若溶剂量达 3 ml 时，该物质仍未溶解或物质溶于 3 ml 以内的沸腾溶剂中，但冷却后无结晶析出，则此溶剂也不适用。若物质能溶于 3 ml 以内的沸腾溶剂中，冷却后能析出大量晶体，这种溶剂可认为适用。如果难以选择一种合适的溶剂，常可使用混合溶剂。混合溶剂一般由两种能以任意比例混溶的溶剂组成。一般常用的混合溶剂有乙醇－水、乙醇－乙醚、乙醇－丙酮、乙醇－氯仿、乙醚－石油醚等。

（2）溶解及滤过。将试样置于锥形瓶中，加入比需要量（根据查得的溶解度数据）稍少的重结晶溶剂，加热到沸腾，若未完全溶解，可再分次添加溶剂，每次加入后均需再加热使溶液沸腾，直至物质完全溶解，趁热滤过。如果此时溶液中含有有色物质，可在溶液中加活性炭脱色。加活性炭时，应将溶液稍放冷，然后加入适量活性炭，再煮沸 5～10 min，趁热滤过。为增加滤过速度，可选用颈短而粗的玻璃漏斗。滤过前，把漏斗放入烘箱中预先烘热，滤过时再将漏斗取出，在漏斗中放一折叠滤纸，先用少量的热溶剂湿润，以免滤纸吸收溶液中的溶剂，使结晶析出而堵塞滤纸的滤过孔隙。滤过时通常只有很少的结晶在滤纸上析出，可用少量热溶剂洗下或弃去。如滤纸上析出的结晶较多，须用刮刀刮下，加少量的溶剂溶解并滤过。滤完后，加塞放置，冷却析晶。

（3）结晶。产生结晶时，如将滤液在冷却过程中不断搅拌，则可得到细小晶体。小晶体中包含的杂质较少，但表面积大，吸附于表面的杂质较多。如将滤液在室温下静置，使之慢慢冷却，则可得到较大晶体。若滤液经冷却后仍无晶体析出，可用玻璃棒摩擦容器内壁以形成粗糙面，使溶质分子呈定向排列而形成结晶，也可投入晶种（若无此物质的晶体时，可用玻棒蘸一些滤液，晾干后摩擦容器内壁），使晶体迅速形成。

（4）减压滤过。为了使滤过迅速，可采用布氏漏斗抽气滤过，简称抽滤（见图 1-21）。抽滤瓶的侧管用较耐压的厚橡皮管与安全瓶相连，再和水泵相连。布氏漏斗配一橡皮塞，塞在抽滤瓶上且必须紧密不漏气，漏斗管下端的斜口要正对抽滤瓶的侧管。布氏漏斗中铺的圆形滤纸要比漏斗内径略小，使之能紧贴于漏斗底壁，但应能盖住所有小孔。

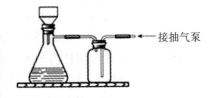

图 1-21 抽滤装置

抽滤前先用少量同一种重结晶溶剂将滤纸润湿，然后打开水泵将滤纸吸紧，避免结晶在抽滤时从滤纸边沿吸入抽滤瓶中。将容器中的液体和结晶倒入布氏漏斗中，进行抽滤。抽尽全部溶液后，可用少量滤液洗出黏附于容器壁上的结晶，以减少损失。洗涤时将抽气暂时停止，在晶体上加少量溶剂，用刮刀或玻璃棒小心搅动（不要使滤纸松动），使所有的结晶湿润。静置，再行抽气，在抽气的同时，将清洁的玻璃塞倒置在结晶表面上，用力挤压，使溶剂和结晶更好地分开。一般重复洗涤 1～2 次即可。每次停止抽气时，必须先将安全瓶上的活塞打开，与大气相通，再关闭水泵。最后取出结晶，置于洁净的表面皿上晾干，或在低于该结晶熔点的温度下烘干。

2. 注意事项

(1) 活性炭可吸附有色杂质、树脂状物质及均匀分散的物质,脱色时应注意以下几点。

① 必须避免活性炭的用量过多,防止吸附样品。活性炭用量应根据杂质颜色深浅而定,一般为干燥粗结晶重量的 1‰～5％。如一次操作不能使溶液完全脱色,则可再用 1‰～5％ 的活性炭重复操作。

② 不能向正在沸腾的溶液中加入活性炭,以免溶液暴沸而溅出。

③ 活性炭在水溶液中脱色效果较好,在非极性溶剂中脱色效果较差。

(2) 如趁热滤过时溶液稍经冷却就很快析出结晶或滤过的液体量较多,则应使用热滤装置(见图1-22),即把玻璃漏斗套在一个金属制的热水漏斗套里。这种滤过方法的好处是,在热水漏斗的保温下,可以防止溶液在滤过过程中因温度降低而在滤纸上析出结晶。在滤过易燃的有机溶剂时,一定要熄灭周围的火焰。

(3) 应用折叠滤纸(又称菊花形滤纸)(见图1-23)时,折纹勿折至滤纸的中心,否则,滤纸中央部易在滤过时破裂。使用时将折好的滤纸翻转并整理好,放入漏斗中,以避免将弄脏的一面接触滤液。

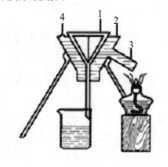

1. 玻璃漏斗 2. 钢制外套 3. 铜支管 4. 注水孔

图 1-22　加热滤过装置

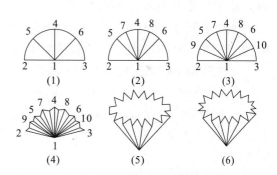

图 1-23　菊花形滤纸折叠顺序

八、液—液萃取、同时蒸馏/萃取、固相萃取和固相微萃取

1. 液—液萃取

液—液萃取是最常用、最普通的一种萃取方法。该方法需要的最简单设备是分液漏斗,常采用少量多次的萃取方法。有条件的话,可采用全自动转盘式连续液—液萃取仪。后者的设备费用要高些,萃取时间较分液漏斗长,但萃取效率高,节省人力。优点:适合于水质样品或水溶性杂质样品,放大倍数高。缺点:极性化合物回收率低,易乳化,可能是由于氧化生成新物质等。遇到化合物发生乳化时,可采用加入 NaCl 和 Na_2SO_4 等盐类(轻溶剂时)电解质、离心或超声波(易燃溶剂不适用)、延长静置时间、慢转动、适当加温等方法破乳化。

图 1-24 是连续液—液萃取仪的示意图。左边烧瓶中加入样品和水,右边烧瓶中加入提取溶剂。溶剂加热后进入冷凝管,冷凝后流入样品瓶。溶剂萃取样品中组分后,通过相分离又回到溶剂瓶。如此反复数次,样品中的组分就转移到溶剂中。

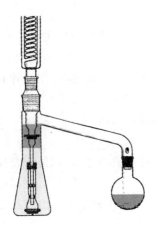
图 1-24　连续液—液萃取仪

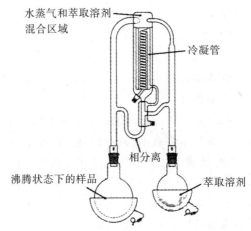
图 1-25　同时蒸馏/萃取装置

2. 同时蒸馏/萃取

优点：容易操作，设备不贵，重现性好，放大倍数高，适用于水质样品或水溶性溶剂样品和含蛋白质、油脂等样品的萃取。

缺点：极性化合物回收率低，这可能是由于溶剂加热会出现基质分解、新物质形成等现象，如糖类生成糠醛，油脂分解为低碳醛等。

一般常用的提取溶剂有乙醚、正戊烷、二氯甲烷等。图 1-25 是同时蒸馏/萃取仪的示意图。将样品和水加入左边的烧瓶，提取溶剂加入右边的烧瓶。两边加热后，样品中的挥发性组分由水蒸气带到中间，并与溶剂在中间交换萃取后，再进行相分离，带样品组分的溶剂进入溶剂烧瓶，而水又回到样品瓶。如此反复进行数次后，样品中的挥发性组分就进入溶剂瓶。

3. 固相萃取

固相萃取（Solid-Phase Extraction, SPE）是由液—固萃取和液相柱色谱技术结合发展起来的一种样品预处理技术，主要用于样品的分离、纯化和浓缩，与传统的液—液萃取法相比较，可以提高分析物的回收率，更有效地将分析物与干扰组分分离，减少样品的预处理过程，其操作简单，省时又省力。固相萃取是一个包括液相和固相的物理萃取过程。在固相萃取过程中，固相对分析物的吸附力大于样品母液，当样品通过固相萃取柱时，分析物被吸附在固体表面，其他组分则随样品母液通过萃取柱，最后用适当的溶剂将分析物洗脱下来。

固相萃取操作步骤如下。

(1) 柱的预处理。为了获得较高的回收率和良好的重现性，固相萃取柱在使用之前必须用适当的溶剂进行预处理。预处理的目的一方面是除去填料中可能存在的杂质，另一方面是使填料溶剂化，提高固相萃取的重现性。

(2) 样品的添加。预处理后，加入试样溶液并保持溶液以一定的流速通过柱子。在该步骤中，分析物被保留在吸附剂上。

(3) 柱的洗脱。在样品通过萃取柱时，不仅分析物被吸附在柱子上，一些杂质也同时被吸附在柱子上。可选择适当的溶剂，将干扰组分洗脱下来，而将分析物留在柱子上。

(4) 分析物的洗脱。用洗脱剂将分析物洗脱在收集管中。为了提高分析物的浓度或方便以后分析、调整溶剂杂质,可以把收集到的分析物用氮气吹干,再溶于体积适当的溶剂中。

4. 固相微萃取

固相微萃取(Solid-Phase Microextraction,SPME)是20世纪90年代兴起并迅速发展起来的、新型的、环境友好型样品前处理技术。该技术使用的是一支携带方便的萃取器,无需使用有机溶剂,适于室内使用和室外的现场取样分析,也易于进行自动操作——这对样品数量多、操作周期短的常规分析极为重要,不仅省时、省力,而且对提高方法的准确度和重现性有重要意义。该技术在一个简单过程中同时完成了取样、萃取和富集三种操作,对液体样品中痕量有机污染物萃取有重要贡献。SPME萃取待测物后可与气相色谱、液相色谱联合使用进行分离。使用的检测器可以是质谱(MS)、氢火焰离子化检测器(FID)、火焰光度检测器(FPD)、电子捕获检测器(ECD)、原子发射光谱检测器(AED)等,该方法的最低检测限可达$ng(10^{-9}g)$甚至$pg(10^{-12}g)$水平。

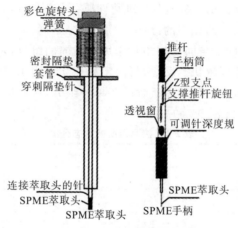

图 1-26 固相微萃取器

SPME有两种萃取方式:一种是将萃取纤维直接暴露在样品中的直接萃取法,该法适用于分析气体样品中的有机化合物;另一种是将纤维暴露于样品顶空中的顶空萃取法,该法采用针头涂敷的吸附剂,对达到气液平衡的气体成分进行吸附后,在气相色谱高温进样口进行解吸附,通过质谱法即可对成分进行定性、定量分析。该方法适用于固体样品中挥发性、半挥发性有机化合物的分析(见图1-26)。

第二章 色谱分离技术

色谱分离技术又称层析分离技术、色谱法等,它是利用不同物质理化性质的差异而建立起来的技术。所有的色谱系统都由两个相组成:一个是固定相,即固体物质或固定于固体物质上的成分;另一个是流动相,即可以流动的物质,如水和各种溶媒。当待分离的混合物随溶媒(流动相)通过固定相时,由于各组分的理化性质存在差异,与两相发生相互作用(吸附、溶解、结合等)的能力不同,在两相中的分配(含量对比)不同,而且随溶媒向前移动,各组分不断地在两相中进行再分配。与固定相相互作用力越弱的组分,随流动相移动时受到的阻滞作用越小,向前移动的速度越快。反之,与固定相相互作用力越强的组分,向前移动的速度越慢。分步收集流出液,可得到样品中所含的各单一组分,从而达到将各组分分离的目的。色谱法的常用分类见表2-1、表2-2和表2-3。

表2-1 按两相所处状态分类

固定相	流动相	
	液体	气体
液体	液—液色谱法	气—液色谱法
固体	液—固色谱法	气—固色谱法

表2-2 按色谱原理分类

名称	分离原理
吸附色谱法	组分在吸附剂表面吸附固定相,吸附能力不同
分配色谱法	各组分在流动相和静止液相(固相)中的分配系数不同
离子交换色谱法	固定相是离子交换剂,各组分与离子交换剂的亲和力不同
凝胶色谱法	固定相是多孔凝胶,各组分的分子大小不同,在凝胶上受阻滞程度不同
亲和色谱法	固定相只能与一种待分离组分专一结合,以此和无亲和力的其他组分分离

表2-3 按操作形式不同分类

名称	操作形式
柱色谱法	固定相装于柱内,使样品沿着一个方向前移而分离
薄层色谱法	将固定相均匀涂铺在薄板上,点样后用流动相展开,使各组分分离
纸色谱法	用滤纸作液体的载体,点样后用流动相展开,使各组分分离
薄膜色谱法	将适当的高分子有机吸附剂制成薄膜,以类似纸色谱的方法进行物质的分离

一、吸附色谱法

吸附色谱法是利用对被分离物质吸附能力不同的吸附剂使组分分离的方法。常用的吸附剂有氧化铝、硅胶、聚酰胺等有吸附活性的物质。液—固吸附色谱法是运用较多的一种方法,特别适用于中等相对分子质量的样品(相对分子质量小于1000Da的低挥发性样品)的分离,尤其是脂溶性成分。一般不适用于高相对分子质量样品的分离,如蛋白质、多糖或离子型亲水性化合物等。吸附色谱法的分离效果决定于吸附剂、溶剂和被分离化合物的理化性质等因素。

1. 吸附剂

常用的吸附剂有硅胶、氧化铝、活性炭、硅酸镁、聚酰胺、硅藻土等。

(1)硅胶。色谱用硅胶为多孔性物质,分子中具有硅氧烷的交链结构,在颗粒表面又有很多硅醇基。硅胶吸附作用的强弱与硅醇基的含量多少有关。硅醇基能够通过氢键的形成而吸附水分,因此,硅胶的吸附力随吸附水分的增加而降低。若吸水量超过17%,吸附力极弱,不能用作吸附剂,但可作为分配色谱中的支持剂。对于硅胶的活化,当硅胶加热至100~110℃时,硅胶表面所吸附的水分即被除去。当温度升高至500℃时,硅胶表面的硅醇基也能脱水缩合转变为硅氧烷键,从而丧失吸附水分的活性,就不再有吸附剂的性质,即使用水处理亦不能恢复其吸附活性。因此,硅胶的活化不宜在较高温度进行(一般在170℃以上即有少量结合水失去)。

硅胶是一种酸性吸附剂,适用于中性或酸性成分的分离。同时,硅胶又是一种弱酸性阳离子交换剂,其表面上的硅醇基能释放弱酸性的氢离子,当遇到较强的碱性化合物,则可因离子交换反应而吸附碱性化合物。

(2)氧化铝。氧化铝可能具有碱性(因其中可混有碳酸钠等成分),对于分离一些碱性天然药物成分,如生物碱类较为理想。但是碱性氧化铝不宜用于醛、酮、酸、内酯等类型化合物的分离,因为碱性氧化铝有时可与上述成分发生次级反应,如异构化、氧化、消除等。除去氧化铝中弱碱性杂质可用水洗法,制成中性氧化铝。中性氧化铝仍属于碱性吸附剂的范畴,适用于酸性成分的分离。用稀硝酸或稀盐酸处理氧化铝,不仅可中和氧化铝中含有的碱性杂质,还可使氧化铝颗粒表面带有 NO_3^- 或 Cl^- 等阴离子,从而具有离子交换剂的性质,适合于酸性成分的分离,这种氧化铝称为酸性氧化铝。供色谱用的氧化铝,用于柱色谱时,其粒度要求在100~160目之间。粒度小于100目时,分离效果差;粒度大于160目时,溶剂流速太慢,易使谱带扩散。样品与氧化铝的用量比一般为1:(20~50),色谱柱的内径与柱长比例为1:(10~20)。在用溶剂冲洗柱时,流速不宜过快,洗脱液的流速一般以每0.5~1 h内流出液体的毫升数与所用吸附剂的重量(g)相等为宜。

(3)活性炭。活性炭是使用较多的一种非极性吸附剂。一般需要先用稀盐酸洗涤,然后用乙醇洗涤,最后用水洗净,于80℃干燥后即可供色谱用。色谱用的活性炭,最好选用颗粒活性炭,若为活性炭细粉,则需加入适量硅藻土作为助滤剂一并装柱,以免流速太慢。活性炭主要用于分离水溶性成分,如氨基酸、糖类及某些苷类化合物。活性炭的吸附作用在水溶液中最强,在有机溶剂中则较弱。故水的洗脱能力最弱,而有机溶剂则较强。如以醇—水进行洗脱时,洗脱力随乙醇浓度的增加而增加。活性炭对芳香族化合物的吸附力大于脂肪族化合物,对大分子化合物的吸附力大于小分子化合物。利用这些吸附性的差别,可将水溶性芳香族物质与脂肪族物质分开、单糖与多糖分开、氨基酸与多肽分开。

2. 溶剂

色谱分离过程中,溶剂的选择对组分分离关系极大。在柱色谱时,所用的溶剂(单一溶剂或混合溶剂)习惯上称洗脱剂,用于薄层色谱或纸色谱时常称展开剂。选择洗脱剂时,须将被分离物质与所选用吸附剂的性质结合起来加以考虑。在用极性吸附剂进行色谱分离时,当被分离物质为弱极性物质时,一般选用弱极性溶剂为洗脱剂;当被分离物质为强极性物质时,则选用极性溶剂为洗脱剂。如果对某一极性物质用吸附性较弱的吸附剂(如以硅藻土或滑石粉代替硅胶),则洗脱剂的极性也应相应降低。

溶解样品时应选择极性较小的溶剂,以便被分离的物质可以被吸附,然后逐渐增大溶剂的极性。这种极性的增大是一个十分缓慢的过程,称为梯度洗脱,即使吸附在色谱柱上的各个物质逐个被洗脱。如果极性增大过快(梯度太大),则不能获得满意的分离效果。溶剂的洗脱能力有时可以用溶剂的介电常数(ε)来表示。介电常数越高,洗脱能力就越大。以上洗脱顺序仅适用于极性吸附剂,如硅胶、氧化铝等。对于非极性吸附剂,如活性炭等,则洗脱顺序正好与上述顺序相反,在水或亲水性溶剂中所形成的吸附作用,比在脂溶性溶剂中强。

3. 被分离物质的性质

被分离物质的性质与吸附剂、洗脱剂共同构成吸附色谱中的三个要素。在指定吸附剂、洗脱剂的情况下,分离效果与被分离物质的结构与性质有关。如对极性吸附剂而言,物质的极性越大,吸附性越强。

当然,天然药物化学成分的整体分子观是很重要的,如极性基团的数目越多,被吸附的可能就越大;在同系物中碳原子数目越少,则吸附力会越强。总之,要根据被分离物质的性质、吸附剂的吸附强度、溶剂性质这三者的相互关系来考虑。操作方法如下。

(1)装柱。将色谱柱洗净、干燥。底部先放数颗已用纱布包着的玻璃珠,再铺一层脱脂棉。装柱方法有两种。

①干装法。将吸附剂通过漏斗倒入柱内,中间不应间断,形成一道细流慢慢加入管内。也可用橡皮锤轻轻敲打色谱柱,使之装填均匀。柱装好后,打开下端活塞,然后倒入洗脱剂,以排尽柱内空气,并保留一定的液面。

②湿装法。将最初准备使用的洗脱剂装入柱内,打开下端活塞,使洗脱剂缓慢流出。然后把吸附剂连续不断地缓慢倒入柱内(或将吸附剂与适量洗脱剂调成混悬液,缓慢加入柱内),吸附剂依靠重力和洗脱剂的带动,在柱内自由沉降。此间要不断把流出的洗脱剂加回柱内,以保持一定的液面高度,直至把吸附剂加完并在柱内不再沉降为止。然后在吸附剂上面加一小片滤纸或少许脱脂棉花。根据加样量控制洗脱剂液面至一定高度。

(2)加样。将欲分离的样品溶于少量装柱时用的洗脱剂中,制成样品溶液,加于色谱柱内吸附剂液面上。如样品不溶于装柱时用的洗脱剂,则将样品溶于易挥发的溶剂中,并加入适量吸附剂(不超过柱中吸附剂总量的1/10)与其拌匀,除尽溶剂,将拌有样品的吸附剂均匀加到柱顶(始终保持洗脱剂有一定的液面),再覆盖一层吸附剂或玻璃珠即可。

(3)洗脱。

①常压洗脱。色谱柱上端不密封,与大气相通。先打开下端活塞,保持洗脱剂流速1~2

滴/秒,等份收集洗脱液。上端不断添加洗脱剂(可用分液漏斗控制添加速度与下端流出速度相近)。如单一溶剂的洗脱效果不好,可用混合溶剂洗脱(一般不超过3种溶剂),通常采用梯度洗脱法。洗脱剂的洗脱能力由弱到强逐渐递增。每份洗脱液采用薄层色谱或纸色谱定性检查,合并含相同成分的洗脱液。经浓缩、重结晶处理往往可得到某一单体成分。如仍为几个成分的混合物,不易析出单体成分的结晶,则需要进一步色谱分离或用其他方法分离。

②低压洗脱。色谱柱上配一个装洗脱剂的色谱球,并将色谱球与氮气瓶相连通,在 $0.5\sim5\ kg/cm^2$ 压强下洗脱。此法所用色谱柱为硬质玻璃柱。使用的吸附剂颗粒直径较小(200~300目),可用薄层色谱用的硅胶H、氧化铝、细颗粒聚酰胺、活性炭等。分离效果较经典柱色谱好。

二、分配色谱法

分配色谱法是利用混合物中各成分在两种不相混溶的液体之间的分布情况不同,而达到分离目的的一种方法。分配色谱法相当于连续逆流萃取分离法,所不同的是前者把其中一种溶剂固定在某一固体物质上,这种固体物质只是用来固定溶剂,本身没有吸附能力,称为支持剂或担体。被支持剂固定的溶剂称为固定相。用来冲洗柱子的溶剂称为流动相。在洗脱过程中,流动相流经支持剂时与固定相发生接触。由于样品中各成分在两相之间的分配系数不同,因而向下移动的速度也不同,易溶于流动相中的成分移动快,而在固定相中溶解度大的成分移动慢,从而得以分离。

1. 支持剂的选择

作为分配色谱的支持剂应具备以下条件:形状为中性多孔粉末,无吸附作用,不溶于色谱分离时所用的溶剂系统;能吸附一定量的固定相,最好能吸附固定相的50%以上,而流动相能自由通过,并不改变其组成。常用的支持剂有以下几种。

(1)含水硅胶。含水量在17%以上的硅胶已失去吸附作用,可作为分配色谱的支持剂。硅胶吸收本身重量50%的水仍呈不显潮湿的粉末状。

(2)硅藻土。硅藻土作为分配色谱的支持剂效果很好,因为硅藻土可吸收其本身重量100%的水,而仍呈粉末状,几无吸附性能,且装柱容易。

(3)纤维素。纤维素能吸收自身重量100%的水,而仍呈粉末状。

2. 固定相的选择

如分离亲水性成分,用正相分配色谱。在正相分配色谱中,所用固定相一般为水及各种水溶液(酸、碱、盐、缓冲液、甲醇、甲酰胺)等。如分离亲脂性成分,则用反相分配色谱。在反相分配色谱中,所用固定相多为亲脂性强的有机溶剂,如硅油、液状石蜡等。

3. 流动相的选择

在正相分配色谱中,流动相常选用石油醚、环己烷、苯、氯仿、乙酸乙酯、正丁醇、异戊醇等与水不相混溶(或少量混溶)的有机溶剂,洗脱时流动相的亲水性由弱到强逐渐增加。在反相分配色谱中,流动相常选用水、甲醇、乙醇等,洗脱时流动相的亲水性由强至弱逐渐减小。

4. 操作方法

(1)装柱。先将选好的固定相溶剂和支持剂放在烧杯内搅拌均匀,在布氏漏斗上抽滤。除去多余的固定相后,再倒入选好的流动相溶剂中,快速搅拌,使两相达到饱和平衡,然后在色谱柱中加入已用固定相溶剂饱和过的流动相,再将载有固定相的支持剂按吸附柱色谱湿装法装入柱中。

(2)加样。样品量与支持剂量的比例为1∶(100～1000),加样量比吸附色谱少。方法是将样品溶于少量流动相中,加于柱的顶端。如样品难溶于流动相,易溶于固定相,则用少量固定相溶解后,用少量支持剂吸附,再装于柱顶。如样品在两相中溶解度均不大,则可溶于其他适宜的易挥发溶剂中,拌以干燥的支持剂,待溶剂挥发尽后,按1∶(0.5～1)(支持剂∶固定相)的量加入固定相,拌匀后上柱。

(3)洗脱。洗脱方法同吸附柱色谱法,但必须注意的是,用作流动相的溶剂一定要事先用固定相溶剂饱和,否则,色谱分离过程中大量的流动相通过支持剂时,就会把支持剂吸附的固定相逐渐溶解去,破坏平衡,甚至最后只剩下支持剂,而达不到分离的目的。

三、离子交换色谱法

离子交换色谱法(Ion Exchange Chromatography,IEC)是利用离子交换剂上的可交换离子与周围介质中被分离的各种离子间的亲和力不同,经过交换平衡达到分离目的的一种柱色谱法。该方法可以同时分离多种离子化合物,具有灵敏度高、重复性、选择性好、分离速度快等优点,常用于多种离子型生物分子的分离,包括蛋白质、氨基酸、多肽及核酸等。

离子交换色谱法对物质的分离通常是在一根充填有离子交换剂的玻璃管中进行的。离子交换剂为人工合成的多聚物,其上带有许多可电离基团,根据这些基团所带电荷的不同,可分为阴离子交换剂和阳离子交换剂。含有待分离离子的溶液通过离子交换柱时,各种离子即与离子交换剂上荷电部位竞争结合。离子通过交换柱时的移动速率取决于与离子交换剂的亲和力、电离程度以及溶液中各种竞争性离子的性质和浓度。

离子交换剂是由基质、荷电基团和反离子构成,在水中呈不溶解状态,能释放出反离子。同时它与溶液中的其他离子或离子化合物相互结合,结合后不改变本身和被结合离子或离子化合物的理化性质。

离子交换剂与水溶液中离子或离子化合物所进行的离子交换反应是可逆的。假定以RA代表阳离子交换剂,在溶液中解离出来的阳离子A^+与溶液中的阳离子B^+可发生可逆的交换反应:$RA + B^+ \leftrightarrow RB + A^+$。该反应能以极快的速度达到平衡,平衡的移动遵循质量作用定律。

溶液中的离子与交换剂上的离子进行交换时,一般来说,电性越强,越易交换。对于阳离子树脂,在常温常压的稀溶液中,交换量随交换剂离子的电价增大而增大,如$Na^+ < Ca^{2+} < Al^{3+} < Si^{4+}$。如价数相同,交换量则随交换离子的原子序数的增大而增大,如$Li^+ < Na^+ < K^+ < Pb^+$。在稀溶液中,强碱性树脂对各负电性基团的离子结合力次序为:$CH_3COO^- < F^- < OH^- < HCOO^- < Cl^- < SCN^- < Br^- < CrO_4^{2-} < NO_2^- < I^- < C_2O_4^{2-} < SO_3^{2-} <$柠檬酸根。弱酸性阴离子交换树脂对各负电性基团结合力的次序为:$F^- < Cl^- < Br^- < I^- < CH_3COO^- < MnO_4^- < PO_4^{3-} < AsO_4^{3-} < NO_3^- <$酒石酸根$<$柠檬酸根$< CrO_4^{2-} < SO_4^{2-} < OH^-$。

两性离子如蛋白质、核苷酸、氨基酸等与离子交换剂的结合力,主要取决于它们的理化性质和特定条件下呈现的离子状态。当pH<pI时,能被阳离子交换剂吸附;反之,当pH>pI时,能被阴离子交换剂吸附。若在相同pI条件下,且pI>pH时,pI越高,则碱性越强,越容易被阳离子交换剂吸附。

选择离子交换剂的一般原则：

(1)选择阴离子交换剂还是阳离子交换剂，取决于被分离物质所带的电荷性质。如果被分离物质带正电荷，应选择阳离子交换剂；如果被分离物质带负电荷，应选择阴离子交换剂；如果被分离物质为两性离子，则一般应根据其在稳定 pH 范围内所带电荷的性质来选择交换剂的种类。

(2)强型离子交换剂使用的 pH 范围很广，所以常用它来制备去离子水和分离一些在极端 pH 溶液中解离且较稳定的物质。

(3)离子交换剂处于电中性时常带有一定的反离子，使用时选择何种离子交换剂，取决于交换剂对各种反离子的结合力。为了提高交换容量，一般应选择结合力较小的反离子。据此，强酸型和强碱型离子交换剂应分别选择 H 型和 OH 型；弱酸型和弱碱型交换剂应分别选择 Na 型和 Cl 型。

(4)疏水性或亲水性的交换剂基质对被分离物质有不同的作用，因此对其稳定性和分离效果均有影响。一般认为，在分离生物大分子物质时，选用亲水性基质的交换剂较为合适，它对被分离物质的吸附和洗脱都比较温和，被分离物质的活性不易被破坏。

四、凝胶色谱法

凝胶色谱法(Gel Chromatography)也称分子筛色谱法，是指混合物随流动相经过凝胶色谱柱时，其中各组分按其分子大小不同而被分离的技术。此法设备简单、操作方便、重复性好、样品回收率高，除用于分离纯化蛋白质、核酸、多糖、激素等物质外，还可以用于测定蛋白质的相对分子质量以及样品的脱盐和浓缩等。

凝胶是一种不带电的具有三维空间的多孔网状结构、呈珠状颗粒的物质，每个颗粒的细微结构及筛孔的直径均匀一致(像筛子)，小的分子可以进入凝胶网孔，而大的分子则被排阻于颗粒之外。当含有分子大小不一的混合物样品加到用此类凝胶颗粒装填而成的色谱柱上时，这些物质即随洗脱液的流动而发生移动。大分子物质沿凝胶颗粒间隙随洗脱液移动，流程短，移动速率快，先被洗出色谱柱；而小分子物质可通过凝胶网孔进入颗粒内部，然后再扩散出来，故流程长，移动速度慢，最后被洗出色谱柱，从而使样品中不同大小的分子分离开来。当两种以上不同相对分子质量的分子都能进入凝胶颗粒网孔时，由于它们被排阻和扩散的程度不同，在凝胶柱中所经过的路程和时间也不同，因此也可以分离开来(见图 2-1)。

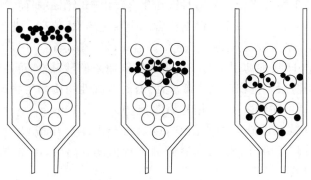

○表示多孔填料颗粒　●表示大分子　•表示小分子

图 2-1　凝胶色谱原理

常用的凝胶类型有交联葡聚糖凝胶、琼脂糖凝胶、聚丙烯酰胺凝胶等。

五、薄层色谱法

薄层色谱法(Thin Layer Chromatography, TLC)是一种简便、快速、微量的色谱方法。一般将柱色谱用的吸附剂撒布到平面如玻璃片上，形成一薄层进行色谱分离，故称薄层色谱，其原理与柱色谱基本相似(见图 2-2)。

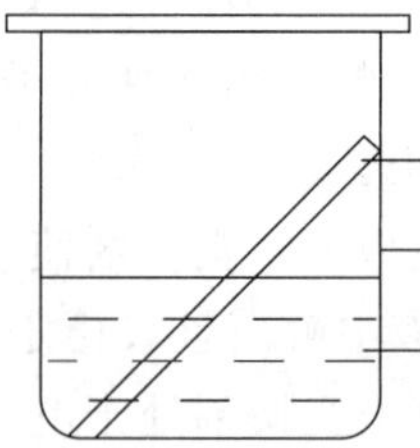

图 2-2 薄层色谱

1. 薄层色谱的特点

薄层色谱在应用与操作方面与柱色谱比较相似。

2. 吸附剂的选择

薄层色谱用的吸附剂及选择原则与柱色谱相似。主要区别在于薄层色谱要求吸附剂(支持剂)的粒度更细，一般应大于 250 目，并要求粒度均匀。用于薄层色谱的吸附剂或预制薄层一般活度不宜过高，以Ⅱ～Ⅲ级为宜。而展开距离则由薄层的粒度粗细而定，薄层粒度越细，展开距离相应越短，一般不超过 10 cm，否则可引起色谱扩散，影响分离效果。

3. 展开剂的选择

当吸附剂活度为一定值时(如Ⅱ级或Ⅲ级)，薄层色谱对多组分的样品能否获得满意的分离，取决于展开剂的选择。天然药物化学成分的脂溶性成分大致可按其极性不同而分为无极性、弱极性、中极性与强极性。

4. 特殊薄层

针对某些性质特殊的化合物的分离与检出，有时需采用一些特殊薄层。

(1)荧光薄层。有些化合物本身无色，在紫外灯下也不显荧光，又无适当的显色剂，则可在吸附剂中加入荧光物质，制成荧光薄层进行分离。展开后置于紫外光下照射，薄层板本身显荧光，而样品斑点处不显荧光，即可检出样品的分离位置。常用的荧光物质多为无机物。其中一种是在 254 nm 紫外光激发下显出荧光的，如锰激化的硅酸锌；另一种为在 365 nm 紫外光激发下发出荧光的，如银激化的硫化锌、硫化镉。

(2)络合薄层。常用的有硝酸银薄层，用来分离碳原子数相等而碳碳双键数目不等的一系列化合物，如不饱和醇、酸等。其主要机理是由于碳碳双键能与硝酸银形成络合物，而饱和的碳碳单键则不与硝酸银络合。分离时饱和化合物由于吸附最弱而 Rf 最高，含一个双键的比含两个双键的 Rf 值高，含一个三键的比含一个双键的 Rf 值高。此外，在一个双键化合物中，顺式的与硝酸银络合较反式的易于进行。因此，络合薄层还可用来分离顺反异构体。

(3)酸碱薄层和 pH 缓冲薄层。为了改变吸附剂原来的酸碱性，可在铺制薄层时采用稀酸或稀碱代替水调制薄层。例如硅胶带微酸性，有时对碱性物质如生物碱的分离效果不好，如不能展开或拖尾，则可在铺薄层时，用稀碱溶液(0.1～0.5 mol/L NaOH 溶液)制成碱性硅胶薄层。如猪屎豆碱在以硅胶为吸附剂，以氯仿－丙酮－甲醇(8∶2∶1)为展开剂时 Rf<0.1，采用碱性硅胶薄层用上述相同展开剂进行色谱分离时，Rf 值增至 0.4 左右，说明猪屎豆碱为碱性生物碱。

5. 应用

薄层色谱法在中药材化学成分的研究中，主要应用于化学成分的预试验、化学成分的鉴定及探索柱色谱分离的条件。

用薄层色谱法进行中药材化学成分预试验时,可依据成分性质及已知条件有针对性地进行。薄层色谱法展开可分离杂质,选择性高,使预试结果更可靠。另外,最好有标准样品用作对照,如用数种溶剂展层后,标准品与鉴定品的 Rf 值、斑点形状以及颜色都完全相同,则可初步认为它们是同一化合物,但一般需要选择化学反应或红外光谱等仪器分析方法加以核对。

用薄层色谱法探索柱色谱分离条件时,首先应考虑选用何种吸附剂与洗脱剂。在洗脱过程中各个成分按何种顺序被洗脱,每一洗脱液中是单一成分还是混合成分,均可用薄层色谱法来判断与检验。薄层色谱法还可以用于了解多组分样品的组成与相对含量。如在薄层色谱上摸索到比较满意的分离条件,即可用于干柱色谱。用薄层色谱法进行某一组分的分离,其 Rf 值范围一般情况下为 $0.85>Rf>0.05$。薄层色谱法亦应用于中药材品种的鉴别、中药材及其制剂真伪的鉴别、质量控制和资源调查。此外,对于控制化学反应的进程,反应副产品产物的检查,中间体分析,化学药品制剂及杂质的检查,临床和生化检验以及毒物分析等,薄层色谱法都是有效的手段。

六、纸色谱法

纸色谱法(Paper Chromatography,PC)是以滤纸作为支持物的分配色谱法。滤纸纤维与水有较强的亲和力,能吸收 22% 左右的水,其中 6%~7% 的水是以氢键形式与纤维素的羟基结合。由于滤纸纤维与有机溶剂的亲和力很弱,故在分离时,以滤纸纤维及其结合的水作为固定相,以有机溶剂作为流动相。

应用纸色谱法对混合物进行分离时,发生两种作用:第一种是溶质在结合于纤维上的水与流过滤纸的有机相之间进行分配(即液-液分离);第二种是滤纸纤维对溶质的吸附及溶质溶解于流动相的不同分配比进行的分配(即固-液分配)。显然,混合物的彼此分离是这两种因素共同作用的结果(见图 2-3)。

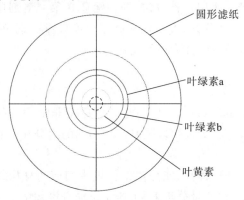

滤纸,展开剂:石油醚-乙醚-甲醇(30∶10∶0.5)

图 2-3　菠菜提取液的辐射纸色谱

在实际操作中,点样后的滤纸一端浸没于流动相液面之下,由于毛细管作用,有机相即流动相开始从滤纸的一端向另一端渗透扩展。当有机相沿滤纸经点样处时,样品中的溶质就按各自的分配系数在有机相与附着于滤纸上的水相之间进行分配。一部分溶质离开原点,随着有机相移动,进入无溶质区,此时又重新进行分配;一部分溶质从有机相进入水相。在有机相不断流动的情况下,溶质就不断地进行分配,沿着有机相流动的方向移动(见图2-4)。

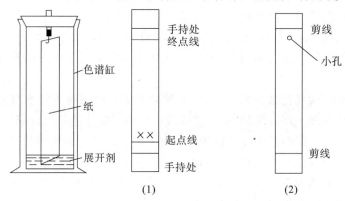

图 2-4　纸色谱垂直展开示意图

可以用相对迁移率(Rf)来表示一种物质的迁移:

　　Rf ＝组分移动的距离/溶剂前沿移动的距离

　　　＝原点至组分斑点中心的距离/原点至溶剂前沿的距离

在滤纸、溶剂、温度等各项实验条件恒定的情况下,各物质的 Rf 值是不变的,不随溶剂移动距离的改变而变化。Rf 与分配系数 K 的关系为:Rf＝1/(1＋αK)。α 是由滤纸性质决定的一个常数。由此可见,K 值越大,溶质分配于固定相的趋势越大,而 Rf 值越小;反之,K 值越小,则分配于流动相的趋势越大,Rf 值越大。Rf 值是定性分析的重要指标。

在样品所含溶质较多或某些组分在单相纸色谱中的 Rf 比较接近,不易明显分离时,可采用双向纸色谱法。该法是将滤纸在某一特殊的溶剂系统中按一个方向展开以后,即予以干燥,再旋转 90°,在另一溶剂系统中进行展层,待溶剂到达所要求的距离后,取出滤纸,干燥显色,从而获得双向色谱谱。应用这种方法,即使溶质在第一溶剂中不能完全分开,经过第二种溶剂的分离也能得以完全分开,大大地提高了分离效率。纸色谱法与区带电泳法结合能获得更好的分离效果,这种方法称为指纹谱法。

七、气相色谱法

气相色谱法(Gas Chromatography,GC)是一种应用非常广泛的分离手段,它是以惰性气体作为流动相的柱色谱法,其分离原理是基于样品中的组分在两相间分配上的差异(见图2-5)。

气相色谱法的优点是:选择性高,能分离结构极为相似的异构体、同位素等;灵敏度高,可分析 10^{-11} 级含量的物质,在痕量分析上,可鉴定出纯有机物中 1 ppm 甚至 1 ppb 的杂质;分离效率高。

气相色谱法虽然可以将复杂混合物中的各个组分分离开,但其定性能力较差,通常只是利用组分的保留特性来定性,这在待定性的组分完全未知或无法获得组分的标准样品时,对组分定性分析就十分困难。随着质谱、红外光谱及核磁共振等定性分析手段的发展,目前主要采用在线的联用技术,即将色谱法与其他定性或结构分析手段直接联机,来解决色谱法定性困难的问题。气相色谱-质谱联用(GC—MS)是最早实现商品化的色谱联用仪器。

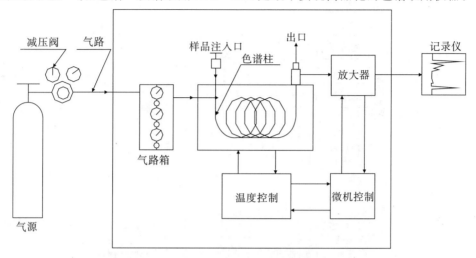

图 2-5　气相色谱仪流程图

现代的气相色谱使用长达 50 m 的毛细管色谱柱(内径为 0.1～0.5 mm)。固定相通常为一种交联的硅多体,附着在毛细管内壁成一层膜。在正常操作温度下,其性质类似于液体膜,但要结实得多。流动相(载气)通常为氮气或氢气。依据不同组分在载气与硅多体之间分配能力的不同而达到选择性分离的目的。大多数生物大分子的分离受柱温的影响。柱温有时在分析过程中维持恒定(等温,通常为 50～250℃),更常见的是设定一个增温的程序(如以每分钟 10℃ 的速度从 50℃ 升高到 250℃)。样品通过一个包含有气紧阀门的注射孔注入柱顶部。柱中的产物可用以下方法检测出。

(1)火焰离子检测法。流出气体通过一种可使任何有机复合物离子化的火焰,然后被一个固定在火焰顶部附近的电极所检测。

(2)电子捕获法。使用一种发射 β 射线的放射性同位素作为离子化的方式。这种方法可以检测极微量(pmol)的亲电复合物。

(3)分光光度计法。分光光度计法包括质谱分析法(GC—MS)和远红外光谱分析法(GC—IR)。

(4)电导法。流出气体中组成成分的改变会引起铂电缆电阻的变化。

八、高效液相色谱法

高效液相色谱法(High Performance Liquid Chromatography, HPLC)是一种多用途的分析方法,可以使用多种固定相和流动相,并可以根据特定类型分子的大小、极性、可溶性或吸收特性的不同将其分离开来。高效液相色谱仪一般由溶剂槽、高压泵(有一元、二元、四元等多种类型)、色谱柱、进样器(手动或自动)、检测器(常见的有紫外检测器、折光检测器、荧光检测器等)、数据处理机或色谱工作站等组成(见图2-6)。

高效液相色谱仪的核心部件是耐高压的色谱柱(HPLC柱)。HPLC柱通常由不锈钢制成,并且所有的组成元件、阀门等都是由耐高压的材料制成。溶剂系统的选择包括:等度(无梯度)洗脱分离,即在整个分析过程中只使用一种溶剂(或混合溶剂);梯度洗脱分离,即使用一种微处理机控制的梯度程序来改变流动相的组分。

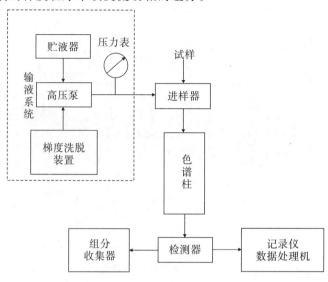

图 2-6　HPLC 仪器组成

由于 HPLC 具有高速、灵敏和用途多等优点,它已成为分离许多生物小分子物质的重要方法,常用的是反相分配色谱法。分离大分子物质(尤其是蛋白质和核酸)通常需要一种"生物适合性"系统,如 Pharmacia FPLC 系统。这类分离用钛、玻璃或氟化塑料代替不锈钢组件,并且使用较低的压力,以避免大分子物质丧失生物活性。这类分离也可以用离子交换色谱、凝胶渗透色谱或疏水色谱等方法来完成。

实验一　四季青中酚类化合物(原儿茶酸、原儿茶醛)的提取和分离

一、实验目的

1. 掌握常压柱色谱的方法和原理。
2. 了解常压柱色谱在天然药物化学成分分离上的应用。

二、实验原理

原儿茶醛(3,4-二羟基苯甲醛)是四季青(见图 2-7)叶中抗心绞痛的主要有效成分之一,具有扩张冠状动脉、增加冠脉血流量的作用。该化合物的熔点为 153~154℃,易溶于乙醇、丙酮、乙酸乙酯、乙醚和热水,可溶于冷水,不溶于苯和氯仿。有引湿性,在水中易氧化变色。

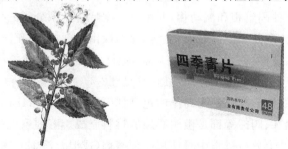

图 2-7　四季青及其药物制剂举例

原儿茶酸（3,4-二羟基苯甲酸）存在于冬青科植物冬青等的叶中，为白色至褐色结晶性粉末，在空气中会变色。该化合物的熔点为 198～200℃，易溶于水、乙醇、乙醚、丙酮和乙酸乙酯，难溶于苯和氯仿。原儿茶酸具有抗菌作用，体外试验时对绿脓杆菌、大肠杆菌、伤寒杆菌、痢疾杆菌、产碱杆菌及枯草杆菌和金黄色葡萄球菌等均有不同程度的抑制作用；亦有祛痰、平喘作用，临床上可用于治疗慢性气管炎。

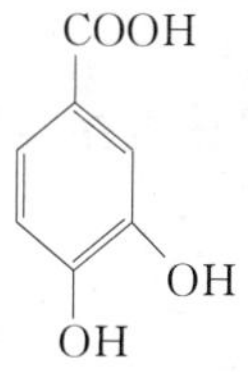

原儿茶酸（$C_7H_6O_4$） 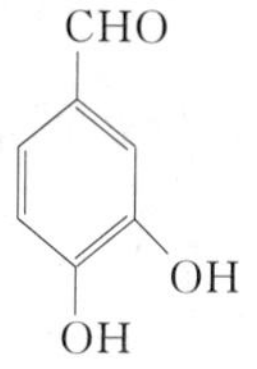　　原儿茶醛（$C_7H_6O_3$） 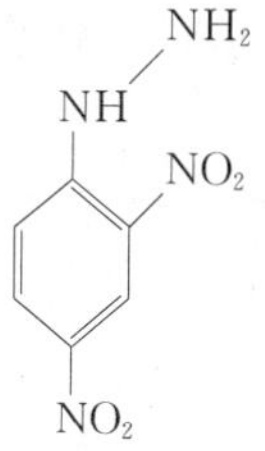　　2,4-二硝基苯肼（$C_6H_6N_4O_4$）

2,4-二硝基苯肼为红色结晶性粉末，熔点为 197～198℃，微溶于水、乙醇，可溶于酸。2,4-硝基苯肼可用于制造炸药，也可用于鉴别醛和酮，与之反应生成的 2,4-二硝基苯腙为黄色或红色晶体，易于观察。按醛的一般检验方法，其反应过程如下：

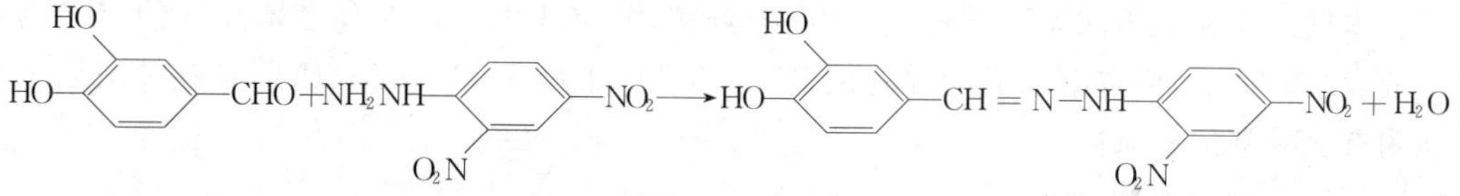

当检测洗脱液出现橙色斑点时，改用氨性硝酸银试剂反应，使银－氨络离子溶液中的银离子被原儿茶酸的邻二酚羟基还原成金属银（$Ag^+ \rightarrow Ag\downarrow$），出现黑色斑点。可通过加热来促进反应的进行。

三、实验步骤

(1) 取四季青药材 20 g，加 70% 乙醇分别回流提取 1 h 和 0.5 h，上 NKA-8 大孔树脂，上样量为 1∶0.5（树脂∶生药），用 70% 乙醇洗脱，洗脱液低温挥发干燥。

(2) 取硅胶（100～160 目，活度 V 级）6 g，干法装柱。

(3) 取样品 5 mg，加洗脱剂 5 ml，加热溶解后过滤，用吸管吸取滤液加入柱顶。

(4) 配制洗脱剂。一般选用石油醚－乙酸乙酯（石油醚∶乙酸乙酯＝4∶6，先配 50 ml，再酌量配少许）。

(5) 收集洗脱液。用小三角瓶收集洗脱液，每份 10 ml，共收集 10 份。

(6) 检出。取 1 块硅胶 CMC-Na 小板（见表 2-4），划小格，用毛细管吸取洗脱液分别滴在各小格内，然后用毛细管吸取检出试剂 2,4-二硝基苯肼、氨性硝酸银试剂滴在检品点处，观察结果，另一格子只滴检出试剂，用作空白对照。

表 2-4　四季青显色反应 CMC-Na 薄层区块

试剂空白											
样品＋试剂											
试剂空白											
样品＋试剂											

从反应结果可判断出哪几个流份含有原儿茶醛，哪几个流份含原儿茶酸，或为空白流

份。将这些流份分别浓缩后点样,进行薄层色谱。薄层色谱的条件:硅胶 CMC-Na 薄层板;展开剂:氯仿－丙酮－甲醇－乙酸(氯仿:丙酮:甲醇:乙酸＝7:2:0.5:0.5);显色剂:2％三氯化铁乙醇溶液。

按薄层结果合并相同流份,常压回收洗脱液至小体积,抽滤后用乙醇为溶剂进行重结晶,得到晶体。取少许晶体,用乙醇溶解后再进行薄层色谱,观察其是否为单体,若是单体,就可测定晶体的熔点,进行初步鉴定。已知化合物可作红外吸收光谱图,并与标准图谱对照来证实。

记录各流份的点滴反应和薄层色谱的结果(绘出图谱),写出所得单体的熔点数据。初步判断分离得到的单体是哪种化合物。

四、注意事项

1. 氨性硝酸银试剂(Tollens 试剂)

取 5％硝酸银溶液 2 ml,置于洁净试管内,先加入 1 滴 10％氢氧化钠溶液,再逐滴加入 20％氨水,同时不断振摇,直到氧化银沉淀恰巧溶解为止。为制得灵敏试剂,氨水的量不可过多。本试剂应在临用前配制,因为它久放会分解,并沉积出一种有高度爆炸性的沉淀物。将试液点在滤纸上,再点上新鲜配制的试剂,于 100℃加热 5～10 min,如果溶液呈深褐色,则证明有含醛基的还原糖。

2. 2,4-二硝基苯肼试剂

取 2,4-二硝基苯肼,配成 0.2％ 2 mol/L 盐酸溶液或 0.1％ 2 mol/L 盐酸乙醇溶液。

五、实验用品与时间安排

实验用品:色谱柱、小三角烧瓶、吸管、移液管、小漏斗、玻棒、NKA-8 大孔树脂、氯仿、丙酮、甲醇、乙酸、乙醇、氨水、2,4-二硝基苯肼、氢氧化钠、石油醚、乙酸乙酯、三氯化铁、硅胶等。

时间安排:要求在 6 学时内完成。

六、思考题

(1)使用 2,4-二硝基苯肼试剂对羰基进行检验需在酸性条件下进行的原因是什么?
(2)薄层色谱中影响被测物质 Rf 值的因素有哪些?

实验二 红辣椒中色素的分离

一、实验目的

掌握用薄层色谱和柱色谱法分离和提取天然产物的原理和实验方法。

二、实验原理

红辣椒中含有多种色素(见图 2-8),已知的有辣椒红、辣椒玉红素和 β-胡萝卜素,它们都属于类胡萝卜素类化合物,从结构上判断都属于四萜化合物。其中辣椒红是以脂肪酸酯的形式存在的,它是红辣椒显深红色的主要原因。辣椒玉红素可能也是以脂肪酸酯的形式存在。

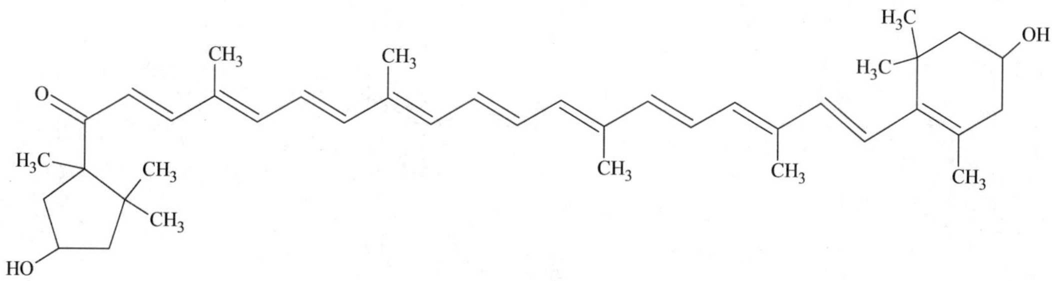

辣椒红

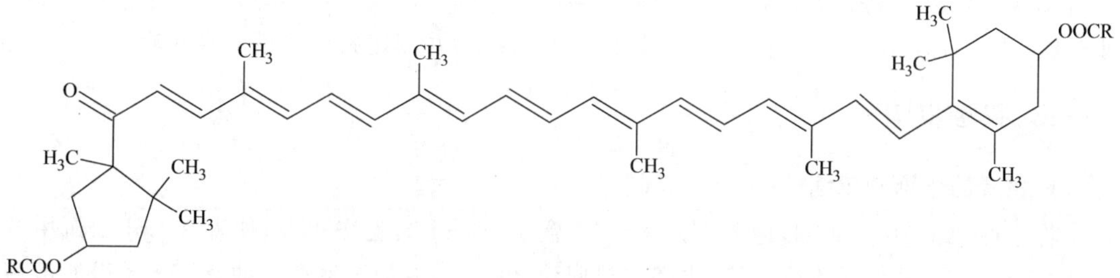

辣椒红脂肪酸酯

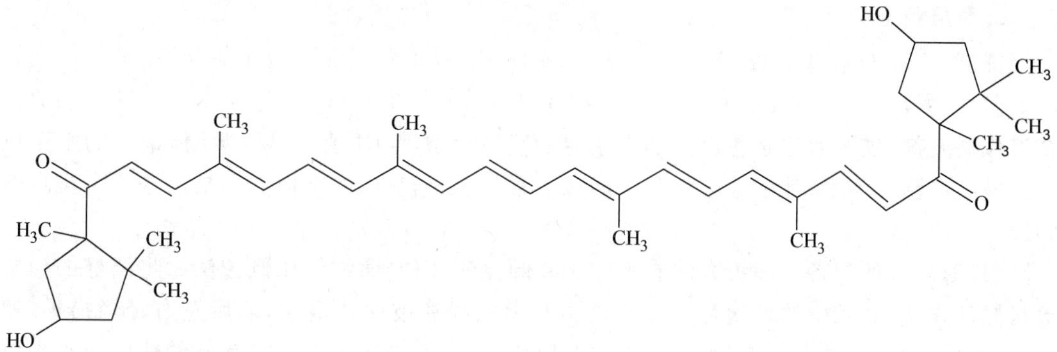

辣椒玉红素

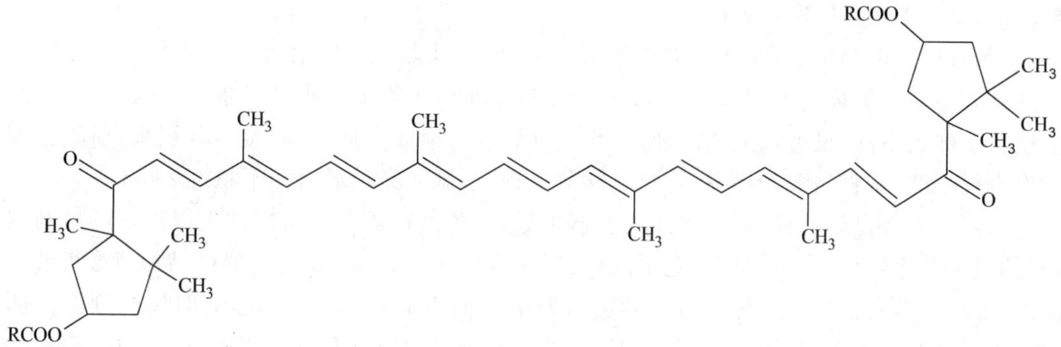

辣椒玉红素脂肪酸酯

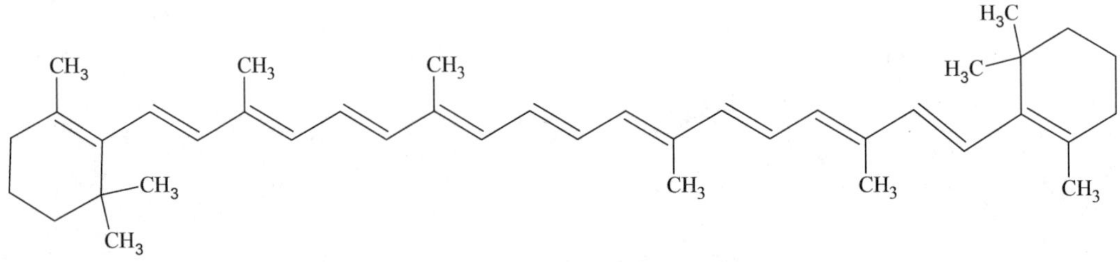

β-胡萝卜素

图 2-8 红辣椒中主要色素成分

本实验是以二氯甲烷为萃取溶剂,从红辣椒中萃取出色素,经浓缩后用薄层色谱法作初步分析,再用柱色谱法分离出红色素,做红外光谱鉴定,并测定紫外光谱的吸收峰。

三、实验步骤

1. 色素的萃取和浓缩

将干红辣椒剪碎、研细,称取 1 g 碎辣椒,置于 50 ml 圆底烧瓶中,加入 10 ml 二氯甲烷和 2～3 粒沸石,装上回流冷凝管,水浴加热回流 20 min,冷却至室温后抽滤。将所得滤液用水浴加热蒸馏,浓缩至剩约 1 ml 残液,即为混合色素的浓缩液。

2. 薄层色谱分析

铺制 CMC 硅胶薄层板(2.5 cm×7.5 cm)6 块,晾干并活化后取出 1 块,用平口毛细管吸取前面制得的混合色素浓缩液点样,用 1 体积石油醚(30～60℃)与 3 体积二氯甲烷的混合液作展开剂,展开后记录各斑点的大小、颜色,并计算其 Rf 值。已知 Rf 值最大的三个斑点是辣椒红脂肪酸酯、辣椒玉红素和 β-胡萝卜素,试根据它们的结构分别指出这三个斑点的归属。

(1)薄层板的制备。铺板方法有平铺法和倾注法 2 种,通常使用倾注法。将调好的匀浆等量倾注在洗净、晾干的玻璃片上。用食指和拇指捏住玻璃片两端,前后左右轻轻摇晃,使流动的匀浆均匀地铺在玻璃片上,即制成薄层板,且表面光洁平整。将铺好的薄层板水平放置晾干,再移入烘箱内加热活化,调节烘箱使其缓缓升温至 105℃,恒温放置 0.5 h 后将薄层板取出,放在干燥器中冷却备用。

(2)点样。取薄层板,在其一端离边沿 1.0 cm 处用软铅笔轻轻画一条点样线。点样时应选择管口平齐的玻璃毛细管,吸取少量所制得的粗红色素置于小锥形瓶中,再加 5～10 滴二氯甲烷配成溶液(也可取上述滤液)。用毛细管吸取溶液点样,轻轻接触薄层板点样处,如一次点样不够,待样品溶剂挥发后,再点样数次,以控制样品扩散直径不超过 2 mm。

(3)展开。薄层色谱需要在密闭的容器中展开(色谱缸或广口瓶),首先将配好的展开剂(石油醚∶二氯甲烷=1∶3)倒入色谱缸(液层厚度约为 0.5 cm)。将点好样品的薄层板放入缸内,点样一端在下(注意:样品点必须在展开剂液面之上)。盖好缸盖,此时展开剂即沿薄层板上升。当展开剂前沿上升到距薄层板顶端 1 cm 左右时,取出薄层板,尽快用铅笔标出前沿位置,然后置通风处晾干,或用电吹风吹干。

(4)Rf 值的计算。一种化合物在薄层板上上升的高度与展开剂上升的高度的比值称为该化合物的 Rf 值,即 Rf 值=化合物移动的距离/展开剂移动的距离。

3. 柱色谱分离

选用内径 1 cm,长约 20 cm 的色谱柱,用硅胶 10 g(100~200 目)在二氯甲烷中装柱(见图 2-9)。柱装好后用滴管吸取混合色素的浓缩液,混合加入柱顶。小心冲洗内壁后改用体积比为 3∶8 的石油醚(30~60 ℃)—二氯甲烷混合液洗脱,用不同的接收瓶分别接收先流出柱子的三个色带。当第三个色带完全流出后停止洗脱。

(1)装柱。可以用湿法装柱,也可以用干法装柱。如果用干法装柱,将 8 g 硅胶(100~200 目)装填到盛有 10 ml 二氯甲烷的带旋塞的滴管或色谱柱中,排出气泡,均匀填平,再加少许干净的砂粒(约 3 mg)。然后旋开旋塞,放出部分二氯甲烷,使其液面降至砂层的上层面。如果用湿法装柱,将 8 g 硅胶用二氯甲烷调成糊状后,徐徐倒入柱中,用橡皮塞轻轻敲打色谱柱下部,使之填装紧密,当装柱至柱高的 3/4 时,再在上面加一层厚约 0.5 cm 的石英砂。注意:操作时,不能使液面低于砂子的上层面。

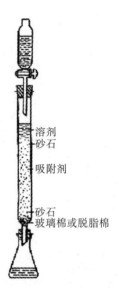

图 2-9 柱色谱装置

(2)加样。当溶剂液面刚好流至石英砂面时,立即沿柱壁加入 1 ml 粗提的辣椒红溶液。当此溶液流至接近石英砂面时,用二氯甲烷洗下管壁的有色物质。

(3)洗脱。用二氯甲烷淋洗色素(色谱柱中会出现色环)。β-胡萝卜素因极性小,故首先向下移动,极性较大的叶绿素、叶黄素和辣椒红色素则留在柱的上端,形成不同的色带。当最先下行的色带快流出时,更换另一接收瓶,继续洗脱,至滴出液近无色为止,收集洗脱液,每份约 2 ml。当红色素洗脱后,可停止淋洗,或继续淋洗,直至洗出第二组分黄色素再停止。将含有相同组分的溶液合并蒸发至干。

4. 柱效和色带的薄层检测

取 3 块硅胶薄层板,画好起始线,用不同的平口毛细管点样。每块板上都点 2 个样,其中一个是混合色素浓缩液,另一个是第一、第二或第三色带。仍选用体积比为 1∶3 的石油醚—二氯甲烷混合液作展开剂。比较各色带的 Rf 值,指出各色带是何种化合物。

5. 红色素的红外光谱鉴定和紫外光谱吸收峰

将柱中分得的红色带浓缩蒸发至干,充分干燥后用溴化钾压片法作红外光谱图,与红色素纯样品的红外光谱图作比较,并说明在 3100~3600 cm^{-1} 区域中为什么没有吸收峰。另外,用自己分离得到的红色素作紫外光谱图,确定 λ_{max} 在 470 nm 和 447 nm 处有两个明显的吸收峰。红外光谱数据表明,该组分含有甲基(2925 cm^{-1}、2850 cm^{-1} 和 1462 cm^{-1})、羰基(1747 cm^{-1})、碳碳双键(3020 cm^{-1} 和 1700 cm^{-1}),且为顺式结构(710 cm^{-1})和碳氧单键(1162 cm^{-1}),见图 2-10 和图 2-11。

四、注意事项

(1)点样时,样品液的浓度要适宜。浓度太高易引起斑点拖尾,浓度太低则会因体积过大而引起斑点扩散。点与点相距 1 cm 左右,斑点大小以直径为 2 cm 左右为宜。

(2)薄层吸附色谱展开剂须根据样品的极性、溶解度和吸附剂的活性等因素综合进行选择。展开剂的极性越大,对化合物的洗脱能力越强,Rf值也越大。

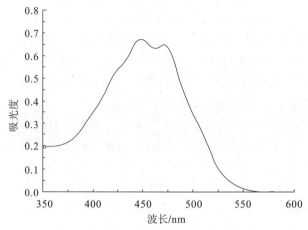

图 2-10　辣椒红紫外-可见光谱图

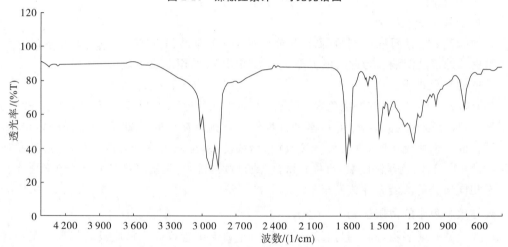

图 2-11　辣椒红色素的红外光谱图

(3)柱子的径高比一般为1:(5~10)。无水无氧柱多用氧化铝作固定相,因为硅胶中有大量的羟基裸露在外,很容易使样品分解,特别是金属有机物和含磷化合物。

(4)柱子下面的活塞一定不要涂润滑剂,否则润滑剂可能会被淋洗剂带入产品中。

(5)干法和湿法装柱没什么区别,关键是要把柱子装实。多数情况下,柱内有些小气泡对分离效果没有很大影响。实验中要避免柱子开裂,竖裂或横裂都会影响分离效果,甚至使柱子作废。

五、实验用品与时间安排

实验用品:色谱柱、小三角烧瓶、吸管、移液管、小漏斗、玻棒、红辣椒、圆底烧瓶、二氯甲烷、薄层板、石油醚、展开槽、滴管、硅胶、红外分光光度计、紫外分光光度计等。

时间安排:要求在6学时内完成。

六、思考题

(1) 提取粗红色素时,在水浴回流中为何要将水温控制在 50℃ 以下?(二氯甲烷的沸点为 39.8℃)

(2) 填充硅胶柱时,为何要在柱子下端塞上脱脂棉?此外,还要注意哪些问题?

实验三　绿叶中色素的提取和分离

一、实验目的

掌握用柱色谱法分离和提取叶绿素的原理和实验方法。

二、实验原理

叶绿素(见图 2-12)存在于多种绿色植物的细胞中。叶绿素在植物细胞中与蛋白质结合成叶绿体,当细胞死亡后,叶绿素即游离出来。绿叶中的色素包括叶绿素和类胡萝卜素两大类,叶绿素总量比胡萝卜素高 4 倍,因而叶子在正常情况下呈现绿色。叶绿素具有促进造血、提供维生素、解毒、抗病等多种作用。

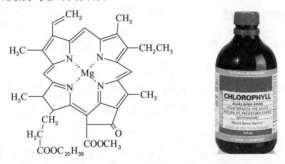

图 2-12　叶绿素及其制剂举例

本实验采用柱色谱法将绿叶中的色素分离成叶绿素、胡萝卜素和叶黄素等几种成分。绿叶中的色素都属于脂溶性色素,可溶于丙酮、乙醇、乙醚、氯仿、石油醚等溶剂,因此,可以用上述溶剂进行提取。游离叶绿素很不稳定,对光和热均敏感,在稀碱溶液中可水解为仍有鲜绿色的叶绿酸盐、叶绿醇和甲醇。在酸性条件下,卟啉环中的镁离子可被氢离子所取代,生成暗绿色或绿褐色的脱镁叶绿素。

三、实验步骤

1. 绿叶中色素的提取

称取绿叶蔬菜 1~2 g,放在研钵中,加少许二氧化硅和碳酸钙研碎,加 1∶1 的石油醚-丙酮混合液 10 ml,研磨成糊状,放置沉淀后,用吸管吸取上清液放入分液漏斗中。加入石油醚(30~60℃)10 ml,再加饱和氯化钠溶液 30 ml,摇匀分层后,分出盐水层。再用 30 ml 饱和食盐水洗涤一次,分去水层,将绿叶色素提取液转移至锥形瓶中,加少许无水硫酸钠干燥 15 min。将滤液倒入蒸发皿中,用水浴加热蒸去溶剂,基本蒸干后,用 2~3 ml 石油醚(60~90℃)溶解,即得到绿叶色素浓缩提取液。

2. 绿叶色素的柱色谱分离

在洗净并干燥的色谱柱底部铺一层脱脂棉,在柱上放一个漏斗,使氧化铝均匀地流经漏斗成一细流,慢慢地装入管内,中间不间断。同时轻轻敲打玻璃管,使之填装均匀,全部装完后,在装好的氧化铝表面覆盖一层无水硫酸钠。

吸取提取液注入柱中,在柱长 1/4 处见到黄色区带时,用 9∶1 的石油醚—丙酮混合液洗脱胡萝卜素,再改用丙酮洗脱叶绿素,将洗脱下的叶绿素接于烧杯中。

3. 叶绿素的性质

(1)与酸作用:取 2～3 ml 丙酮提取液加 5 滴稀盐酸,振荡,观察现象。
(2)与碱作用:取 2～3 ml 丙酮提取液加 5 滴稀碱液,振荡,观察现象。

四、注意事项

(1)盐水的作用是萃取出可溶于水及丙酮而不溶于石油醚的物质,加食盐是为了避免石油醚的乳化。
(2)色谱柱的径高比一般为 1∶(20～30)。
(3)分离 1 g 样品需用 20～50 g Al_2O_3,Al_2O_3 的高度一般为玻璃管高度的 3/4。

五、实验用品与时间安排

实验用品:绿叶蔬菜、玻璃粉(将碎玻璃放在铁研钵中研细后,经 20 目筛分出,用浓盐酸进行去铁处理,然后用氢氧化钠中和酸,最后用蒸馏水洗至中性后,再在烘箱中烘干)、石油醚(30～60℃)、石油醚(60～90℃)、中性氧化铝(100～200 目)、无水硫酸钠、丙酮、饱和氯化钠溶液、0.5 mol/L 盐酸、0.5 mol/L 氢氧化钠、研钵、分液漏斗、蒸发皿、色谱柱、锥形瓶和漏斗。

时间安排:要求在 6 学时内完成。

六、思考题

(1)为什么要选用新鲜浓绿的叶片?
(2)研磨时加入二氧化硅和碳酸钙的目的是什么?

第三章 结构鉴定技术

一、概述

20世纪下半叶,光谱学已成为有机结构化学的基础课程。20世纪30年代发展起来的紫外(UV)光谱和20世纪40年代发展起来的红外(IR)光谱为化学家提供了识别有机化合物生色基团和官能团的有效方法。研究者可以采用极少量的样品,用非破坏性的实验得到有关结构的信息。20世纪50年代发展起来的质谱(MS)方法进一步给有机结构化学带来革命性的影响,MS实验可以给出化合物的分子式,并且通过裂解方式提供分子的结构信息。

对有机结构化学影响最大的波谱学方法当推核磁共振(NMR),它对有机化学的影响是迅速的并且是震撼性的。近50年来,有机波谱学尤其是NMR技术的发展革新了天然产物结构鉴定的方法。波谱技术已成为探究大自然中分子内部秘密的最可靠和最有效的手段。

20年前,无论是HMBC、COSY等2D NMR技术,还是波谱学家刚开发的脉冲序列,都是应用较少的高新技术,但是,在近些年市售的NMR波谱仪器上,这些技术已成为常规方法。众所周知的吗啡(Morphine)是1806年由Serturner分离得到的,可直到1952年人工合成成功,用了150年时间,才确定了吗啡的化学结构。番木鳖碱(Strychnine,士的宁)的结构确定用了半个多世纪(1891-1946年),耗费了几代杰出化学家的心血,原因就是当时确定结构的主要方法是湿法化学。

严格地说,UV和IR属于光谱,MS不是光谱,而是物质粒子的质量谱,NMR属于波谱。早年习惯将以上四者称为四大光谱。

1. 样品结构的背景信息

从各种植物中分离出来的成分可以说大部分是已知化合物,只要文献充足,这些已知物的结构鉴定一般都是比较快捷和容易进行的。只有小部分是未知化合物,且这些化合物大多仅仅是骨架上的取代基或立体结构与已知的有所不同。

(1)样品来源和参考文献。参考文献与样品来源有关,如植物界、门、纲、目、科、属、种,已知化合物波谱数据是研究该种属植物成分结构必备的参考文献,但是要注意文献的年代、仪器及测定结构方法学。

(2)样品化合物的物性。由样品的物性,如液体、固体、结晶形态、熔点、沸点、颜色、荧光、柱色谱特性、TLC特性、纸色谱特性、HPLC特性、显色反应、旋光性、溶解度、纯度等,再结合文献背景来推断所测定样品的化合物类型,这是获得样品骨架信息的重要方法。

(3)样品化合物的骨架信息。样品分子骨架类型的信息可以从上述资料和实验结果中得到,这为研究者迅速进入结构鉴定程序提供了方便。如果得不到结构骨架类型的信息,那就需要从多种波谱数据入手获得结构骨架的信息。

2. 结构鉴定的化学方法(湿法化学)

鉴于波谱技术已经改变天然产物结构鉴定的方法,采用化学方法测定天然产物结构已退居很次要的位置。通常用波谱方法可以准确无误地测定比较复杂的结构,包括立体化学结构。但在不少情况下,进行化学转化和衍化是很有益处的,甚至是很有必要的。天然药物化学不单单是天然药物的提取、分离和结构鉴定,还应包括结构修饰以及合成等多个领域。

3. 紫外可见光谱和红外光谱

(1)紫外可见(UV/Vis)光谱。UV/Vis 光谱方法比较简单,由光谱提供的结构信息也比较少,UV/Vis 光谱可给出有关共轭生色团和助色团的信息。一般情况下,由 UV/Vis 光谱推断可靠的分子骨架是比较困难的,这是因为即使碳骨架相同,当共轭体系中断时,其 UV 吸收峰也会有很大区别。即使两个化合物结构并非属于一类,并且相对分子质量相差甚远,只要生色团相同,就会有几乎相同的 UV 谱线。

(2)红外光谱(IR)。20 世纪 50～70 年代,IR 一直是有机化合物结构鉴定最重要的方法,如对黄酮、蒽醌、三萜、甾体苷元等类型的化合物进行了 IR 特征吸收谱带的规律性研究。现在主要是对重要官能团的鉴别有重要意义,如羰基的鉴定,羧酸和酸酐的鉴定,羰环大小的鉴定,CN、NCO、NCS 和 SH 的鉴定,砜、亚砜、磺酸基和硝基的鉴定以及判断有无羟基等。值得强调的是,在有标准谱图和对照品存在的情况下,IR 用于化合物的鉴定是既方便而又可靠的,这是由于 IR 具有指纹鉴定功能。

在天然产物结构鉴定中,最重要和最常用的是 FT-IR 和光栅 IR,早期的标准图谱基本上都是光栅 IR 图谱。

分析 IR 图谱应注意的问题包括峰位、峰形、峰强和测定条件。峰位是指峰的吸收频率,用 cm^{-1} 表示;峰形是指峰的形状,也就是胖、瘦、钝、锐的问题;峰的强度(即"峰强")一般分为强(s)、中强(m)和弱(w);测定条件有液膜涂片、KBr 压片等。

4. 质谱法

质谱(MS)法是鉴定有机物结构的重要方法,其灵敏度之高,远远超过 NMR 和 IR。MS 可以测定相对分子质量和分子式。天然产物结构测定中常用的 MS 方法按电离方式可分为以下几种。

(1)电子轰击质谱(EIMS)和高分辨电子轰击质谱(HREIMS)。EIMS 和 HREIMS 是天然化合物结构测定中应用最多的 MS 方法,可以用其测定相对分子质量、分子式、碎片离子的元素组成和分子的裂解方式。但 EIMS 也有不尽如人意的地方,如对于热不稳定的化合物、极性较大的化合物以及相对分子质量较大的化合物往往得不到分子离子峰,或分子离子峰很弱,以至于难以判断。

(2)快速原子轰击谱(FAB)和高分辨快速原子轰击谱(HRFAB)。FAB 和 HRFAB 适用于测定挥发性极低、强极性有机化合物,热不稳定的化合物和相对分子质量较大的化合物。

(3)场解吸(FD)。场解吸谱中通常为 M 峰和 MH 峰,一般适用于相对分子质量较小而极性较强的化合物。

(4)化学电离(CI)。化学电离与电子轰击源的相同之处是都为热源,因此,容易挥发、受热不易分解的样品才适合用 CI 源测定。在 EIMS 观察不到分子离子峰时,用 CI 源常常可以得到相对分子质量信息。

(5)电喷雾电离(ESI)。电喷雾电离适用于多肽、蛋白质、糖蛋白、核酸等的分析。

(6)大气压化学电离(APCI)。大气压化学电离适用于小分子化合物的定性分析和药代动力学研究。

(7)基质辅助激光解吸电离(MALDI)。MALDI 适用于多肽、蛋白质、糖蛋白、DNA 片段和多糖等的分析。

在多种电离源获得的 MS 中,以 EIMS 提供的结构信息最多。如果我们想用最少的样品获得最多的结构信息,首当选择 EIMS。在大多数情况下,用 EIMS 不仅可以得到样品的相对分子质量和分子式,还可以得到丰富的裂解碎片信息,这些碎片离子的元素组成亦可由 HREIMS 测得。如果所测样品的分子骨架比较稳定,并且有明确的裂解规律,则 EIMS 推断分子结构往往是很奏效的。

(8)气相色谱-质谱联用(GC-MS)。气相色谱-质谱联用已成为鉴定天然有机混合物中各组分结构的有力手段之一,几乎所有用 GC 可分离的组分都可以用 GC-MS 得到比较满意的图谱,哪怕组分的含量只有纳克级。

(9)液相色谱-质谱联用(LC-MS,HPLC-MS)。液相色谱-质谱联用适合于极性分子的分离和结构鉴定。液相色谱-质谱联用仪是分析相对分子质量大、极性强的化合物时不可缺少的分析仪器。

5. 核磁共振法

(1)NMR 溶剂问题。测定 NMR 图谱要使用氘代试剂,这些溶剂和其中水峰的化学位移值在常见的相关教科书中可以查到。

(2)一维核磁共振(1D NMR)。多种 1D NMR 图谱中,最常见的是 ^{1}H NMR、^{13}C NMR、DEPT 和 NOE 差谱。

①活泼氢的识别方法。在 1H NMR 图谱中,活泼氢信号变化多端,有的峰尖锐,有的峰较宽,有的峰积分面积明显较小,有的峰和其他信号重叠,有的峰几乎和基线一致等。产生上述现象有两个原因:内因是由分子结构引起,外因是与样品的浓度、温度、溶剂以及样品中的水分等因素有关。下面介绍几种识别活泼氢信号的方法。

Ⅰ.重水交换。重水交换是最经典和常用的识别活泼氢的方法。

Ⅱ.由 H-C COSY 谱识别活泼氢信号。因为活泼氢不与碳直接相连,所以和碳没有相关峰的质子信号应是活泼氢的峰。

Ⅲ.变温实验识别活泼氢。在活泼氢信号和其他信号发生重叠或部分重叠时,此时接着做升温实验,温度升高时活泼氢信号会向高场位移。通过将常温测定的图谱与升温测定的图谱进行比较,来识别活泼氢的信号。

②水峰压制(Water Peak Suppression)。用重水做溶剂测定 ^{1}H NMR 时,溶剂信号往往很强,会干扰化学位移、水峰化学位移以及与样品接近的信号。当样品浓度较低时,溶剂信号和溶剂中的水峰也会很强,会干扰样品信号,这时可以采用水峰压制技术来压制或消去水峰和溶剂峰。

③质子同核自旋去偶(Proton Homonuclear Spin Decoupling)谱。质子同核自旋去偶是

一种常用且重要的双共振实验。当谱线分裂比较复杂时,采用此技术可简化图谱,确定相互偶合信号之间的关系,发现隐藏的信号和得到偶合常数等。

④1D NOE 差谱(1D NOE Difference Spectra)。在差谱图中,所有未受影响的信号消失,而显示的是增强的信号,以及在照射频率处的一个强信号。

⑤测定数据与文献数据或图谱比较时应注意的问题。比较时首先要注意氘代试剂是否相同,如果溶剂不同,由于溶剂效应,化学位移会有一定的差别;其次要看内标是否一致,内标不一致会直接造成化学位移差别。

⑥常规 ^{13}C NMR 谱。在 ^1H 宽带去偶条件下,可常规测定 ^{13}C NMR 谱,因为消除了 ^1H 核和 ^{13}C 核间的偶合产生的裂分,从而使非灵敏度 ^{13}C 的信号变成窄的单峰,同时使连接质子的 ^{13}C 信噪比大大提高。

⑦偏共振去偶谱。偏共振去偶谱是早期用来测定碳上连接氢数目的技术。

⑧无畸变极化转移技术(DEPT)谱。DEPT 谱是目前最理想的鉴别碳上连氢数目的常规技术。

(3) 二维核磁共振(2D NMR)。

①同核相关谱。

Ⅰ. H-H COSY。H-H COSY 是确定质子间偶合关系的有力工具,它相当于多次质子同核自旋去偶实验。H-H COSY 中的相关峰(或称交叉峰)主要反映的是 2J 和 3J 偶合关系,偶尔会出现远程相关峰。

Ⅱ. 相敏 H-H COSY。与 H-H COSY 相比,相敏 H-H COSY 谱是纯吸收线型,分辨率和信噪比都大为改善。

Ⅲ. TOCSY。可以找到同一偶合体系中所有氢核的相关信息,也就是说,从某一个氢核信号的出现,能找到与它处在同一个自旋系统中所有质子的相关峰。

②异核相关谱。

Ⅰ. H-C COSY 谱。H-C COSY 谱是相关 ^1H NMR 和 ^{13}C NMR 信号的常规图谱,比较直观,容易分析。其作用与 HMQC 和 HSQC 相同。

Ⅱ. HMQC 和 HSQC。这两种图谱的作用与 H-C COSY 相当,由于是反向实验,故灵敏度高。HMQC 和 HSQC 相比,HSQC 的优点更多一些。而当样品量较多时,宜做 H-C COSY。

Ⅲ. HMBC。HMBC 一般反映不出单键相关峰,只能区分出双键和三键谱相关峰。

Ⅳ. COLOC 谱。远程相关峰的强度取决于相应的偶合常数值,对于偶合常数较小的,往往检测不到相关峰,因此,要适当改变实验参数才能得到理想的图谱。

(4) 液相色谱-核磁共振(LC-NMR,HPLC-NMR)的应用。近些年来,LC-NMR 联机仪器进入了化学实验室,它包含了 HPLC 强有力的分离功能和 NMR 图谱,由这些图谱提供的大量结构信息有助于进行结构鉴定。

二、结构鉴定方法

1. 背景信息的搜索和验证

来源于文献检索和化学实验结果的有关样品结构的各种背景信息,以及从各种波谱实验得到的信息是非常重要的,但必须经过反复证实才能得出可靠的结论。

从图谱中可以判断化合物的类型,若分子结构是已知的,则主要是信号归属问题,应当从化学位移或偶合类型容易归属的信号开始,然后逐步展开。对于初步解析得到的结论,在随后的解析过程中必须加以确证。最后,各种信息必须相互符合,一系列论证符合逻辑才能得到正确结论。某一特征结构信息时常具有各种独立的实验数据和(或)证据,这些实验数据和(或)证据是互相支持的。随着分子结构复杂性的增加,将会出现更多的特征信息。

2. 结构鉴定

(1)天然药物结构骨架类型的背景知识。天然药物化学研究者应当养成阅读专著、跟踪阅读天然药物化学相关文献、不断学习各种波谱新技术的习惯,积累特征化合物的波谱数据和图谱特征资料。

(2)关于分子式。通常,并非要先测定分子式,由各种波谱图的解析也可直接推出结构式。有了分子式就有了元素组成和不饱和度的信息,查阅结构文献资料可以为解析带来方便和依据。分离得到的样品量太少或样品纯度欠佳时,最好不要作燃烧分析,最好采用适当电离源的高分辨质谱测定分子式。

(3)测定结构从哪种波谱方法入手。最好先测定 ^1H NMR、^{13}C NMR、MS,认真分析并与文献对照,如果很快鉴定出是已知化合物,则不必进行过多的测试。如果尚不能断定是已知物或是新化合物,就需要进行多种波谱的测定。某些情况下得到的样品量只有几毫克,这就需要异常小心。用几毫克样品进行结构测定时,建议用 HREIMS 或 HRFAB 测定分子式而不是进行燃烧分析。测定了几种常规的 NMR 图谱后,小心保存好 NMR 样品管,以备进一步测定。最后回收 NMR 样品管中的样品,测定 IR 和比旋光度等,保存好测定 IR 的溴化钾片或涂膜片以及测定比旋光度的样品溶液,以备回收。

(4)推断分子骨架,提出"工作结构"(或称假定结构)是结构测定的关键。

①通常根据样品来源、颜色反应、色谱行为、参考文献和波谱数据等分析判断样品属于何种骨架。

②与收集到的相似结构和特征光谱数据对照分析,找出相同点,处理不同点。

③如何由化合物的图谱获得结构骨架信息。各种波谱图,尤其是 ^1H NMR 和 ^{13}C NMR 图谱,可以揭示天然物骨架的信息,在由图谱得到波谱数据的同时,图谱的"谱线分布特征"是识别化合物骨架类型的重要依据。

(5)利用 NMR 寻找目的骨架化合物。采用 NMR 寻找目的化合物既快捷又实用,特别是对于没有专属颜色反应的化合物。

(6)对映体和非对映异构体。NMR 不能区分对映体,但可以区分和鉴定非对映异构体。

(7)对映体过量。当一种对映体过量时,采用手性 NMR 位移试剂可将两种对映体各自的 NMR 信号分开。

(8)结构的最后确证。对于已知化合物的结构鉴定,有对照品时鉴定比较容易,没有对照品时最好与原始文献数据对照。

对于新化合物,除方法可靠、数据确凿外,应当引用相似化合物的文献数据给予支持。所有 NMR 信号应当全部准确归属或尽可能全部归属,而 IR 和 MS 数据则不一定要全部进行解释。

第四章 各类成分的提取和分离实例

第一节 糖 类

实验一 香菇多糖的提取

香菇来源于口蘑科香菇（*Lentinus edodes*（Berk.）*sing*）的子实体（见图4-1），是世界第二大食用菌，也是我国特产之一，在民间素有"山珍"之称。它是一种生长在木材上的真菌，味道鲜美，香气沁人，营养丰富，素有"植物皇后"的美誉。香菇中麦角甾醇含量很高，对防治佝偻病有效；香菇多糖是β-1,3-葡聚糖，能增强细胞免疫能力，从而抑制癌细胞的生长；其分子式为$(C_{42}H_{70}O_{35})_n$，香菇含有六大酶类的40多种酶，可以纠正人体酶缺乏症；香菇中含有脂肪酸，对人体降血脂有益。

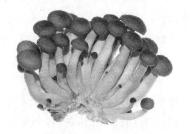 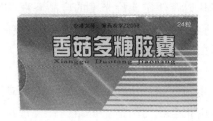

图4-1 香菇及其制剂举例

一、实验目的

掌握热水煮沸法分离多糖类化合物的原理和方法。

二、实验原理

多糖可溶于热水，不溶于60%以上乙醇，所以可用热水提取多糖。乙醇沉淀可除去部分醇溶性杂质。

三、实验步骤

1. 制作标准曲线

采用苯酚硫酸法，以葡萄糖为标准物，称取在105℃条件下干燥至恒重的葡萄糖

14.8 mg,置于100 ml容量瓶中,加水溶解并稀释至刻度,分别取 0 ml,0.4 ml,0.6 ml, 0.8 ml,1.0 ml,1.2 ml,1.4 ml,1.6 ml,1.8 ml,加水补充至 2.0 ml,再加 1 ml 5%苯酚溶液,迅速加入5 ml浓硫酸,摇匀,静置 20 min,冷却至室温。以蒸馏水为空白,在 490 mm 波长处测定吸光度,绘制标准曲线,得到回归方程为:$y=0.006x+0.032,R=0.9991$,线性范围为 $0\sim266.4\ \mu g$。数据如表4-1所示。

表 4-1 标准曲线的绘制

葡萄糖溶液的量/ml	0	0.4	0.6	0.8	1.0	1.2	1.4	1.6	1.8
A_{490}	0.005	0.016	0.020	0.019	0.029	0.031	0.041	0.044	0.049

2. 提取

取干香菇粉碎,称取 20 g 置于 250 ml 烧杯中,加入 100 ml 蒸馏水,在石棉网上加热至沸腾,并不断搅拌,30 min 后抽滤,滤渣再用 100 ml 蒸馏水煮沸 30 min。合并两次滤液,加热浓缩至 20 ml,溶于 95%乙醇中,搅拌并冷却至室温,静置 1 h,以 4000 r/min 离心 10 min,将沉淀物真空干燥,得到香菇多糖粗品。

3. 除蛋白

加入 50 ml 100℃热水溶解粗糖,加 Sevag 溶液 10 ml,剧烈振荡 10 min,静置 10 min,以 4000 r/min 离心 10 min,取上清液,加 Sevag 溶液反复操作 5 次。

4. 纯化

将粗糖置于烧杯中,加蒸馏水 50 ml 溶解,加入等体积的 0.15 mol/L 十六烷基三甲基溴化铵(CTAB)与硼酸缓冲溶液,静置 10 min,以 4000 r/min 离心得沉淀,用 1%乙醇溶解,静置 10 min,以 4000r/min 离心后取上清液,加等体积的甲醇,静置 24 h,抽滤,得精品香菇多糖。

5. 实验结果

(1)香菇多糖粗品的质量约为 3.46 g。

(2)取 0.01 g 干燥的香菇多糖,配制成 100 ml 溶液,取 1 ml 溶液按照制作标准曲线的操作过程,以蒸馏水为空白,在 490 mm 波长处测定吸光度,利用标准曲线计算香菇多糖的含量。

四、注意事项

(1)若得到的香菇多糖有点发灰,则可能是由杂质导致的。

(2)Sevag 法:将三氯甲烷按照多糖水溶液的 1/5 体积加入,然后加入三氯甲烷 1/5 体积的正丁醇,剧烈振摇 20 min,离心,除去水层与溶液层交界处的变性蛋白。此法温和,但需重复 5 次左右才能除去大部分蛋白质。

(3)0.15 mol/L 十六烷基三甲基溴化铵与硼酸缓冲溶液:先配制硼酸缓冲液,由 1 g 硼酸溶于 100 ml 水中制成,其 pH 约为 5.0,可直接作溶剂。另称取 5.5 g CTAB,加入硼酸缓冲液 100 ml,溶解均匀。

五、实验用品与时间安排

实验用品:香菇,葡萄糖,乙醇,苯酚,浓硫酸,紫外可见分光光度计,恒温浴槽,三氯甲烷,正丁醇,十六烷基三甲基溴化铵,硼酸。

时间安排:要求在 6 学时内完成。

六、思考题

(1)香菇多糖的提取原理是什么?
(2)影响香菇多糖提取收率的因素有哪些?

实验二 麻黄多糖的提取

麻黄(见图 4-2)是我国使用历史比较悠久的中药材,来源于麻黄科植物草麻黄(*Ephedra sinica* Stapf)、中麻黄(*E. intermedia* Schrenk et C. A. Mey.)或木贼麻黄(*E. equisetina* Bge.)的干燥草质茎。麻黄具有发汗解表、宣肺平喘和利尿的功效,主治感冒风寒、水肿以及肺气不宣导致的咳嗽。麻黄含有生物碱、黄酮、挥发油、有机酸和多糖等成分,其中,多糖是麻黄的主要有效成分之一,具有降血脂和保护肝脏等作用。

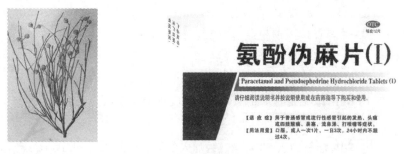

图 4-2 麻黄及其制剂举例

一、实验目的

掌握水提醇沉法提取麻黄多糖类化合物的原理和方法。

二、实验原理

多糖溶于热水,不溶于 60% 以上乙醇,所以可用热水提取多糖。乙醇沉淀可除去部分醇溶性杂质,热水同时会将蛋白质类物质提取出来,可用木瓜蛋白酶－Sevag 法除去多余的蛋白质。

三、实验步骤

1. 标准曲线的制备

采用苯酚－硫酸法,以葡萄糖为标准物,精密称取葡萄糖 4 mg,置于 100 ml 容量瓶中,加蒸馏水溶解并稀释至刻度。精密量取 0.4 ml、0.6 ml、0.8 ml、1.0 ml、1.2 ml、1.4 ml、1.6 ml、1.8 ml 溶液,加水补充至 2.0 ml,再加 1 ml 6% 苯酚溶液,摇匀,迅速加入浓硫酸 5.0 ml,即刻摇匀,放置 5 min 后,置沸水浴加热 15 min,取出冷却至室温(25℃)。另以蒸馏水 2.0 ml,同上操作,作为空白对照,在 490 mm 波长处测定吸光度值。以葡萄糖含量为横坐标,吸光度值为纵坐标,绘制标准曲线,得回归方程(见图 4-3)。

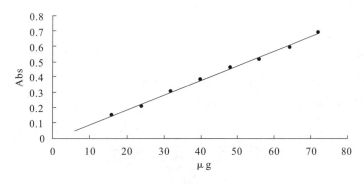

图 4-3 葡萄糖标准曲线

2. 提取

取干燥寸断的麻黄药材 20 g,置于 1000 ml 圆底烧瓶中,加 14 倍体积的蒸馏水,在 100℃的条件下水浴回流提取 4 h,冷却至室温。过滤得滤液和滤渣,再向滤渣中加入同初次等量的蒸馏水,重复上述操作 2 次。最后合并 3 次回流所得的滤液,在 50℃条件下减压浓缩至 20 ml。在不断搅拌下,向上清液中加入 3 倍量左右的 95%乙醇,使其终浓度为 75%。4℃下静置 24 h 后,以 3000 r/min 离心 20 min(4℃),收集沉淀,用无水乙醇洗涤,再在 4℃下以 3000 r/min 离心 20 min。除去不溶物后,收集上清液,进行低温干燥,得麻黄多糖冻干品。

3. 脱蛋白质

称取麻黄多糖并溶解成 5%水溶液,加入一定量的木瓜蛋白酶,使酶的终浓度为 1%(W/V),酶解 2 h。滤液以体积比 1∶3 加入 Sevag 试剂,充分振荡 30 min,静置分层至水层与有机层交界处基本无白色蛋白质沉淀,以 2000 r/min 离心除去变性蛋白质。然后加入 3 倍量乙醇进行醇沉,离心分离后取醇沉物,用水复溶,低温干燥即得精品麻黄多糖。

4. 实验结果

精密称取 60℃干燥至恒重的麻黄多糖 8 mg,溶解于双蒸水中,定容至 100 ml,样品溶液各 2 ml。按标准曲线制备项下方法操作,平行测量 3 次,从回归方程中求出供试液中葡萄糖的含量,按下式计算样品中多糖含量,多糖含量(%)=C×D×f×100/W。式中:C—供试液中葡萄糖浓度(mg/ml);D—多糖的稀释倍数(ml);f—换算因子;W—供试样品的质量(mg)。

四、实验注意

(1)脱蛋白质的方法还有三氯乙酸法、酶解法等。

(2)换算因子的测定:精密称取 60℃干燥至恒重的麻黄多糖 25 mg,置于 100 ml 容量瓶中,加水溶解并稀释至刻度。然后分别取 2 ml 溶液置于 5 个 25 ml 容量瓶中,用水稀释至刻度。分别按标准曲线制备项下方法测定其吸光度,由回归方程计算出 5 份麻黄多糖中葡萄糖的含量和平均值,再计算出换算因子 f=W/(C×D),式中 W 为多糖质量(mg),C 为多糖溶液中葡萄糖浓度(mg/ml),D 为多糖的稀释倍数。

五、实验用品与时间安排

实验用品:麻黄,葡萄糖,乙醇,苯酚,浓硫酸,紫外可见分光光度计,恒温浴槽,三氯甲烷,正丁醇,木瓜蛋白酶。

时间安排:要求在6～9学时内完成。

六、思考题

(1)加入乙醇沉淀麻黄提取液时为什么需要不断搅拌?
(2)还有哪些提取麻黄多糖的方法?

第二节 苯丙素类

实验一 秦皮中七叶苷、七叶内酯的提取、分离和鉴定

秦皮为木樨科植物苦枥白蜡树(*Fraxinus rhynchophylla* Hance)、白蜡树(*F. chinensis* Roxb.)、尖叶白蜡树(*F. szaboana* Lingelsh.)或宿柱白蜡树(*F. stylosa* Lingelsh.)的干燥枝皮或干皮(见图4-4)。味苦,性微寒,具有清热、燥湿、收涩等作用,主治温热痢疾、目赤肿痛等症。

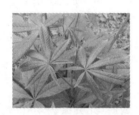 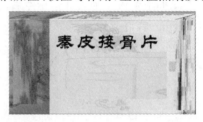

图4-4 秦皮及其制剂举例

秦皮中含有多种内酯类成分及皂苷、鞣质等,其中主要有七叶苷、七叶内酯、秦皮苷及秦皮素等。其成分多有抗菌消炎的生理活性,七叶内酯对细菌性痢疾、急性肠炎有较好的治疗效果,兼有退热作用,毒副作用小,几乎无苦味,适于小儿服用。秦皮中主要化学成分(见图4-5)如下。

七叶苷　　七叶内酯

秦皮苷　　秦皮素

图4-5 秦皮中主要化学成分

(1)七叶苷:又称马栗树皮苷,白色粉末状结晶,熔点205～206℃。易溶于热水(1∶15),

可溶于乙醇(1∶24),微溶于冷水(1∶6 或 1∶10),难溶于乙酸乙酯,不溶于乙醚、氯仿,在稀酸中可水解。水溶液中有蓝色荧光。

(2)七叶内酯:黄色针状结晶,熔点 276℃,易溶于沸乙醇及氢氧化钠溶液,可溶于乙酸乙酯,稍溶于沸水,几乎不溶于乙醚、氯仿。

(3)秦皮苷:熔点 205℃。

(4)秦皮素:熔点 227~228℃。

一、实验目的

1. 掌握液－液萃取法在分离香豆素苷和苷元中的作用。
2. 熟悉重结晶的基本操作。

二、实验原理

七叶苷、七叶内酯均能溶于沸乙醇,可用沸乙醇将二者提取出来,再利用二者在乙酸乙酯中的溶解性不同而分离之。

三、实验步骤

1. 提取

取秦皮粗粉 150 g,置于索氏提取器中,加 400 ml 95％乙醇,回流 2 h,得乙醇提取液,减压回收溶剂至浸膏状,即得总提取物。

2. 分离

在上述浸膏中加 40 ml 水,加热使其溶化。移于分液漏斗中,以等体积氯仿萃取 2 次,将氯仿萃取过的水层蒸去残留氯仿后,加等体积乙酸乙酯萃取 3 次。合并乙酸乙酯液,以无水硫酸钠脱水,减压回收溶剂至干,将残留物溶于温热甲醇中,浓缩至适量,放置析晶,即有黄色针状结晶析出。滤出结晶,以甲醇、水反复重结晶,即得七叶内酯。

将乙酸乙酯萃取过的水层浓缩至适量,放置析晶,即有微黄色晶体析出。滤出结晶,以甲醇、水反复重结晶,即得七叶苷。

3. 鉴定

(1)化学检验知识。

①取七叶苷、七叶内酯各少许,分别置于试管中,加乙醇 1 ml 溶解。加 1％$FeCl_3$ 溶液 2~3 滴,显暗绿色,再滴加浓氨水 3 滴,加水 6 ml,日光下观察显深红色。

②取七叶苷、七叶内酯各少许,分别置于试管中,加入盐酸羟胺甲醇溶液 2~3 滴,再加 1％NaOH 溶液 2~3 滴,水浴加热数分钟至反应完全,冷却,再用盐酸调至 pH 为 3~4,加 1％$FeCl_3$ 溶液 1~2 滴,溶液呈红色至紫红色。

③Gibb's 或 Emerson 反应:见第五章香豆素类成分预试验项下试验。

(2)观察荧光。取七叶苷、七叶内酯的甲醇溶液,分别滴 1 滴于滤纸上,于 254nm 紫外灯下观察荧光颜色,然后在原斑点上滴加 1 滴 NaOH 溶液,观察荧光有何变化。

(3)薄层鉴定。

吸附剂:硅胶 G。

样品:七叶苷、七叶内酯标准品及自制七叶苷、七叶内酯的醇溶液。

展开剂:乙酸乙酯－甲醇－1％乙酸水溶液(7∶3∶0.1)。
显色:
①UV$_{254nm}$灯下观察,七叶苷为灰色荧光,七叶内酯为灰褐色荧光。
②以重氮化对硝基苯胺喷雾显色,七叶苷和七叶内酯均呈玛瑙色。
结果:七叶苷 Rf≈0.04,七叶内酯 Rf≈0.28。

四、注意事项

(1)秦皮的混杂品较多,有些伪品不含香豆素,应注意与原植物品种进行区分。
(2)萃取振摇时,注意防止乳化,以轻轻旋转式萃取为宜。
(3)香豆素在薄层色谱紫外灯下观察通常具有荧光,可以用来鉴别。

五、实验用品与时间安排

实验用品:回流装置,溶剂回收装置,过滤装置,250 ml 分液漏斗,锥形瓶(500 ml,250 ml,50 ml),展开槽,色谱板,滤纸,沸石,秦皮,95％乙醇,三氯甲烷,乙酸乙酯,甲醇,异羟肟酸铁试剂,Gibb's 试剂,Emerson 试剂。
时间安排:要求在 6 个学时内完成。

六、思考题

(1)在色谱图谱上出现两个主要荧光斑点,试判断哪个是七叶苷?哪个是七叶内酯?为什么?
(2)如何用最简便的方法确定天然药物中有香豆素类成分?

实验二 丹皮酚的提取、分离和鉴定

牡丹皮为毛茛科植物牡丹(*Paeonia suffruticosa* Andr.)的干燥根皮(见图 4-6)。丹皮酚是牡丹皮的主要有效成分之一。此外,含丹皮酚的植物还有矮牡丹(*P. suffruticosa* Andr. var spontanea Rehd.)、紫斑牡丹(*P. papaveracea* Andr.)、黄丹皮(*P. potanini* Kom.)、四川牡丹(*P. szechuanica* Fang.)以及徐长卿(*Cynanchum paniculatum*(Bge) Kitag.)等。

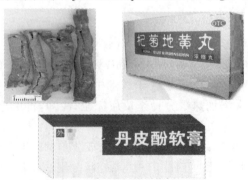

图 4-6 牡丹皮及其制剂举例

本品具有清热凉血、活血化瘀的作用,用于温毒发斑、吐血、夜热早凉、无汗骨蒸、经闭痛经、肿痛疮毒、跌打损伤等症。其主要成分有丹皮酚(含量 1.9％~2％)、牡丹酚苷(丹皮酚苷)、丹皮酚原苷、丹皮酚新苷等。此外,尚含挥发油(0.15%~0.4%)及植物甾醇等。

(1)丹皮酚。分子式为$C_9H_{10}O_3$,白色针状结晶,熔点49.5~50.5℃,稍溶于水,具有挥发性,能随水蒸气蒸馏,可溶于乙醇、乙醚、丙酮、氯仿、苯等。

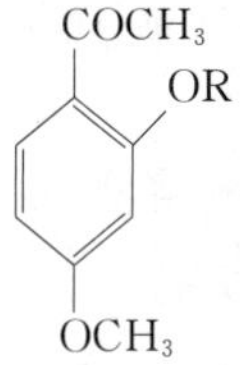

丹皮酚　　　R＝H

丹皮酚苷　　R＝葡萄糖

丹皮酚原苷　R＝葡萄糖－阿拉伯糖

(2)丹皮酚苷。分子式为$C_{15}H_{20}O_8$,无色柱状结晶(乙醇),熔点81~82℃,可溶于水、醇、丙酮、乙酸乙酯等,微溶于氯仿、苯等。

(3)丹皮酚原苷。分子式为$C_{20}H_{28}O_{12}$,无色柱状结晶(乙醇－乙酸乙酯),熔点157~158℃,可溶于水、乙醇、丙酮、乙酸乙酯等,难溶于苯、石油醚等。

一、实验目的

(1)掌握用水蒸气蒸馏法提取丹皮酚的方法。

(2)熟悉丹皮酚的色谱检识和定性检识方法。

(3)了解杞菊地黄丸中主要成分丹皮酚的鉴别方法。

二、实验原理

(1)丹皮酚具有挥发性,可随水蒸气蒸馏,又因在冷水中难溶,故放冷后即析出结晶。

(2)杞菊地黄丸中含有8味中药,丹皮酚为有效成分之一。利用丹皮酚溶于乙醚的性质,用乙醚提取,并将乙醚提取液用酚类的显色反应检识,与丹皮药材提取液和丹皮酚标准品对照鉴别。

三、实验步骤

1. 丹皮酚的提取分离

取市售丹皮150 g,粉碎,加入700 ml蒸馏水、10 ml乙醇和40 g氯化钠。浸润后,进行水蒸气蒸馏,收集蒸馏液约300 ml,将蒸馏液放冷,静置过夜,有白色针状结晶析出,滤取结晶,干燥,称重。如结晶不纯,可加入95%乙醇至全部溶解(约为粗晶的15倍),抽滤,滤液中加入4倍量的蒸馏水,使溶液呈乳白色,静置后则有大量白色针状结晶析出。若在提取过程中得不到白色结晶,只有油珠状物质沉出,可在蒸馏液中加入少量晶种,摩擦瓶壁后,即有较大量的丹皮酚结晶析出。也可用乙醚萃取蒸馏液几次,合并萃取液后,加无水硫酸钠脱水,回收乙醚至少量,放置析晶,抽滤,结晶用少量水洗2~3次,置干燥器中干燥后称重。

2. 丹皮酚的鉴定

(1)显色反应。

①三氯化铁反应。取丹皮酚结晶少许,加1 ml乙醇溶解,滴加5%三氯化铁醇溶液,观察现象。

②与浓硝酸反应。取丹皮酚结晶少许,加 1 ml 乙醇溶解,滴加浓硝酸数滴,观察现象。
(2)薄层色谱鉴别。
薄层板:硅胶 G-CMC-Na 板。
点样:丹皮酚供试品和对照品的乙醇溶液 10 μl。
展开剂:环己烷－乙酸乙酯(3:1)。
显色:喷以盐酸酸化的 5% 三氯化铁醇溶液,用热风吹至斑点显色清晰。

3.杞菊地黄丸中丹皮酚的薄层色谱鉴别

本品为蜜丸或水蜜丸,具有滋肾养肝的功效,由枸杞子、菊花、熟地黄、山茱萸(制)、牡丹皮、山药、茯苓和泽泻共八味中药组成。

(1)预处理。
①供试液的制备。取本品大蜜丸 9 g(水蜜丸 6 g),切碎,加硅藻土 4 g,研匀,加乙醚 40 ml,水浴加热回流 1 h,过滤,滤液挥去乙醚,残渣加乙醇 1 ml 使之溶解,即为供试液。
②对照液的制备。自制丹皮酚及丹皮酚对照品加乙醇,各制成 1 ml 含 1 mg 丹皮酚的溶液。

(2)薄层色谱鉴别。同丹皮酚的鉴定项下内容。

四、注意事项

(1)丹皮因产地、采收季节的不同,丹皮酚含量差异较大,春秋季节采收含量高,以四川产的含量较高,实验时可以根据丹皮酚的含量,加减提取的药材量。
(2)丹皮酚易溶于热水而难溶于冷水,由于初馏液中的丹皮酚浓度过大,遇冷易析出结晶,固着于冷凝管内壁,可加入乙醇使之溶解而流入接收瓶中。
(3)加入氯化钠可明显提高蒸馏的速度,缩短提取时间。

五、实验用品与时间安排

实验用品:丹皮,杞菊地黄丸,95%乙醇,氯化钠,三氯化铁,丹皮酚对照品,环己烷,乙酸乙酯,硅藻土,乙醚;水蒸气蒸馏装置,回流提取装置,展开槽,薄层板。
时间安排:要求在 6 学时内完成。

六、思考题

(1)水蒸气蒸馏法适用于提取什么样的成分?
(2)如何鉴定中成药中某一类化学成分?

第三节 醌 类

实验一 大黄中蒽醌类化合物的提取和分离

大黄为蓼科大黄属植物掌叶大黄(*Rheum palmatum* L.)、唐古特大黄(*R. tanguticum* Maxim.ex Balf.)或药用大黄(*R.officinale* Baill.)的干燥根和根茎(见图 4-7),主要含蒽醌

类化合物,有泻下和抗菌作用,为常用中药之一。

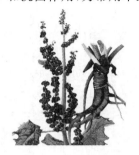
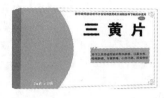

图 4-7　大黄及其制剂举例

大黄中具有泻下作用的成分是几种蒽醌类衍生物(羟基蒽醌苷类成分见图 4-8),其中苷是主要的成分,大黄的致泻效力与其中的结合性大黄酸含量成正比。具有较强致泻作用的蒽醌苷有以下几种:大黄酚-1-葡萄糖苷、大黄素-6-葡萄糖苷、芦荟大黄素-8-葡萄糖苷、大黄酸-8-葡萄糖苷、大黄素甲醚葡萄糖苷。还有蒽醌衍生物双糖苷,如大黄素双葡萄糖苷、芦荟大黄素双葡萄糖苷、大黄酚双葡萄糖苷以及番泻苷 A、番泻苷 B、番泻苷 C、番泻苷 D。番泻苷的泻下作用比蒽醌苷强,但含量远比后者少。近年来,从大黄中分离出四种新的大黄泻下成分,称大黄酸苷 A、大黄酸苷 B、大黄酸苷 C、大黄酸苷 D。除此之外,还含有大黄鞣酸及相关物质,如没食子酸(一部分是游离的,一部分是结合成没食子酰葡萄糖苷)、儿茶素,此类鞣质及相关物质有止泻作用,与蒽醌衍生物的苷类的泻下作用恰恰相反。

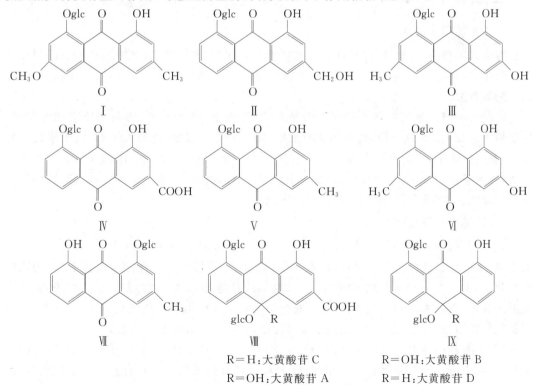

Ⅰ:大黄素甲醚葡萄糖苷　Ⅱ:芦荟大黄素葡萄糖苷　Ⅲ:大黄素葡萄糖苷　Ⅳ:大黄酸葡萄糖苷
Ⅴ:大黄酚葡萄糖苷　Ⅵ:大黄素-1-O-β-D-葡萄糖苷　Ⅶ:大黄酚-1-O-β-D-葡萄糖苷

图 4-8　大黄中羟基蒽醌苷类成分

大黄苷元主要包括大黄酚、大黄素、大黄酸、芦荟大黄素和大黄素甲醚共 5 种蒽醌苷元，基本上无致泻作用。蒽醌苷元的主要成分结构如下：

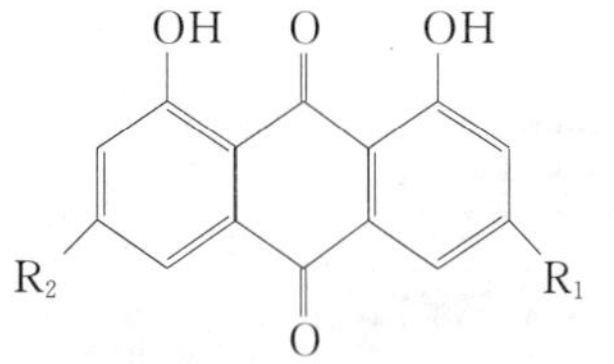

大黄酚　　　$R_1=CH_3$　　　$R_2=H$
大黄素　　　$R_1=CH_3$　　　$R_2=OH$
大黄酸　　　$R_1=COOH$　　　$R_2=H$
大黄素甲醚　$R_1=CH_3$　　　$R_2=OCH_3$
芦荟大黄素　$R_1=CH_2OH$　　$R_2=H$

一、实验目的

(1) 掌握 pH 梯度萃取法提取和分离大黄中各种蒽醌苷元的原理及实验方法。
(2) 了解蒽醌类化合物的颜色反应及色谱检查方法。

二、实验原理

在酸性条件下，大黄中的蒽醌苷类加热可水解成游离羟基蒽醌和糖，而游离羟基蒽醌不溶于水，可溶于乙醚、氯仿等亲脂性有机溶剂，从水解物中将游离羟基蒽醌提取出，再利用游离羟基蒽醌的酸性不同，采用 pH 梯度萃取法将其分离。也可利用游离蒽醌的极性不同，采用硅胶柱色谱方法进行分离。

三、实验步骤

1. 游离蒽醌的提取

称取大黄粗粉 25 g，加 20% H_2SO_4 水溶液 150 ml，直火加热 1 h，放冷，抽滤。滤饼用水洗至近中性，抽滤，于 70℃ 干燥后研碎，置索氏提取器中，加入乙醚 150 ml，回流提取 2 h，得到乙醚提取液。

乙醚提取液经薄层色谱可检测到大黄酸、芦荟大黄素、大黄素、大黄素甲醚和大黄酚。薄层板为硅胶-CMC 黏合板，展开剂为石油醚（60～90℃）－乙酸乙酯（7:3），近水平或直立展开，在可见光下，可看到四个斑点。其中 Rf=0.9 的黄色斑点为大黄酚和大黄素甲醚的混合物，在此条件下，二者不能分开，其余 3 个斑点依 Rf 值由大到小的顺序是：大黄素（橙色斑点）、芦荟大黄素（黄色斑点）、大黄酸（黄色斑点）。

2. pH 梯度萃取分离

(1) 大黄酸的分离。将乙醚提取液加入 250 ml 分液漏斗中，用 40 ml 5% $NaHCO_3$ 水溶液萃取，水层呈紫红色。分出水层，再重复萃取数次至不显红色。合并水层提取液，用浓盐酸酸化至 pH=3，可得大黄酸沉淀（注意：加酸时应缓慢加入，以防酸液溢出）。过滤，先用水洗沉淀数次，再用冰冷的丙酮洗，以除去有色杂质。干燥后用冰乙酸或吡啶结晶 2～3 次，得到黄色针状结晶。经熔点测定、纸色谱或薄层色谱检测，与标准品对照鉴定。

(2) 大黄素的分离。经 5% $NaHCO_3$ 水溶液萃取后的乙醚层，继以 5% Na_2CO_3 水溶液萃取，每次 40 ml，水层呈红色。分出水层，再重复萃取数次至不显红色。合并水层提取液，加盐酸至酸性，得黄色沉淀，过滤，用水洗沉淀，再用冰冷丙酮洗，在冰乙酸或吡啶中结晶数次，得到橙色针状结晶。经熔点测定、纸色谱或薄层色谱检测，与标准品对照鉴定。

(3) 芦荟大黄素的分离。经 5% Na_2CO_3 水溶液萃取后的乙醚层，继以 2.5% NaOH 水溶液萃取，每次 40 ml，水层呈红色。分出水层，再重复萃取数次至不显红色。合并水层提取液，加盐酸至酸性，得到橙色沉淀，过滤，用水洗沉淀，在冰乙酸或乙酸乙酯中结晶数次，得到橙色针状结晶。经熔点测定、纸色谱或薄层色谱检测，与标准品对照鉴定。

(4) 大黄酚和大黄素甲醚的分离。经 2.5% NaOH 水溶液萃取后的乙醚层，继以 5% NaOH 水溶液萃取至碱水层无色，每次 50 ml，合并 NaOH 萃取液，酸化得沉淀。过滤，用水洗至洗出液呈中性。低温干燥后得大黄酚与大黄素甲醚混合物，溶于乙酸乙酯，用硅胶柱色谱分离，洗脱剂为石油醚（沸程 60～90℃）-乙酸乙酯（15∶1）混合液。先洗脱下的化合物为大黄酚，后洗脱下的为大黄素甲醚，再分别进行乙酸乙酯结晶纯化、熔点测定和薄层鉴别。也可以溶于小体积石油醚中，改用下述纸色谱条件将两者分开。

纸色谱条件：滤纸（7 cm×20 cm）。

展开剂：水饱和石油醚（沸点 60～90℃）。

展开方式：上行法。

显色剂：4% NaOH 乙醇溶液。

3. 用纤维素粉柱色谱法分离大黄酚和大黄素甲醚

(1) 纤维素粉的制备：将滤纸（或其边角纸屑）剪成小片，称取 15 g，加入稀硝酸（每 100 ml 水中加 65%～68% 硝酸 5 ml）300 ml，加热水解（约 2 h），抽滤（G3 号耐酸漏斗），滤饼用蒸馏水洗至中性，再依次加少量乙醇、乙醚各洗涤 1 次，待挥发掉残存的乙醚后，低温烘干，粉碎，过 120 目筛备用。

(2) 装柱：取纤维素粉约 8 g，用水饱和石油醚（沸点 60～90℃）按湿法装柱。

(3) 样品上柱：将样品溶液用移液管小心加入色谱柱柱床顶端。

(4) 洗脱：用水饱和石油醚（沸程 60～90℃）洗脱，分段收集，每份 10 ml，分别浓缩。经纸色谱检查（纸色谱条件同上），将相同者合并，分别收集大黄酚和大黄素甲醚。大黄酚用乙酸乙酯重结晶后测熔点。

4. 硅胶柱色谱精制大黄素

(1) 装柱：取 100～200 目硅胶约 10 g，按干法装柱（柱长 1.5 cm×8.5 cm）。

(2) 加样：将大黄素粗提取物溶解于 5 ml 石油醚（沸程 60～90℃）-乙酸乙酯（7∶3）混合液中，用吸管吸取样品溶液，滴于色谱柱顶端。

(3) 洗脱：用石油醚（沸程 60～90℃）-乙酸乙酯（7∶3）混合液进行洗脱，分段收集，每份 10 ml，用硅胶薄层板追踪检查。

5. 大黄酚的鉴定

(1) 在薄层板上用点滴反应检查大黄酚对 NaOH、$MgAc_2$ 试液的反应。

(2) 测定大黄酚的紫外光谱。

(3) 用溴化钾压片法测定大黄酚的红外光谱。

四、注意事项

(1) 大黄中蒽醌的存在形式以结合状态为主，游离状态的仅占小部分。为了提高游离蒽醌的得率，提取时采用酸水解和萃取相结合的方法。

(2) 两相萃取时，不可猛力振摇，只能轻轻旋转摇动，时间可长一些，以免造成严重乳化而影响分层。例如，氯仿液用水洗时，容易乳化，可加入氯化钠进行盐析，使两层分离。

五、实验用品与时间安排

实验用品:500 ml 圆底烧瓶、烧杯、滴管、橡皮管、球形冷凝管(30 cm)、色谱缸、广口瓶、索氏提取器一套、250 ml 分液漏斗、布氏漏斗、抽滤瓶、普通滤纸、薄层板、色谱柱、喷雾器、广谱 pH 试纸;大黄 10~20 g, $NaHCO_3$、Na_2CO_3、NaOH、硫酸、氨水、盐酸、乙醚、石油醚、乙酸乙酯。

时间安排:要求在 6 学时内完成。

六、思考题

(1) 简述大黄中 5 种游离羟基蒽醌类化合物的酸性与结构的关系。

(2) pH 梯度萃取法的原理是什么?如何利用该方法分离大黄中的 5 种游离羟基蒽醌类化合物?

实验二　虎杖中大黄素的提取、分离和鉴定

虎杖又名阴阳莲、土地榆、苦杖,为蓼科植物虎杖(*Polygonum cuspidatum* Sieb. et Zucc.)的根茎和根(见图 4-9)。虎杖具有活血化瘀、清热解毒、祛痰止咳等功用,近年来用于治疗急性黄疸,降低血脂,增加白细胞和血小板数量,并可治疗慢性气管炎等多种炎症及烧伤等。其中大黄素是其蒽醌类成分之一,具有较广泛的生物活性。

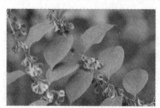 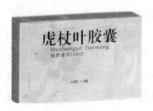

图 4-9　虎杖及其制剂举例

虎杖根茎中已知主要成分见图 4-10,其理化性质如下:

	R_1	R_2	R_3
大黄酚	—CH_3	—H	—H
大黄素	—CH_3	—OH	—H
大黄素甲醚	—CH_3	—OCH_3	—H
大黄素葡萄糖苷	—CH_3	—OH	—glc

白藜芦醇　R=H
虎杖苷　R=glc

图 4-10　虎杖中主要化学成分

(1) 大黄酚:金黄色片状结晶(丙酮)或针状结晶(乙醇),熔点 196~197℃,能升华;可溶

于苯、氯仿、乙酸、乙醇、NaOH 水溶液及热的 Na_2CO_3 水溶液，微溶于石油醚和乙醚，不溶于水、$NaHCO_3$ 和 Na_2CO_3 水溶液。

(2) 大黄素：橙黄色针状结晶，熔点 256～257℃，能升华；易溶于乙醇，可溶于 NH_4OH、Na_2CO_3 和 NaOH 水溶液，几乎不溶于水。

(3) 大黄素甲醚：砖红色针状结晶，熔点 206℃，能升华；易溶于 NaOH 溶液，可溶于苯、氯仿、吡啶、甲苯，微溶于乙酸、乙酸乙酯、乙醚，不溶于水。

(4) 大黄素葡萄糖苷：浅黄色针状结晶（在稀乙醇中析出，含结晶水），熔点 190～191℃。

(5) 白藜芦醇：无色针状结晶，熔点 256～257℃、216℃、264℃，能升华；易溶于乙醚、氯仿、甲醇、乙醇、丙酮等。

(6) 虎杖苷（白藜芦醇葡萄糖苷）：无色针状簇晶，熔点 223～226℃（分解）；易溶于甲醇、乙醇、丙酮、热水，可溶于乙酸乙酯、Na_2CO_3 和 NaOH 水溶液，微溶于冷水，难溶于乙醚。

一、实验目的

(1) 掌握从虎杖中提取羟基蒽醌类成分的方法。
(2) 熟悉用硅胶柱色谱方法分离混合羟基蒽醌类成分的一般操作技术。
(3) 熟悉羟基蒽醌类化合物的主要检识反应。

二、实验原理

本实验根据游离蒽醌类成分能溶于含水氯仿的性质，将原料用浓酸溶液湿润后，加入含水氯仿进行回流提取，在回流过程中即可将结合态的蒽醌（苷类）类成分水解成为游离蒽醌，这样就可连同原来存在的游离态蒽醌成分一并被含水氯仿提取出来。也可根据虎杖中的蒽醌类成分能溶于乙醇的性质，采用乙醇提取，再利用游离蒽醌类物质可溶于热的含水氯仿的性质，将乙醇提取物用含水氯仿加热回流，使游离蒽醌与蒽醌苷及其他极性较大的醇溶性杂质分离。

羟基蒽醌类化合物可以利用化合物酸碱强弱不同进行分离，含羧基或多个 β 位酚羟基的化合物可溶于碳酸氢钠溶液，具有一个 β 位酚羟基的化合物可溶于碳酸钠溶液，故可以用 pH 梯度法进行分离。另外，也可根据化合物极性大小不同，用硅胶柱色谱法进行分离。例如，大黄素的极性比大黄素甲醚大，在吸附色谱中吸附较牢，在大黄素甲醚之后洗脱下来。

三、实验步骤

1. 游离蒽醌的提取

方法一：称取虎杖粗粉 50 g，加 10% 硫酸溶液 50 ml，充分搅拌混匀，加氯仿 200 ml，在热水浴上回流提取 1 h，过滤得氯仿滤液。药渣用氯仿 200 ml 回流 1 h，过滤，合并两次氯仿提取液，置于圆底烧瓶中，加数粒沸石，水浴上蒸馏回收氯仿至干（可减压抽干氯仿），得红棕色残留物。再加苯 30 ml 于圆底烧瓶中，水浴加热，回流 0.5 h，过滤得苯滤液，置于蒸发皿中，加柱色谱用硅胶粉 3～5 g，搅拌均匀后于通风处晾干，得均匀样品粉末，供作柱色谱分离用。

方法二：取虎杖粗粉 50 g，加 95% 乙醇 500 ml，加热回流 1 h，倒出液体，再加 400 ml 乙醇，回流 0.5 h，合并两次提取液，过滤，滤液回收乙醇至无醇味，加入含水氯仿 100 ml，加热回流提取 1 h，倾出氯仿（如果氯仿提取液颜色较深，则再提 1 次）。合并提取液，用水

50 ml分2~3次在分液漏斗中洗涤,洗后回收氯仿至剩约 10 ml,趁热倒入一小锥形瓶中,放置析晶,抽滤,得橙黄色总游离蒽醌。

2. 大黄素柱色谱分离

(1)装硅胶色谱柱。取 100~160 目柱色谱用硅胶粉 10~15 g,装入底部垫有少许精制棉花的 20 mm×300 mm 色谱柱内。轻轻敲击色谱柱,使硅胶粉在柱内均匀充实后,即得干硅胶色谱柱。

(2)柱色谱分离。取上述提取项下所得游离蒽醌与硅胶粉混合的样品粉末,仔细加入硅胶色谱柱的上端,轻敲色谱柱,使样品粉末平整,打开色谱柱的下端活塞。缓缓加入适量苯于色谱柱中,使苯慢慢渗入柱内,然后用苯作为洗脱剂进行洗脱,柱下用锥形瓶收集洗脱液。经过一段时间的洗脱之后,可以看到在硅胶柱的上段逐渐形成清晰的红色和棕色两个色带,继续用苯洗脱,使两个色带分开至较大距离(2 cm 左右)时,改用乙酸乙酯—苯(2∶8)混合溶剂继续洗脱。更换收集容器,直至柱上第一段色带开始流出,控制流量并收集流出液(每 15 ml 为一流分),顺次编号,直到色谱柱上的两个色带全部洗脱下来为止。每个流分经薄层色谱检查,将相同斑点者合并,并分别蒸馏回收溶剂并浓缩。放置析晶,分别滤集结晶。先被洗脱下来的为大黄素甲醚,后被洗脱下来的为大黄素。

3. 大黄素 pH 梯度分离

将总蒽醌加入乙醚约 100 ml,使其完全溶解(或用上述氯仿提取液),加 5%碳酸钠溶液萃取数次(每次 20~30 ml),至萃取碱水液呈淡红色为止。合并萃取碱液,加盐酸至溶液呈酸性(pH 2~3),析出全部大黄素沉淀。抽滤,水洗,再滴稀乙醇抽洗。所得粗制大黄素可用吡啶或冰乙酸重结晶。用碳酸钠液萃取后的乙醚液(方法同上述碳酸钠溶液的处理方法)经酸化后,可得大黄素甲醚等弱酸性蒽醌类成分。

4. 大黄素的检识

(1)熔点。大黄素的熔点为 256~257℃。

(2)碱液反应。取大黄素少许,加 2 ml 乙醇溶解,继续加氢氧化钠试液 2~3 滴,溶液立即产生红色,继续加稀盐酸酸化,红色即褪去。

(3)乙酸镁反应。取大黄素少许,加 2 ml 乙醇溶解,加数滴乙酸镁试液,即产生橙红色(或紫红色)。

(4)薄层色谱检识。

吸附剂:硅胶-CMC 薄层板。

展开剂:苯-乙酸乙酯(8∶2)。

对照品:1%大黄素醇溶液或1%大黄素甲醚醇溶液。

供试品:分离后的1%大黄素和1%大黄素甲醚醇溶液。

显色剂:先在自然光下观察,再用氨气熏后观察。

四、注意事项

(1)游离蒽醌的提取方法中,结合状态的羟基蒽醌类成分不溶于氯仿,故未被提出。方法一中先用10%硫酸与氯仿共同回流,其目的是使结合状态蒽醌水解为游离状态蒽醌,易被氯仿提取出来,这样提取出的蒽醌类成分较为完全。

(2)柱色谱的硅胶用量应视样品量的多少而定,一般样品与吸附剂之比为1:100,若用量少则分离效果差,用量过多时易使柱体加长、洗脱速度减慢。

(3)如采用湿法装柱,可先在色谱柱中加入苯液,再通过漏斗将硅胶加入柱中,并始终保持硅胶面上有苯存在。样品上柱时也可采用干法加样,即将总蒽醌溶于少量丙酮,加降活性的硅胶,拌匀放置,待溶剂自然挥发或低温去掉溶剂,小心将其加入柱顶,再用苯洗脱。

(4)由于大黄酚和大黄素甲醚的极性接近,用硅胶柱色谱分离的效果不够理想,若采用磷酸氢钙作为吸附剂,以石油醚为洗脱剂,则大黄酚和大黄素甲醚可依次洗脱下来。

(5)按照一般常规柱色谱分离操作,本实验应先用苯洗脱大黄素甲醚,后用苯、乙酸乙酯混合液洗脱大黄素。为了保证实验进度,不致拖延时间,不必全部洗脱大黄素甲醚之后才改换溶剂,只要能看出两个色带明显分离一定距离时,即可更换溶剂进行下一步的洗脱。

(6)本实验需要多次使用乙醚,因此要特别注意防火安全,绝对禁止在有明火的情况下使用乙醚。

五、实验用品与时间安排

实验用品:虎杖粗粉、含水氯仿(水饱和)、苯、乙醇、柱色谱用硅胶(100~160目)、硅胶—CMC硬板、苯—乙酸乙酯(8:2)、乙醚、碳酸钠、氢氧化钠、盐酸、点滴板、1000 ml圆底烧瓶、蒸发皿、色谱柱、试管、梨形分液漏斗、精制棉、循环水泵、旋转蒸发器、电热套、水浴锅。

时间安排:要求在6学时内完成。

六、思考题

(1)羟基蒽醌类成分具有哪些性质?根据它的性质,说明其提取与分离的原理。

(2)大黄素的碱液反应和乙酸镁反应的原理是什么?

第四节　黄酮类

实验　芦丁的提取、分离和鉴定

芦丁(Rutin)亦称芸香苷(Rutinoside),广泛存在于植物界中。槐花米和荞麦叶含有较多量的芦丁,可作为提取芦丁的原料。槲皮素即芦丁苷元,可经芦丁水解制得。

槐花米系豆科植物 *Sophora japonica* L. 的花蕾(见图4-11),可作为止血药。槐花米的主要成分芦丁有减小毛细血管通透性的作用,临床上常作为防治高血压的辅助治疗药物。此外,芦丁对于放射性伤害所引起的出血症亦有一定治疗作用。

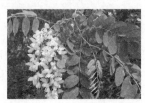
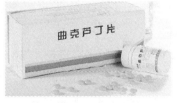

图4-11　槐花及其制剂举例

槐花米中芦丁的含量高达20%,另外还含有少量皂苷,皂苷水解后,可得到桦皮醇(Betulin,$C_{30}H_{50}O_2$)及槐二醇(Sophoradiol,$C_{30}H_{50}O_2$)。

(1)芦丁。芦丁为淡黄色细小针状结晶,分子式为$C_{27}H_{36}O_{16} \cdot 3H_2O$,熔点为177～178℃,无水物熔点为190℃(不完全),214～215℃时发泡分解。芦丁可溶于热水(1∶200),难溶于冷水(1∶8000);可溶于热甲醇(1∶7)、冷甲醇(1∶100)、热乙醇(1∶30)、冷乙醇(1∶300),难溶于乙酸乙酯、丙酮,不溶于苯、氯仿、乙醚及石油醚等溶剂。芦丁溶于碱液中呈黄色,酸化后又析出。

(2)槲皮素(Quercetin)。槲皮素为黄色结晶,分子式为$C_{15}H_{10}O_7 \cdot 2H_2O$,熔点为313～314℃,无水物熔点为316℃。槲皮素可溶于热乙醇(1∶23)、冷乙醇(1∶300),可溶于冰乙酸、乙酸乙酯、丙酮等溶剂,不溶于石油醚、苯、乙醚、氯仿和水。

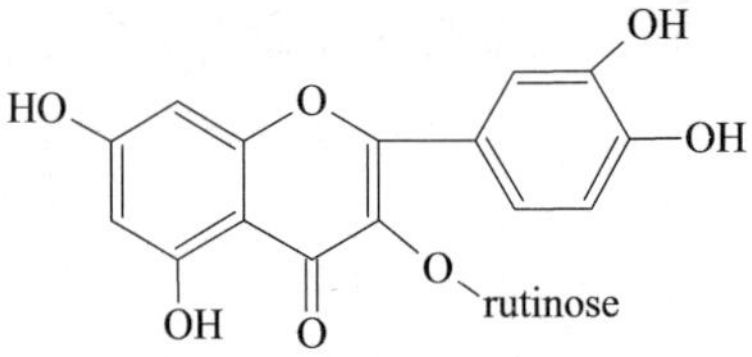

芦 丁

一、实验目的

(1)掌握碱溶酸沉法提取黄酮苷的原理和方法。
(2)以芦丁为实例,熟悉黄酮类成分的提取与分离方法。
(3)了解黄酮类成分的主要性质及黄酮苷、苷元和糖部分的鉴定方法。

二、实验原理

根据芦丁结构中含多个酚羟基,显酸性,能溶于碱水而难溶于酸水的特性,将其从植物材料中提出。也可根据芦丁在水中和乙醇中的溶解度,用水或醇提取。

三、实验步骤

1. 提取方法

称取1～1.5 g石灰粉(CaO),置于干燥的小研钵中,加入10 ml水后研成乳液备用。取槐花米20 g,置于干燥的研钵中用钵棒挤压成粗粉,置于500 ml烧杯中,加0.4%硼砂水的沸腾溶液400 ml,在搅拌下用石灰乳调至pH 8～9。加热微沸30 min,补充失去的水分,静置5～10 min,倾出上清液,用纱布过滤。残渣重复提取一次,合并滤液,冷却至60～70℃,用浓盐酸调至pH 4～5,再加8滴氯仿,放置过夜,抽滤,水洗3～4次,放置于空气中自然干燥,可得粗制芦丁。

2. 重结晶方法

取粗制芦丁2 g,加去离子水或蒸馏水400 ml(比例为1∶200),加热煮沸15 min,趁热抽滤,放置过夜析晶(或放冷析晶),抽滤,晾干或在60～70℃条件下干燥,得精制芦丁。

3. 芦丁的水解

取芦丁 1 g,加 2% H_2SO_4 80 ml,小火加热微沸回流 30 min 至 1 h。加热 10 min 后变为澄清溶液,逐渐析出黄色小针状结晶,即槲皮素。抽滤取结晶(保留滤液 20 ml,以检查其中所含单糖),用少许水洗去酸,干燥称重,然后用 95% 乙醇约 10 ml 进行重结晶,用薄层色谱鉴定。

4. 芦丁、槲皮素和糖的鉴定

(1)理化反应。芦丁属黄酮苷,具有黄酮苷的反应通性。

①Molisch 反应。取少量芦丁于试管中,加 0.5 ml 乙醇溶解,加等量 1% α-萘酚乙醇液,摇匀,再沿试管壁加入 0.5 ml 浓硫酸(小心使用,加后勿振摇),观察两液面有无紫色环出现。

②Fehling's 反应。取少许芦丁于试管中,加少量热水溶解,加入斐林试剂 1 ml,沸水浴加热,观察有无砖红色沉淀产生。如无沉淀,则加入浓盐酸 1 ml,水浴加热 0.5 h,再观察有无沉淀;如有沉淀,过滤除去,滤液加入氢氧化钠溶液,调至弱碱性,再加入斐林试剂 1 ml,沸水浴加热,观察有无砖红色沉淀产生。

③盐酸-镁粉反应。取芦丁少许,置于试管中,加乙醇 5 ml,水浴热溶,加镁粉少许,再滴加浓盐酸数滴,略微加热,观察颜色变化。

④三氯化铁反应。取芦丁少许,溶于水或乙醇中,加入 1% 三氯化铁乙醇溶液 1 滴,观察颜色变化。也可以在滤纸上进行。

⑤三氯化铝反应。取芦丁乙醇液滴于滤纸上,在紫外灯下观察荧光,然后喷 1% 三氯化铝甲醇液,再在紫外灯(365nm)下观察荧光。

(2)薄层色谱。

样品:自制芦丁、槲皮素。

对照品:芦丁、槲皮素。

展开剂及显色:正丁醇-乙酸-水(4∶1∶5 上层或 4∶1∶1),在可见光或紫外光下观察;25% 乙酸水溶液,经氨气熏后观察;85% 乙酸水溶液,喷三氯化铝试剂后观察。

(3)糖的检出。

①薄层色谱法。取上述滤除槲皮素时保留的水解滤液 20 ml,加 $Ba(OH)_2$ 的细粉(约 2.6 g)中和至 pH 为 7,滤除生成的 $BaSO_4$ 沉淀,滤液浓缩至约 1 ml,供薄层点样用。

展开剂:正丁醇-乙酸-水(4∶1∶5 上层或 4∶1∶1)。

对照品:葡萄糖、鼠李糖水溶液。

显色剂:苯胺-邻苯二甲酸(试剂喷后,105℃烘 10 min,显棕色或棕红色斑点)。

②圆形滤纸法。取上述水解母液 10 ml,小心用 $Ba(OH)_2$(1~1.5 g,并预先用 10 ml 水调成乳液)中和至中性,过滤出生成的 $BaSO_4$ 沉淀,滤液用热水浴小心浓缩至小体积(约 1 ml)备用。取一张圆形滤纸,用铅笔画出通过圆心的三条直线,将滤纸等分为 6 份,用对角点样法,将样品、葡萄糖、鼠李糖标准品分两次点于距圆心一定距离(>0.5 mm)处。用其他滤纸卷成的滤纸芯通过圆滤纸的圆心,借助滤纸芯的毛细管作用,用正丁醇-乙酸-水(4∶1∶5 上层)溶液作径向展开。

显色剂:苯胺-邻苯二甲酸,喷洒后在 105℃下加热数分钟,观察结果并记录。

四、实验用品与时间安排

实验用品：烧杯(100 ml,500 ml)、圆底烧瓶(100 ml,150 ml)、冷凝管、抽滤瓶、循环水泵、紫外灯、0.4%硼砂水、石灰乳、乙醇、甲醇、2%硫酸、盐酸、氢氧化钡、三氯化铝、正丁醇—乙酸—水(4∶1∶5上层或4∶1∶1)、25%乙酸、85%乙酸、芦丁、槲皮素、葡萄糖、鼠李糖。

时间安排：要求在9~12学时内完成。

五、思考题

(1) Molisch反应鉴别的是芦丁的什么结构特征？
(2) 如果某化合物的上述检识反应都呈阳性，能否证明它就是芦丁？为什么？
(3) 芦丁水解不完全时将产生什么结果？水解的产物是什么？
(4) 提取芦丁工艺中影响产量与质量的因素是什么？为什么要加硼砂水溶液？

第五节 萜类和挥发油

实验一 橙皮中柠檬烯的提取

橙皮又称黄果皮，是芸香科植物香橙(*Citrus junos* Sieb. ex Tanaka.)的干燥果皮(见图4-12)。橙皮很早就是中药的一种，味辛、微苦，入脾、肺二经，有止咳化痰的功效。橙皮含挥发油1.5%~2%，其主要成分为正癸醛、柠檬醛、柠檬烯和辛醇等，另含枸橘苷、橙皮苷、柚皮苷。柠檬烯又名苧烯、香芹烯。纯柠檬烯是无色液体，沸点176~178℃，有一种令人愉快的柠檬样香气，是生产软饮料、冰淇淋、糖果以及烘烤食品的添加剂之一。另外，柠檬烯具有良好的镇咳、祛痰、抑菌作用，复方柠檬烯在临床上可用于利胆、溶石、促进消化液分泌和排除肠内积气。

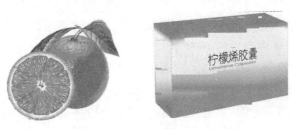

图4-12 香橙及其制剂举例

柠檬烯

一、实验目的

(1) 掌握从橙皮中提取柠檬烯的方法。
(2) 熟悉单萜的研究和鉴别方法。

二、实验原理

柠檬烯具有挥发性,能随水蒸气被蒸馏出来,可应用水蒸气蒸馏法进行提取。

三、实验步骤

取 2~3 个橙子的皮剪碎,放入 500 ml 三颈烧瓶中,加热水 200~250 ml 进行蒸馏,直到馏出液体达 60 ml 左右停止蒸馏。此时可见馏出液上面有一层薄油状物。将馏出液转入分液漏斗中,用 10 ml 二氯甲烷萃取 3 次,合并萃取液于 50 ml 干燥锥形瓶中,加无水硫酸钠 2~3 g 干燥。将干燥好的溶液滤入 50 ml 烧瓶中,进行蒸馏。水浴加热蒸去二氯甲烷。见二氯甲烷蒸完时,再接水泵,减压蒸去瓶中残余的二氯甲烷,瓶中留下的少量橙黄色液体即是橙油。对橙油进行气相色谱测定,其中柠檬烯的含量约为 95%。同时可测定折光率和旋光度。

四、注意事项

(1) 橙皮以新鲜的为好,干的也可以用作实验,但柠檬烯的产率低。
(2) 测旋光度时,应用 95% 乙醇配成 5% 橙油溶液进行测定。橙油的量不够时,可将几份合在一起配置测定液。必要时可取纯样配成溶液对比。

五、实验用品与时间安排

实验用品:二氯甲烷、无水硫酸钠、柠檬烯对照品、2~3 个橙子、500 ml 三颈烧瓶、50 ml 锥形瓶、水浴锅、水蒸气蒸馏装置、气相色谱仪、折光仪、旋光仪、真空泵、抽滤瓶、50 ml 烧瓶、布氏漏斗、分液漏斗。

时间安排:要求在 6 学时内完成。

六、思考题

将 d-柠檬烯催化加氢(两分子)后产物是什么?产物还有光学活性吗?为什么?

实验二　穿心莲中穿心莲内酯的提取、分离和鉴定

穿心莲为爵床科植物穿心莲(*Andrographis paniculata*（Burm. f.）Nees)的干燥地上部分(见图 4-13),有清热解毒、消炎、消肿止痛的作用。内服主治细菌性痢疾、尿路感染、急性扁桃体炎、肠炎、咽喉炎、肺炎和流行性感冒等;外用可治疗疮疖肿毒、外伤感染等。穿心莲含有多种二萜类化合物,主要为穿心莲内酯、去氧穿心莲内酯、新穿心莲内酯、脱氧穿心莲内酯等,它们的结构与性质如下。

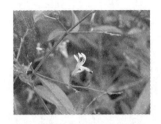
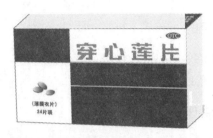

图 4-13 穿心莲及其制剂举例

(1) 穿心莲内酯。分子式为 $C_{20}H_{30}O_5$，相对分子质量为 350.44；无色方形或长方形结晶，味极苦；熔点为 230～231℃，易溶于甲醇、乙醇、丙酮、吡啶，微溶于氯仿、乙醚，难溶于水、石油醚、苯。

(2) 新穿心莲内酯。分子式为 $C_{26}H_{40}O_8$，相对分子质量为 480.58；无色柱状结晶，无苦味；熔点为 167～168℃，易溶于甲醇、乙醇、丙酮、吡啶，微溶于水，较难溶于苯、乙醚、氯仿及石油醚。

(3) 去氧穿心莲内酯。分子式为 $C_{20}H_{30}O_4$，相对分子质量为 334.44；无色片状（丙酮、乙醇或氯仿）或无色针状结晶（乙酸乙酯）；味稍苦；熔点为 174～175℃，易溶于甲醇、乙醇、丙酮、吡啶、氯仿，可溶于乙醚、苯，微溶于水。

(4) 脱水穿心莲内酯。分子式为 $C_{20}H_{28}O_4$，相对分子质量为 332.42；无色针状结晶（30% 或 50% 乙醇）；熔点为 204℃，易溶于乙醇、丙酮，可溶于氯仿，微溶于苯，几乎不溶于水。

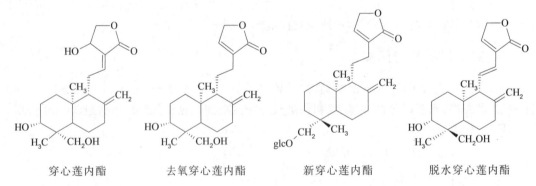

穿心莲内酯　　　　去氧穿心莲内酯　　　　新穿心莲内酯　　　　脱水穿心莲内酯

一、实验目的

(1) 掌握从穿心莲药材中提取亲脂性成分的原理和方法。
(2) 熟悉除去叶绿素的原理和方法。
(3) 了解内酯类成分的主要理化性质及鉴别方法。

二、实验原理

本实验是利用穿心莲内酯类成分易溶于甲醇、乙醇、丙酮等溶剂的性质，选用乙醇为提取溶剂进行提取。穿心莲中含有大量叶绿素，故要用活性炭吸附除去叶绿素等脂溶性杂质。根据穿心莲内酯与去氧穿心莲内酯在氯仿中溶解度不同而对它们进行分离。另外，也可利用穿心莲内酯、去氧穿心莲内酯及新穿心莲内酯因结构上的差异所表现的极性不同，用氧化铝柱色谱进行分离。

三、实验步骤

1. 提取

方法1：

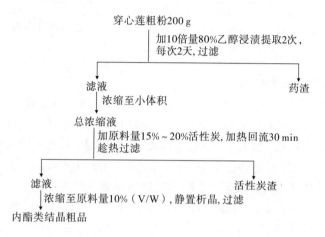

方法2：

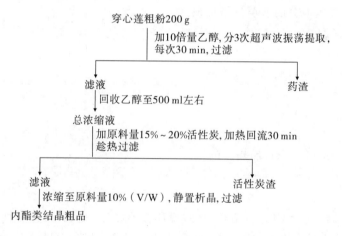

2. 精制

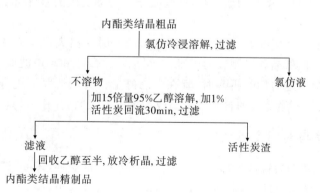

3. 分离

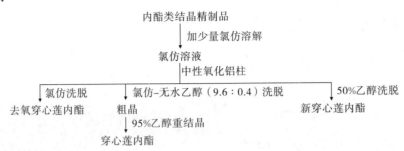

4. 穿心莲内酯类成分的检识

(1)异羟肟酸铁反应。取穿心莲内酯结晶数毫克,加乙醇 1 ml 溶解,加 7% 盐酸羟胺甲醇溶液 2~3 滴,加 10% 氢氧化钾甲醇溶液 1~2 滴使其呈碱性,于水浴上加热 2 min。放冷后,加稀盐酸使溶液呈酸性,加 1% 三氯化铁溶液 1~2 滴,混匀,此时溶液呈紫红色。

(2)Legal 反应。取穿心莲内酯结晶少许,加乙醇 1 ml 溶解,加 0.3% 亚硝酰铁氰化钠溶液 2~4 滴,加 10% 氢氧化钠溶液 1~2 滴,此时溶液呈紫色。

(3)Kedde 反应。取穿心莲内酯结晶少许,加乙醇 1 ml 溶解,加碱性 3,5-二硝基苯甲酸试剂 2 滴,此时溶液呈紫色。

(4)穿心莲内酯类成分的薄层色谱检识。
薄层板:硅胶 H-CMC-Na。
试样:自制穿心莲内酯乙醇溶液。
对照品:穿心莲内酯对照品乙醇溶液。
展开剂:
①氯仿-甲醇(9:1)。
②氯仿-正丁醇-甲醇(2:1:2)。
显色剂:喷雾 Kedde 试剂,加热显色。

四、注意事项

(1)穿心莲内酯类化合物为二萜类内酯,性质极不稳定,易氧化、聚合而树脂化。因此,提取所用的穿心莲应是当年产的新药材,并且要用未受潮变质的茎叶部分,否则内酯含量明显下降,难以提取得到。

(2)用热乙醇加热回流提取穿心莲总内酯时,能同时提出大量穿心莲中的叶绿素、树脂以及无机盐等杂质,使析晶和精制较为困难,故可以用冷浸法和超声波振荡法提取。

(3)分离项下穿心莲内酯的析晶时,宜在含乙醇量稍高的情况下进行,因为此时结晶形状与结晶纯度都较好。当溶液的含水量较高或黏稠度太大时,往往不易析出结晶。

五、实验用品与时间安排

实验用品:减压浓缩装置,1000 ml、500 ml、100 ml、10 ml 烧杯,10 ml 试管,试管架,托盘天平,量筒,三角漏斗,洗瓶,布氏漏斗,水浴锅,10 cm×20 cm 薄层板,10 cm×20 cm 薄层色谱缸,点样毛细管,紫外灯,玻棒,牛骨匙,纱布,脱脂棉,显色剂喷瓶,小型空压机,超声波振荡器,色谱柱(φ1.5 cm),穿心莲粗粉,滤纸,pH 试纸,活性炭,氯仿,中性氧化铝(柱色谱用),7% 盐酸羟胺甲醇溶液,氢氧化钾甲醇溶液,稀盐酸,1%三氯化铁溶液,0.3%亚硝酰铁氰化钠溶液,10%氢氧化钠溶液,碱性3,5-二硝基苯甲酸试剂,薄层色谱用硅胶H,0.2%CMC-Na,甲醇,穿心莲内酯对照品,展开剂氯仿—甲醇(9∶1)和氯仿—正丁醇—甲醇(2∶1∶2)。

时间安排:要求在9学时内完成。

六、思考题

(1)叶绿素除用活性炭吸附法去除外,还可采用哪些方法去除?

(2)穿心莲总内酯的分离可采用哪些方法?试比较各种方法的优缺点。

(3)Legal反应和Kedde反应的机理是什么?什么样的结构才有阳性反应?

实验三　八角茴香挥发油的提取和鉴定

八角茴香为木兰科八角茴香(*Illicium verum* Hook.f.)的干燥成熟果实(见图4-14),分布于广西、贵州、云南等省区;含挥发油4%～9%,脂肪油约22%(主要存在于种子中),还含有蛋白质、树胶、树脂等。挥发油的主要成分是茴香醚,为总挥发油含量的80%～90%,冷时常自油中析出,故称茴香脑。此外,挥发油中尚含莽草酸及少量甲基胡椒酚、茴香醛、茴香酸等,其结构和理化性质如下。

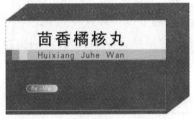

图4-14　八角茴香及其制剂举例

(1)茴香醚。分子式为$C_{10}H_{12}O$,相对分子质量为148.21;白色结晶,熔点21.4℃,沸点235℃;与乙醚、氯仿混溶,溶于苯、乙酸乙酯、丙酮、二硫化碳及石油醚,几乎不溶于水。

(2)莽草酸。莽草酸又称毒八角酸,分子式为$C_7H_{10}O_5$,相对分子质量为174.15;无色针状结晶(甲醇—乙酸乙酯),熔点190～191℃;易溶于水,可溶于乙醇,几乎不溶于氯仿、苯、石油醚。

莽草酸

(3)甲基胡椒酚。分子式为$C_{10}H_{12}O$;无色液体;沸点215～216℃。

(4)茴香醛。分子式为$C_8H_8O_2$,有两种状态:棱晶,熔点36.3℃,沸点236℃;液体,熔点0℃,沸点248℃。

(5)茴香酸。分子式为$C_8H_8O_3$;针状结晶;熔点184℃,沸点275～280℃。

一、实验目的

(1)掌握挥发油的水蒸气蒸馏提取法。

(2)熟悉挥发油中化学成分的薄层定性检识。

(3)了解挥发油的一般检识和挥发油单向二次薄层色谱检识。

二、实验原理

水蒸气蒸馏法是提取挥发油的通法。挥发油的组成成分较复杂,常含有烷烃、烯烃、醇、酚、醛、酮、酸、醚等官能团。因此,可以用一些检出试剂在薄层板上进行点滴试验,从而了解组成挥发油的成分类型。挥发油中各类成分的极性互不相同,一般不含氧的烃类和萜类化合物极性较小,在薄层色谱板上可被石油醚较好地展开;而含氧的烃类和萜类化合物极性较大,不易在石油醚中展开,但可在石油醚与乙酸乙酯的混合溶剂中较好地展开。为了使挥发油中各成分能在一块薄层色谱板上进行分离,常采用单向二次色谱法展开。

三、实验步骤

1. 茴香脑的提取分离

取八角茴香粗粉50 g,置于圆底烧瓶中,加适量水浸泡湿润,按一般水蒸气蒸馏法进行蒸馏提取。也可将捣碎的八角茴香置于挥发油测定器的烧瓶中,加蒸馏水500 ml与数粒玻璃珠,连接挥发油测定器与回流冷凝管,自冷凝管上端加水,使之充满挥发油测定器的刻度部分,直至溢流入烧瓶时为止。缓缓加热至沸,至测定器中油量不再增加,停止加热,放冷,分取油层。置冰箱中冷却1 h,即有白色结晶析出,趁冷滤过,用滤纸压干。结晶为茴香脑,滤液为八角茴香油。

2. 检识

(1)油斑试验。取八角茴香油适量,滴于滤纸片上,常温下(或加热烘烤)观察油斑是否消失。

(2)薄层色谱板点滴反应。取硅胶G薄层色谱板1块,用铅笔按表4-2画线。将挥发油试样用5～10倍量乙醇稀释后,用毛细管分别滴加于每排小方格中,再将各种检识试剂用滴管分别滴于各挥发油试样斑点上,观察颜色变化。初步推测每种挥发油中可能含有的化学成分的类型。

表4-2 挥发油薄层板点滴反应

试剂 试样	1	2	3	4	5	6
八角茴香油						
柠檬油						
丁香油						
薄荷油						
樟脑油						
桉叶油						
松节油						
空白对照						

试剂
1. 三氯化铁试剂
2. 2,4-二硝基苯肼试剂
3. 碱性高锰酸钾试剂
4. 香草醛－浓硫酸试剂
5. 0.05%溴酚蓝试剂
6. 硝酸铈铵试剂

(3)薄层色谱单向二次展开。取硅胶H-CMC-Na薄层板(6 cm×15 cm)一块,在距底边1.5 cm及8 cm处分别用铅笔画起始线和终点线。将八角茴香油溶于丙酮,用毛细管点于起始线上呈一长条形,先用石油醚(30～60℃)－乙酸乙酯(85∶15)为展开剂,展开至终点线处取出,挥去展开剂,再放入石油醚(30～60℃)中展开,至接近薄层板顶端时取出,挥去展开剂后,分别用下列几种显色剂喷雾显色。

①1%香草醛－硫酸试剂:可与挥发油产生紫色、红色反应等。

②荧光素－溴试剂:如挥发油产生黄色斑点,表明含有不饱和化合物。

③2,4-二硝基苯肼试剂:如挥发油产生黄色斑点,表明含有醛类或酮类化合物。

④0.05%溴甲酚绿乙醇试剂:如挥发油产生黄色斑点,表明含有酸性化合物。

四、注意事项

(1) 通过观察馏出液的混浊程度来判断挥发油是否提取完全。最初的馏出液中含油量较多,明显混浊,随着馏出液中油量的减少,混浊度也随之降低,至馏出液变为澄清甚至无挥发油气味时,停止蒸馏。

(2) 提取完毕后须放冷,待油水完全分层后,再将油层放出,尽量不带出水分。

(3) 进行单向二次展开时,先用极性较大的展开剂展开至终点线,然后再用极性较小的展开剂展开。在第一次展开后,应将展开剂完全挥干,再进行第二次展开,否则将影响第二次展开剂的极性,从而影响分离效果。

(4) 挥发油易挥发逸失,因此进行色谱检识时,操作应迅速及时,不宜久放。

(5) 喷洒香草醛一浓硫酸显色剂时,应在通风橱内进行;用溴甲酚绿试剂显色时,应避免在酸性条件下进行。

五、实验用品与时间安排

实验用品:100 ml、10 ml 烧杯,250 ml 三角烧瓶,10 ml 试管,试管架,托盘天平,量筒,洗瓶,蒸馏装置,电热套,10 cm×20 cm 薄层板,展开槽,点样毛细管,紫外灯,玻棒,牛骨匙,显色剂喷瓶,小型空压机。八角茴香粗粉,滤纸,三氯化铁试剂,2,4-二硝基苯肼试剂,碱性高锰酸钾试剂,香草醛一浓硫酸试剂(临时配制),0.05%溴酚蓝试剂,柠檬油,丁香油,薄荷油,樟脑油,桉叶油,松节油,丙酮,石油醚(30~60℃),乙酸乙酯。

时间安排:要求在 6 学时内完成。

六、思考题

(1) 从八角茴香中提取、分离茴香脑的原理是什么?

(2) 利用点滴反应检识挥发油组成的优点是什么?

(3) 单向二次展开薄层色谱法检识挥发油中各成分时,为什么第一次展开所用的展开剂极性最好大于第二次展开所用的展开剂的极性?单向二次展开薄层色谱法有什么优点?

实验四　栀子中京尼平苷的提取、分离和纯化

栀子是茜草科植物栀子(*Gardenia jasminoides* Ellis)的干燥成熟果实(见图4-15);性苦寒,无毒;能清热泻火,凉血,主治热病虚烦不眠、黄疸、目赤、咽痛、尿血、扭伤肿痛等症。栀子的主要化学成分有三类:环烯醚萜苷类、有机酸类及色素类等。栀子中含有大量的环烯醚萜类化合物,主要是京尼平苷,具有抗炎、解热、利胆和缓泻等作用。

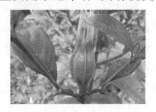 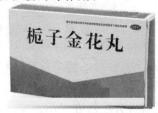

图 4-15　栀子及其制剂举例

京尼平苷,分子式为 $C_{17}H_{24}O_{10}$,无色针晶(四氯化碳),味苦,熔点 161℃~162℃,可溶于乙醇、水,微溶于乙酸乙酯、丙酮、乙醚、四氯化碳,不溶于氯仿、石油醚。

京尼平苷

一、实验目的

(1)掌握大孔吸附树脂柱色谱分离化合物的原理和方法。
(2)了解利用氧化镁吸附分离化合物的方法。

二、实验原理

大孔吸附树脂是一种不含交换基团的、具有大孔结构的高分子吸附剂,也是一种亲脂性物质。利用大孔吸附树脂吸附极性较小的化合物的特性除去糖类等水溶性杂质,再通过梯度醇洗脱达到分离纯化的目的。

吸附法对中药成分进行分离纯化有两种类型。一种是吸附要分离得到的物质,不吸附杂质;另一种是吸附杂质,不吸附要分离得到的物质。氧化镁是常用的吸附剂之一,本实验是利用氧化镁吸附所需物质,再用洗脱剂洗脱下来。

三、实验步骤

1. 提取分离流程(见图 4-16)

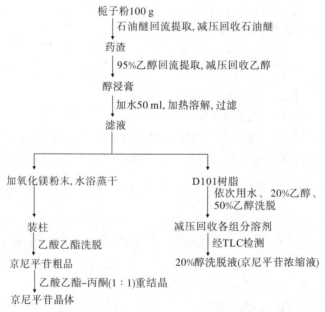

图 4-16 栀子中京尼平苷的提取和分离

(1)提取。取栀子粉 100 g,置于 1000 ml 圆底烧瓶中,加入 200 ml 石油醚回流提取 0.5 h,抽滤。药渣加 95% 乙醇 200 ml 回流提取 3 次,每次 30 min,合并提取液,减压回收乙醇得醇浸膏。浸膏用 60℃ 水浴加热溶解,抽滤。滤液可用于做下面两个实验之一。

(2)大孔吸附树脂柱色谱。

预处理:取 1.8 cm×28 cm 玻璃色谱柱 1 根,称取 25 g D101 大孔吸附树脂,加水浸湿

30 min,倒入柱中。用 95%乙醇洗柱,至流出液加 2 倍水不浑浊为止,再用水洗柱除尽乙醇,备用。

上样:将制备好的样品加入柱顶。

洗脱:先用水洗脱,流出液用 Molisch 反应检测糖类,至反应检测无糖类成分或显色很弱时,停止洗脱。再用 20%乙醇、50%乙醇依次洗脱,Molisch 反应呈阴性时更换洗脱液。减压浓缩收集的三个组分,并与标准品经 TLC 检测。京尼平苷主要集中于 20%醇洗脱液中,即得京尼平苷浓缩液。另外,水中还有少量京尼平苷,50%乙醇洗脱液中则没有。

(3)氧化镁吸附。将滤液倒入蒸发皿中,加入氧化镁 30 g,60℃水浴蒸干,得吸附有样品的氧化镁粉末。再将氧化镁装入色谱柱中,用乙酸乙酯洗脱 500 ml,减压回收溶剂,浓缩得京尼平苷粗品。在乙酸乙酯—丙酮(1:1)中重结晶得京尼平苷纯品。

2. 硅胶薄层色谱鉴别

样品:自制京尼平苷及京尼平苷对照品。

展开剂:乙酸乙酯—丙酮—甲酸—水(5:3:1:1 或 5:5:1:1)。

显色剂:

①50%硫酸乙醇溶液。

②艾氏试剂:将对二甲氨基苯甲醛 0.25 g 溶于 50 g 冰乙酸、5 g 85%磷酸和 20 ml 水中,用棕色瓶保存。

四、实验用品与时间安排

实验用品:栀子粉,圆底烧瓶,石油醚,真空泵,95% 乙醇,玻璃色谱柱,D101 大孔树脂,乙酸乙酯,丙酮,甲酸,硫酸,冰乙酸,磷酸。

时间安排:要求在 6 学时内完成。

五、思考题

(1)大孔吸附树脂分离化合物的原理是什么?

(2)为什么在水洗脱液中还含有京尼平苷?

(3)氧化镁分离纯化的原理是什么?

第六节 三萜苷类

实验一 甘草酸的提取和鉴定

甘草酸又称甘草皂苷,是豆科植物甘草(*Glycyrrhiza uralensis* Fisch.)、胀果甘草(*G. inflata* Bat.)或光果甘草(*G. glabra* L.)的干燥根和根茎(见图 4-17)中的主要活性成分,其含量为 7%~10%,味极甜,故又称甘草甜素。甘草中还含有多种黄酮成分,如甘草素、异甘草素、甘草苷、新甘草苷、新异甘草苷等。现代药理学研究表明,甘草制剂及甘草酸具有肾上腺皮质激素样作用,还具有解毒作用。解毒作用的机制为甘草酸对毒物有吸附作用,其水解产生的葡萄糖醛酸能与毒物结合,临床上可利用此机制治疗消化性溃疡。

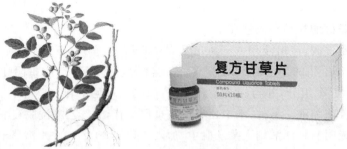

图 4-17　甘草及其制剂举例

一、实验目的

(1)掌握甘草酸的提取原理和方法。
(2)熟悉皂苷的性质和鉴定方法。

二、实验原理

甘草酸为白色柱状结晶(冰乙酸),熔点220℃;易溶于热水、热稀乙醇、丙酮,不溶于无水乙醇、乙醚等;在加热、加压及稀酸作用下,可水解为甘草次酸及二分子葡萄糖醛酸。

甘草酸分子式

甘草酸的提取精制原理:甘草酸在原料中以钾盐或钙盐形式存在。甘草酸盐易溶于水,因此可用水温浸,提出甘草酸盐,再加硫酸,因甘草酸难溶于酸性冷水,而析出游离。甘草酸可溶于丙酮,加氢氧化钾后,生成甘草酸三钾盐结晶。此结晶极易吸潮,不便保存,加冰乙酸后,转变为甘草酸单钾盐,具有完好的晶形,易于保存。

三、实验步骤

1. 甘草酸的提取

取甘草粗粉 20 g,加水 150 ml,于水浴上温浸 30 min,用棉花过滤,药渣再用 100 ml 水按同法提取 1 次。合并滤液,水浴浓缩至 40 ml,滤除沉淀物,放冷后加入浓 H_2SO_4 并不断搅拌,至不再析出甘草酸沉淀为止。放置片刻,倾出上清液,下层棕色黏性沉淀用水洗涤 4 次,室温放置干燥,磨成细粉,得甘草酸粗品。

将粗制甘草酸置于圆底烧瓶中,用 50 ml 乙醇回流 1 h,过滤,残渣再用 30 ml 乙醇回流 30 min,过滤,合并滤液,浓缩至 20 ml,放冷。在搅拌下加入 20%KOH 乙醇溶液至不再析出沉淀,使溶液 pH 为 8 左右,静置,抽滤。沉淀为甘草酸三钾盐结晶,于干燥器内干燥,称重。

将甘草酸三钾盐置于小烧杯中,加 15 ml 冰乙酸,水浴上加热溶解,热过滤,再用少量热冰乙酸淋洗滤纸上吸附的甘草酸,滤液放冷后,有白色的结晶析出,抽滤,用无水乙醇洗涤,得乳白色甘草酸单钾盐。

2. 性质实验及色谱检查

(1)泡沫实验。取甘草酸单钾盐水溶液 2 ml,置试管中用力振摇,放置 10 min 后观察泡沫。

(2)醋酐—浓硫酸反应(Liebermann-Burchard reaction)。取甘草酸单钾盐少量,置白瓷板上,加乙酸酐 2~3 滴使其溶解,再加半滴浓硫酸观察颜色变化。

(3)氯仿—浓硫酸反应。取甘草酸单钾盐少量,加 1 ml 氯仿,再沿试管壁滴加浓硫酸 1 ml,观察两层的颜色变化及荧光。

(4)薄层色谱。

吸附剂:硅胶 G 板(105℃活化 0.5 h)。

展开剂:正丁醇—乙酸—水(6∶1∶3 上层)。

样品:甘草酸单钾盐标准品,甘草酸单钾盐 70%乙醇液。

显色剂:磷钼酸。

四、注意事项

(1)甘草酸三钾盐极易吸潮,因此必须在干燥器中保存。

(2)薄层鉴定中显色前,薄层板上的展开剂需挥干。

五、实验用品与时间安排

实验用品:甘草,棉花,浓硫酸,圆底烧瓶,回流装置,KOH,乙醇,pH 试纸,烧杯,冰乙酸,水浴锅,真空泵,氯仿。

时间安排:要求在 6 学时内完成。

六、思考题

(1)甘草酸的显色反应有哪些?

(2)甘草酸的提取中,水提液中加入浓 H_2SO_4 的目的是什么?

实验二 齐墩果酸的提取、分离和鉴定

女贞子为木犀科植物女贞(*Ligustrum lucidum* Ait.)的干燥成熟果实(见图 4-18),为常用扶正固本中药。其促进免疫功能的成分为齐墩果酸、熊果酸及乙酰齐墩果酸,此外,还含有橄榄苦苷、D-甘露醇、硬脂酸、植物蜡等。齐墩果酸属于五环三萜类化合物,广泛分布于植物界,以游离态、酯、苷或兼有的形式存在于 150 多种植物中。例如,齐墩果酸以游离态和结合成苷的形式同时存在于女贞子中。经检测发现,其含量以幼果期(8 月份)最高,可达

8.04%,随着果实发育成熟逐渐下降到 2.5%左右。

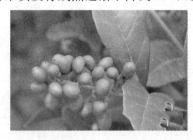 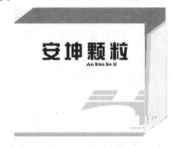

图 4-18 女贞子及其制剂举例

另外,齐墩果酸也是一种广谱抗变态反应药,对Ⅰ型、Ⅱ型变态反应均有抑制作用,是一种良好的免疫调节剂,具有抑制肿瘤,降低转氨酶,防治肝炎、肝硬化,降血糖,升高白细胞和增强机体免疫功能等功效。

女贞子中的主要有效成分和理化性质如下。

A   B   C

(1)齐墩果酸(A)。分子式为 $C_{30}H_{48}O_3$,白色针状结晶(95%乙醇),熔点 305~306℃;可溶于热甲醇、乙醇、乙醚、氯仿、丙酮等,不溶于水。

(2)乙酰齐墩果酸(B)。分子式为 $C_{32}H_{50}O_5$,白色簇晶,熔点 258~260℃;溶于氯仿、乙醚、无水乙醇,不溶于水。

(3)熊果酸(C)。分子式为 $C_{30}H_{48}O_3$,白色针状结晶(95%乙醇),熔点 286~287℃;易溶于二氧六环、吡啶,可溶于热乙醇,微溶于苯、氯仿、乙醚,不溶于水。

一、实验目的

(1)掌握三萜皂苷元的提取、分离和鉴定技术。
(2)熟悉三萜皂苷元的性质。
(3)了解两相溶剂水解方法。

二、实验原理

根据女贞子中齐墩果酸以游离型和结合成苷的形式共存于果实中的性质,采用酸水解、氯仿同步萃取法提取齐墩果酸。

三、实验步骤

1. 提取

称取女贞子果皮粗粉 50 g,置于圆底烧瓶内,加 15%盐酸溶液 350 ml、氯仿 250 ml,

70 ℃水浴回流水解 2 h,过滤,分取氯仿提取液(用水洗至中性,用无水硫酸钠脱水干燥,过滤)另存。药渣用水洗至中性,抽干,干燥药渣,使其含水量小于 10%。将干燥药渣置于圆底烧瓶内,加氯仿 250 ml 回流 1 h,合并二次氯仿提取液,取出 2 ml 提取液留待薄层检识,其余减压回收氯仿至糖浆状,趁热转移至烧杯中,冷后成半固状物。

2. 分离与精制

方法 1:取上述半固状物,以少量苯洗涤,除去脂溶性较大的成分,即有固体析出,抽干,得浅黄色析出物。用 1∶100 倍量(W/V)95%乙醇回流 10 min,过滤,滤液浓缩至小体积,放置析出粗晶,抽滤得齐墩果酸粗品。反复用 90%乙醇重结晶,可得较纯的齐墩果酸。

方法 2:浅黄色析出物的制备方法同方法一。用苯处理得浅黄色析出物,加 10 倍量 5%氢氧化钠溶液,煮沸 10 min。放冷后抽滤,用适量热水洗涤 1~2 次,抽干得类白色析出物,用 95%乙醇回流溶解,趁热过滤,用盐酸调至 pH 为 1~2,放置析晶。抽滤得齐墩果酸粗品,用正己烷-乙醇(1∶1)重结晶,可得较纯的齐墩果酸。

3. 鉴定

(1)呈色反应。取齐墩果酸少许置于试管中,加乙酸酐 1 ml,使其溶解后,沿试管壁加硫酸数滴,在两液层交界处出现紫红色环。

(2)薄层色谱鉴别。

薄层板:硅胶 G-CMC-Na 板。

点样:女贞子氯仿提取液、自制齐墩果酸乙醇溶液、齐墩果酸对照品乙醇溶液(1 mg/ml)。

展开剂:氯仿-丙酮(95∶5)和环己烷-乙酸乙酯(8∶2)任选一种。

显色:喷 10%硫酸甲醇溶液,105 ℃烘至显色,在日光灯和紫外光灯(365 nm)下检识。

四、注意事项

(1)女贞子中齐墩果酸的含量因采收季节、产地不同而有较大差异,可根据原料含量酌情增加药材量。

(2)用苯洗涤时应控制苯的用量,以防主成分的损失,也可用适量石油醚替代。

五、实验用品与时间安排

实验用品:女贞子果皮粗粉,圆底烧瓶,盐酸,氯仿,回流装置,水浴锅,真空泵,烧杯,苯,pH 试纸,乙酸酐,齐墩果酸,丙酮,环己烷,甲醇,紫外灯。

时间安排:要求在 6 学时内完成。

六、思考题

(1)采用果皮作为原料的优点是什么?

(2)两相溶剂水解法的原理是什么?

(3)本实验中采用皂化反应有何意义?

(4)齐墩果酸和熊果酸在结构上有何差异?在薄层色谱中如何区分?如何分离?

第七节 甾体类

实验 薯蓣皂苷元的提取和鉴定

薯蓣皂苷元,俗称"薯蓣皂素",存在于薯蓣科植物中,含量为1‰~3‰。我国薯蓣科植物资源丰富,种类亦多,分布于南北各地,其中作为薯蓣皂苷元生产原料的植物主要有盾叶薯蓣(*Dioscorea zingiberensis* C. H. Wright),俗称"黄姜";穿龙薯蓣(*D. nipponica* Makino),俗称"穿山龙"(见图4-19),两者的根茎常作为提取薯蓣皂苷元的原料。

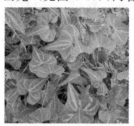
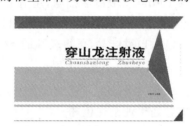

图4-19 薯蓣及其制剂举例

薯蓣皂苷属于甾体皂苷,水解可得薯蓣皂苷元,这种甾体皂苷元是近代制药工业中合成甾体激素和甾体避孕药的重要原料。薯蓣皂苷为无定形粉末或针状结晶,熔点288℃;可溶于甲醇、乙醇、甲酸,难溶于丙酮和弱极性有机溶剂,不溶于水。薯蓣皂苷元为白色粉末,熔点204~207℃;可溶于有机溶剂及甲酸,不溶于水。

一、实验目的

(1)掌握甾体皂苷元的理化性质。
(2)熟悉甾体皂苷元(亲脂性、中性成分)的提取和分离方法。
(3)了解甾体皂苷元的检识方法。

二、实验原理

本实验以穿山龙为原料提取薯蓣皂苷元。穿山龙中含有多种甾体皂苷,根据其水溶性分为水溶性皂苷和水不溶性皂苷。总皂苷水解可得薯蓣皂苷元,其含量为1.5%~2.6%。利用薯蓣皂苷元不溶于水而溶于有机溶剂的性质,用石油醚连续回流提取,可将其从植物中提取出来。

三、实验步骤

1. 预试验

在研究天然药物或中药化学成分时,应首先了解其所含化学成分类型,以便选择一种适当的提取分离方法,这就需要进行化学成分的预试验。预试验分为系统预试验和单项预试验。系统预试验旨在全面检查各类成分,单项预试验则是重点检查某类成分,本试验即选用此法。要寻找含皂苷的天然药物或中药,可单纯进行皂苷的预试验,具体试验方法采用泡沫试验和溶血试验。

(1)泡沫试验。取穿山龙粗粉 1 g,加水浸泡(1∶10)1 h 或置 80℃水浴上温浸 30 min,过滤得滤液供以下试验。

取供试液 2 ml 于试管中,塞紧试管口后猛力振摇,试管内液体产生大量的持久性的似蜂窝状泡沫,则说明有皂苷。

(2)溶血试验。取 2%血细胞悬浮液 1 ml,加生理盐水 8 ml,再加用于泡沫试验的滤液 1 ml,混合均匀后放置,几分钟内溶液由红色混浊变成红色透明,产生溶血现象,则说明有皂苷。

2. 薯蓣皂苷元的提取、分离

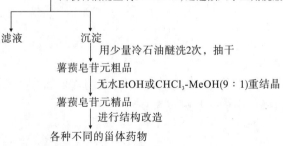

3. 薯蓣皂苷元的鉴定

(1)物理常数的测定。测定熔点和旋光。

(2)化学检识。

①乙酸酐-浓硫酸反应(Liebermann-Burchard 反应)。取样品适量,加冰乙酸 0.5 ml,使其溶解,继续加乙酸酐 0.5 ml,搅匀,再于溶液的边沿滴加 1 滴浓硫酸,观察并记录现象。

②三氯甲烷-浓硫酸反应(Salkowski 反应)。取样品适量,加三氯甲烷 1 ml,使其溶解,

沿试管壁加等量的浓硫酸,分别置于可见光及紫外灯下观察,并记录现象。

(3)UV鉴定。

UV $\lambda_{H_2SO_{4\,max}}$,nm(logε):334(3.68),412(4.1),512(3.52)。

(4)薄层色谱。

吸附剂:硅胶－CMC-Na薄层板。

样品:5%自制薯蓣皂苷元乙醇液。

对照品:5%薯蓣皂苷元标准品乙醇液。

展开剂:苯－乙酸乙酯(8∶2)。

显色剂:5%磷钼酸乙醇溶液,105℃加热至斑点显色清晰。

四、注意事项

(1)原料经酸水解后应充分洗涤至中性,以免烘干时炭化。

(2)在干燥水解原料的过程中,应注意压散团块和勤翻动,以利于快干。

(3)在连续提取过程中,欲检查有效成分是否提取完全,可取提取器中提取液数滴,滴于白瓷盘中,挥散溶剂,观察有无残留物,然后进行乙酸酐－浓硫酸反应。若反应呈阴性,说明已提尽。

(4)含蛋白质和黏液质的水溶液虽然也能产生泡沫,但不持久,放置时很快消失。

(5)所得薯蓣皂苷元粗品可作熔点测定,若测定不合格,再进行重结晶处理。

(6)溶血试验可同时作空白对照,以使比较现象更为明显,操作方法相同,只以生理盐水1 ml代替供试液即可。

五、实验用品与时间安排

实验用品:穿山龙,圆底烧瓶,浓硫酸,回流装置,研钵,碳酸钠,索氏提取器,石油醚,三角烧瓶,三氯甲烷,甲醇,乙酸酐,紫外分光光度计,硅胶－CMC-Na薄层板,薯蓣皂苷元标准品,乙酸乙酯,磷钼酸。

时间安排:要求在6学时内完成。

六、思考题

(1)甾体皂苷可用哪些反应进行鉴定?

(2)试设计一种从穿山龙中提取薯蓣皂苷元的工艺流程,并说明提取和分离原理。

(3)使用石油醚作提取溶剂时,操作中应注意哪些事项?

第八节 生物碱类

实验一 氧化苦参碱的提取、分离和鉴定

中药苦参是豆科植物苦参(*Sophora flavescens* Ait.)的干燥根,有清热燥湿、杀虫、利尿的功效。苦参在临床上用于杀虫,治疗痢疾、肝炎、荨麻疹、湿疹、气管炎等。药理实验证明,

苦参总生物碱有抗心律失常及抗癌活性等,氧化苦参碱有抗癌、抗衰老等作用。苦参中主要含生物碱和黄酮类成分,主要生物碱有苦参碱、氧化苦参碱、槐定、槐果碱(见图4-20)等,其理化性质见表4-3。

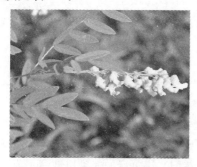
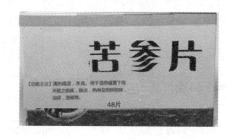

图4-20 苦参及其制剂

氧化苦参碱 ^{13}C-NMR 数据:68.7(C-2),17.0(C-3),25.9(C-4),34.3(C-5),66.6(C-6),42.4(C-7),24.4(C-8),17.0(C-9),69.1(C-10),52.8(C-11),28.3(C-12),18.5(C-13),32.7(C-14),169.8(C-15),41.6(C-17)。

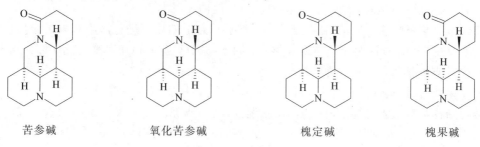

苦参碱　　　　　氧化苦参碱　　　　　槐定碱　　　　　槐果碱

表4-3　苦参中生物碱的理化性质

物质	分子式	性状	熔点(℃)	旋光性	溶解度
苦参碱	$C_{15}H_{24}N_2O$	白色针状结晶	76	+39.11°	易溶于醇、氯仿,溶于乙醚、苯、水
氧化苦参碱	$C_{15}H_{24}N_2O_2$	白色方晶	207~208	+47.7°	易溶于水、乙醇、甲醇、氯仿,不溶于乙醚、苯
槐定碱	$C_{15}H_{24}N_2O$	白色棱晶	106~108	-63.45°	易溶于水、甲醇、乙醇、四氯化碳等
槐果碱	$C_{15}H_{22}N_2O$	白色棱晶	80~81	-29.44°	易溶于水、甲醇、乙醇、四氯化碳等

从苦参中提取生物碱一般用水、酸水或醇提法,粗提物用树脂法或酸碱法纯化,分离方法多用氧化铝或硅胶柱色谱。

一、实验目的

(1)掌握渗漉法的原理、操作与影响因素。
(2)掌握连续回流提取法的原理、特点及仪器的使用方法。
(3)学习粗提物的纯化方法,学会分析纯化过程中所应用的原理。

二、实验原理

苦参中生物碱主要有苦参碱和氧化苦参碱。分子结构中均有两个氮原子,一个为叔胺,一个为酰胺。苦参生物碱可与酸结合成盐,因此用酸水提取后,生物碱呈阳离子状态而被阳离子交换树脂所交换,再用氨水碱化后使生物碱游离,用有机溶剂回流提取之。

三、实验步骤

1. 离子交换树脂的预处理

将 70 g 聚苯乙烯磺酸型树脂(交联度 3%)放入烧杯中,加 200 ml 80℃蒸馏水溶胀 30 min,倾出蒸馏水后加入 2 mol/L 盐酸 300 ml,充分搅拌,放置 0.5 h(静态转型),然后装入树脂柱(2 cm×100 cm),并使全部酸水溶液通过树脂柱(动态转型),流出液的速度以液滴不成串为宜。然后用蒸馏水洗至中性,待用。注意:从装柱到洗涤过程中始终保持液面高于树脂床。

2. 总生物碱的提取与纯化

称取苦参根的粉末 200 g,加入 260 ml 左右 0.5%盐酸湿润,搅匀,放置 20 min 后装入渗漉筒,加入适量 0.5%盐酸至下口有溶液流出且筒内无气泡。

将渗漉筒与树脂柱相连,计算渗漉速度。然后以合适的流速进行渗漉和离子交换,实验开始时及每过 1 h 检查渗漉液和交换液的 pH 和生物碱反应,并讨论其变化的原因。当生物碱提取完全或树脂完全饱和时终止实验。

停止渗漉后,用蒸馏水洗树脂至中性,倾出水层,将树脂倒入搪瓷盘中,铺平,晾干。将晾干的树脂称重后放入烧杯中,加 14%氨水湿润(使树脂充分溶胀又无过剩的水),加盖,静置 20 min,装入索氏提取器,用 300 ml 95%乙醇回流提取生物碱约 6 h,中间注意检查生物碱是否已被提取完全。停止实验后,将树脂回收,提取液置 500 ml 三角瓶中保存。

3. 氧化苦参碱粗品的获得

将乙醇提取液常压回收乙醇至小体积(6 ml 左右),加入 70～80 ml 氯仿溶解,转入分液漏斗中,静置分层,分出氯仿层,油状物另外保存。氯仿溶液用无水硫酸钠干燥 1~2 h(注意干燥过程中经常振摇),回收氯仿至干。残留物用丙酮析晶,即析出黄白色固体,放置,抽滤。用少量丙酮洗涤,得氧化苦参碱粗品,放到干燥器中干燥,母液放置待用。氧化苦参碱粗品用丙酮重结晶可得其精品。

4. 氧化苦参碱的分离

(1)粗品的检识(分离条件的寻找)。

方法:硅胶 HF_{254}－CMC 碱性薄层。

黏合剂:0.5%CMC 溶液－4%NaOH(9∶1)。

玻璃板:5 cm×15 cm,4 块/人。

展开剂:

①氯仿－甲醇(4∶1)。

②氯仿－甲醇－氢氧化铵(5∶0.6∶0.3下层)。

③氯仿－甲醇－氢氧化铵(10 ml∶1.2 ml∶2 滴)。

④苯－丙酮－乙酸乙酯－氢氧化铵(2∶3∶4∶0.2)。

(2)氧化苦参碱的分离。

①制备性薄层色谱法。

玻璃板:20 cm×20 cm。

硅胶 HF_{254}:20 g。

黏合剂:同粗品检识项下,用量为 60 ml 左右。

样品:氧化苦参碱粗品 300 mg。

展开剂:自选,用量 250 ml/4 人。

显色方法:自选。

洗脱:将氧化苦参碱色带刮下,装入洗脱柱,用氯仿-甲醇(7:3)混合溶剂洗脱至无生物碱为止,回收溶剂。残留物用丙酮溶解,过滤,回收丙酮至少量,放置待析晶完全,滤集结晶,干燥(注:将氧化苦参碱后面色带刮下,交给老师)。

②闪柱色谱法。

色谱柱规格:2 cm×50 cm。

吸附剂:230~400 目闪柱硅胶 35 g。

压力:0.3~0.5 kg/cm^2。

样品:120 mg 氧化苦参碱精品溶于 1 ml 氯仿中,湿法上样。

洗脱剂:氯仿-甲醇-氢氧化铵(5:0.6:0.3)(充分振摇后,静置,用下层)。

洗脱:每 5 ml 一流份,用硅胶碱性薄层检识,合并单一色点流份,回收溶剂,得氧化苦参碱纯品。

5. 氧化苦参碱的结构鉴定

(1)纯度检查:用 TLC 法,条件自选。

(2)测定熔点。

(3)测定产品的 IR、MS、^{1}H-NMR 谱。

四、注意事项

(1)苦参粗粉过 10 目筛即可,不宜太粗或太细。

(2)树脂使用前应用水充分膨胀,否则交换效率低,重现性差。

(3)喷改良碘化铋钾试液前,薄层板上残留展开剂要挥干。

五、实验用品与时间安排

实验用品:索氏提取器,渗漉筒,阳离子交换树脂,500 ml、100 ml、10 ml 烧杯,10 ml 试管,试管架,托盘天平,量筒,三角漏斗,洗瓶,布氏漏斗,水浴锅,10 cm×20 cm 薄层板,10 cm×20 cm 薄层色谱缸,点样毛细管,紫外灯,玻棒,牛骨匙,脱脂棉,显色剂喷瓶,小型空压机,色谱柱(ϕ1.5 cm),苦参粗粉,滤纸,pH 试纸,盐酸,丙酮,改良碘化铋钾试剂,薄层用硅胶 H,0.5%CMC-Na,4%氢氧化钠,甲醇,苦参碱、氧化苦参碱对照品。苦参碱展开剂:甲苯-乙酸乙酯-甲醇-水(2:4:2:1)10℃下放置的上层溶液。氧化苦参碱展开剂:氯仿-甲醇-浓氨试液(5:0.6:0.3)10℃下放置的下层溶液,氯化钠,无水硫酸钠。

时间安排:要求在 12 学时内完成。

六、思考题

(1)叙述酸水法及离子交换法提取纯化生物碱的原理。
(2)应如何检查：①渗漉液中是否含有生物碱？②渗漉液中生物碱是否被交换在树脂上？③离子交换树脂是否已饱和？
(3)简述索氏提取器的提取原理及特点。
(4)什么叫闪柱色谱？其有何优缺点？
(5)制备性薄层色谱的特点是什么？
(6)简述提取、分离和鉴定生物碱的程序，并分析所测氧化苦参碱的各种波谱数据。

实验二　黄柏中小檗碱的提取、分离和鉴定

黄柏为芸香科植物黄皮树(*Phellodendron chinense* Schneid.)的干燥树皮。小檗碱属于季铵型生物碱，为黄色针晶，能溶于水，在热水和乙醇中溶解度较大，难溶于丙酮、氯仿或苯；其盐在水中溶解度较小，尤其是盐酸小檗碱，难溶于冷水(1∶500)而易溶于热水。小檗碱及其盐类有较好的抗菌作用，临床上用以治疗菌痢和一般炎症。

小檗碱主要存在于黄连、黄柏、三颗针等中草药中(见图4-21)，本实验从黄柏中提取、分离小檗碱。小檗碱含量为1.4%～4%(川黄柏中含量较高)。性状：黄色结晶，含5.5分子结晶水，熔点145℃。溶解性：能缓缓溶于冷水中(1∶20)，微溶于冷乙醇(1∶100)，易溶于热水和热乙醇，微溶或不溶于苯、氯仿和丙酮，硝酸盐极难溶于水，盐酸盐微溶于冷水(1∶500)但较易溶于沸水，硫酸盐和枸橼酸盐在水中溶解度较大(1∶30)。盐酸小檗碱为黄色结晶，含2分子结晶水，220℃时分解并转变为棕红色小檗红碱，285℃时完全熔融。

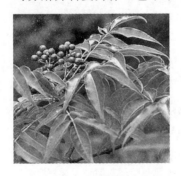
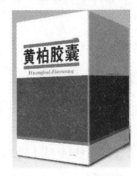

图 4-21　黄柏及其制剂举例

小檗碱

一、实验目的

(1)掌握从黄柏中提取、分离、检识小檗碱的原理和方法。
(2)熟悉渗漉法、柱色谱在提取中草药有效成分中的应用。

二、实验原理

小檗碱属季铵碱,其游离型在水中溶解度较大,其盐酸盐在水中溶解度小。利用小檗碱的溶解性及根据黄柏中富含黏液质的特点,首先用石灰乳沉淀黏液质,用碱水自黄柏中提出小檗碱,再加盐酸使其转化为盐酸小檗碱而沉淀析出。

三、实验步骤

1. 提取

装渗漉筒:渗漉筒用纱布垫底,用铁圈、铁夹将渗漉筒固定在铁架台上,旋紧下口和乳胶管上的螺旋夹。

称取黄柏粗粉(若为饮片应适当破碎)50 g,置烧杯中,加入石灰乳搅拌均匀(加入量:使药材刚好被润湿而无多余液体为宜)。装筒时边装边用玻棒压紧,平整,使筒内药材均匀一致。装筒后表面上盖一片圆形滤纸,滤纸上面用几块干净的小石块压住,加 500 ml 饱和石灰水(缓慢沿器壁加入,尽量保持高于药材部分的液体无色)。浸泡 2 h 后渗漉,控制流速为 5 ml/min,收集渗漉液 500 ml,加入渗漉液体积 7%(W/V)的食盐,搅拌后放置过夜,析出沉淀,抽滤(抽滤前勿摇动沉淀,可先用滴管将绝大多数上清液吸出后再抽滤)。沉淀用蒸馏水洗至中性,抽干后于 80 ℃ 干燥,即得盐酸小檗碱粗品。

2. 精制

(1)将粗品加入适量沸水中(60～80 ml,可逐渐加,以粗品刚好全部溶解为度),于水浴上溶解,趁热过滤。滤液于水浴上加热至澄清后,加浓盐酸调 pH 为 2～3,搅拌后放冷,用滤纸抽滤,沉淀用蒸馏水洗至中性,80 ℃ 干燥,即得盐酸小檗碱结晶。

(2)柱色谱。

吸附剂:中性氧化铝。

洗脱剂:95%乙醇。

样品液:取盐酸小檗碱结晶溶于少量 95%乙醇中。

干法装柱(装柱量为柱长的 2/3),上样,用 95%乙醇洗脱至无色,将洗脱液置于水浴中浓缩(勿用电炉)至小体积(约 10 ml),放置析晶。

3. 检识

(1)生物碱的一般鉴别反应。取少量精制盐酸小檗碱,用酸水溶解,分成四份,分别滴加以下试剂。

①碘化铋钾试剂(Dragendorff 试剂),观察产生沉淀的颜色。
②碘化汞钾试剂(Mager 试剂),观察产生沉淀的颜色。
③碘—碘化钾试剂(Wagner 试剂),观察产生沉淀的颜色。
④硅钨酸试剂(Bertand 试剂),观察产生沉淀的颜色。

(2)小檗碱的特殊鉴别反应。

①取盐酸小檗碱少许,加漂白粉(或次氯酸钠)少许,即显樱红色。

②取盐酸小檗碱少许,加稀硫酸 2 ml 使其溶解,加浓硝酸 1~2 滴,即显樱红色。

③取盐酸小檗碱约 0.05 g,溶于 5 ml 热水中,加入 10% NaOH 溶液 2 ml,显橙色。溶液放冷,加入丙酮约 0.5 ml,静置,有黄色丙酮小檗碱结晶析出。

④取盐酸小檗碱少许,加水 2 ml 溶解,加锌粉少许,再分数次加入浓硫酸数滴,振摇,每隔 10 min 加一次,观察其黄色是否消退。

四、注意事项

(1)实验原料尽可能选用小檗碱含量较高的川黄柏。

(2)加入氯化钠的目的是将小檗碱转化成盐酸小檗碱,并利用盐析作用,降低其在水中的溶解度。其用量不宜过少,否则盐析效果不好,收率过低。

(3)精制盐酸小檗碱时,因盐酸小檗碱几乎不溶于冷水,放冷易析晶,所以水浴加热溶解后,要趁热过滤,防止盐酸小檗碱在过滤时析晶,使过滤困难,产量降低。

五、实验用品与时间安排

实验用品:渗漉筒、水浴锅、真空泵、温度计、小色谱柱、烘箱、烧杯、胶头滴管、抽滤装置、玻璃棒。黄柏、石灰、中性氧化铝、95%乙醇、丙酮、盐酸、食盐、漂白粉、碱式硝酸铋、碘、碘化钾、氯化汞、冰乙酸、氢氧化钠、硅钨酸、蒸馏水、氢氧化钙或氧化钙(可用桶或盆子加水配成石灰乳,静置后即为饱和石灰水)。纱布、滤纸、卷纸、乳胶管、pH 试纸。

时间安排:要求在 6 学时内完成。

六、思考题

(1)如何测定所得到的小檗碱的纯度?

(2)如何鉴定小檗碱的化学结构?

(3)怎样从黄柏中提取分离盐酸小檗碱?原理是什么?为什么加石灰乳?

(4)用薄层色谱法检识盐酸小檗碱时,选用氧化铝或硅胶作吸附剂,二者有何区别?展开剂有何不同?

实验三 茶叶中咖啡因的提取及其红外光谱测定

咖啡因又叫咖啡碱,是一种生物碱,存在于茶叶、咖啡、可可等植物中(见图 4-22)。例如茶叶中含有 1%~5% 的咖啡因,同时还含有单宁酸、色素、纤维素等物质。

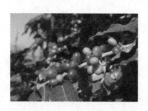
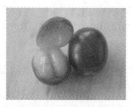
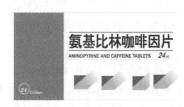

图 4-22 咖啡及其制剂举例

咖啡因是弱碱性化合物,可溶于氯仿、丙醇、乙醇和热水,难溶于乙醚和苯(冷)。纯品熔点 235～236℃,含结晶水的咖啡因为无色针状晶体,在 100℃时失去结晶水,并开始升华,120℃时显著升华,178℃时迅速升华。利用这一性质可纯化咖啡因。

咖啡因

咖啡因(1,3,7-三甲基-2,6-二氧嘌呤)是一种温和的兴奋剂,具有刺激心脏、兴奋中枢神经和利尿等作用。工业上咖啡因主要是通过人工合成制得,是复方阿司匹林(阿司匹林,非那西汀和咖啡因)等药物的组分之一。

一、实验目的

(1)掌握索氏提取器的原理及其应用。
(2)掌握升华法的原理及操作。
(3)了解傅立叶变换红外光谱仪的工作原理和使用方法。
(4)熟悉固态物质红外制样方法——溴化钾压片法。
(5)了解利用红外吸收光谱进行定性结构鉴定的方法。

二、实验原理

提取咖啡因的方法有碱液提取法和索氏提取器提取法。本实验以乙醇为溶剂,用索氏提取器提取,再经浓缩、中和和升华,得到含结晶水的咖啡因。

三、实验步骤

1. 实验流程

茶叶末 —95%乙醇回流提取→ 提取液 —蒸干→ 粗提取液 —蒸干→ 粗提取物 —(1)升华/(2)收集→ 咖啡因

2. 咖啡因的提取

称取 5 g 干茶叶,装入滤纸筒内,轻轻压实。滤纸筒上口塞一团脱脂棉,置于索氏提取器中,圆底烧瓶内加入 60～80 ml 95% 乙醇,加热乙醇至沸,连续抽提 2 h,待冷凝液刚刚虹吸下去时,立即停止加热。

将仪器改装成蒸馏装置(见图 4-23),加热回收大部分乙醇。然后将残留液(10～15 ml)倾入蒸发皿中,用少量乙醇洗涤烧瓶,洗涤液也倒入蒸发皿中,蒸发至近干。加入 4 g 生石灰粉,搅拌均匀,用电热套加热(100～120V),蒸发至干,除去全部水分。冷却后,擦去沾在蒸发皿边上的粉末,以免升华时污染产物。

将一张刺有许多小孔的圆形滤纸盖在蒸发皿上,取一只大小合适的玻璃漏斗罩于其上,漏斗颈部疏松地塞一团棉花。

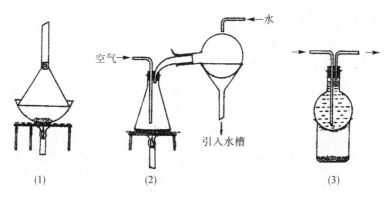

图 4-23 咖啡因升华装置

用电热套小心加热蒸发皿,慢慢升高温度,使咖啡因升华。咖啡因通过滤纸孔遇到漏斗内壁凝为固体,附着于漏斗内壁和滤纸上。当纸上出现白色针状晶体时,暂停加热,冷却至100℃左右,揭开漏斗和滤纸,用小刀仔细把附着于滤纸及漏斗壁上的咖啡因刮入蒸发皿中。将蒸发皿内的残渣加以搅拌,重新放好滤纸和漏斗,用较高的温度再加热升华一次。此时,温度也不宜太高,否则蒸发皿内大量冒烟,产品既遭受污染又蒙受损失。合并两次升华所收集的咖啡因,测定熔点。

3. 咖啡因的鉴定

(1)沉淀反应。取咖啡因结晶的一半于小试管中,加 4 ml 水,微加热,使固体溶解并分装于 2 支试管中:一支加入 1～2 滴 5% 鞣酸溶液,记录现象;另一支加 1～2 滴 10% 盐酸(或 10% 硫酸),再加入 1～2 滴碘-碘化钾试剂,记录现象。

(2)氧化反应。在蒸发皿剩余的咖啡因中,加入 30% H_2O_2 8～10 滴,置于水浴上蒸干,记录残渣颜色。再加一滴浓氨水于残渣上,观察并记录颜色的变化。

(3)其他鉴别方法。咖啡因可以通过测定熔点或采用光谱法加以鉴别。此外,还可以通过制备咖啡因水杨酸盐衍生物进一步确证。咖啡因可与水杨酸反应生成咖啡因水杨酸盐衍生物,此盐的熔点为137℃。其反应式如下:

咖啡因水杨酸盐衍生物的制备方法:在试管中加入 50 mg 咖啡因、30 mg 水杨酸和 2.5 ml 甲苯,在水浴上加热摇振使其溶解,然后加入约 1.5 ml 石油醚(60～90℃),在冰浴中冷却结晶。如无晶体析出,可以用玻璃棒或刮刀摩擦管壁。用玻璃漏斗过滤并收集产物,测定产物的熔点。纯盐的熔点为137℃。

(4)红外吸收光谱测定。固态样品一般可采用压片法和糊状法制样。压片法是将样品与溴化钾粉末混合,磨细研匀后,压制成厚度约为 1 mm 的透明薄片;糊状法是将样片研磨成足够细的粉末,然后用液状石蜡或四氯化碳调成糊状,然后将糊状物薄薄地均匀涂布在溴化钾晶片上。

①开启仪器,启动计算机并进入 OMNIC 窗口。

②压片法制样。取 1~2 mg 干燥试样放入玛瑙研钵中,加入 100 mg 左右的溴化钾粉末,磨细研匀。按照图 4-24 所示顺序放好压模的底座、底模片、试样纸片和压模体,然后将研磨好的含试样的溴化钾粉末小心放入试样纸片中央的孔中,将压杆插入压模体,再插到底,轻轻转动,使加入的溴化钾粉末铺匀。把整个压模放到压片机的工作台垫板上(见图 4-24 和图 4-25),旋转压力丝杆手轮,压紧压模,顺时针旋转放油阀到底,缓慢上下压动压把,观察压力表。当压力达到时,停止加压,维持 2~3 min,逆时针旋转放油阀,压力解除,压力表指针回到"0",旋松压力丝杆手轮,取出压模,即可得到固定在试样纸片孔中的透明晶片。将试样纸片小心放在磁性样品架的正中间,供下一步测定样品图时使用。

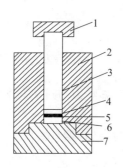

1. 压杆帽 2. 压模体 3. 压杆 4. 顶模片
5. 试样纸片 6. 底模片 7. 底座

图 4-24　压模结构

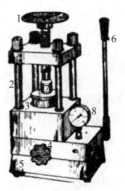

1. 压力丝杆手轮 2. 拉力螺栓 3. 工作台垫板
4. 放油阀 5. 机座 6. 压把 7. 压模 8. 压力表

图 4-25　压片机

③绘制红外光谱图并进行标准谱库检索。整个过程包括:设定收集参数;收集背景资料;收集样品图;对所得试样谱图进行基线校正、标峰等处理;标准谱库检索;打印谱图。

④收集样品图完成后,即可从样品室中取出样品架。并用浸有无水乙醇的脱脂棉将用过的研钵、镊子、刮刀、压模等清洗干净,置于红外干燥灯下烘干,以备制下一个试样。

四、注意事项

(1)加入生石灰起中和作用,以除去单宁酸等酸性物质。生石灰一定要研细。

(2)乙醇将要蒸干时,固体易溅出皿外,应注意防止着火。

(3)升华前,一定要将水分完全除去,否则在升华时漏斗内会出现水珠。遇此情况,则用滤纸迅速擦干水珠,并继续焙烧片刻而至升华。提取时,如烧瓶里留有少量水分,升华开始时,将产生一些烟雾,会污染器皿和产品。

(4)在升华过程中必须始终严格控制加热温度,温度太高,将导致被烘物和滤纸炭化,一些有色物质也会被带出来,影响产品的质量。升华过程中,始终都需用小火间接加热。如温度太高,会使产物发黄。注意温度计应放在合适的位置,才能正确反映出升华的温度。如无砂浴,也可以用简易空气浴加热升华,即将蒸发皿底部稍离开石棉网进行加热,并在附近悬挂温度计指示升华温度。

(5)在无索氏提取器的情况下,可采用回流提取装置。但一般回流提取装置所用溶剂量较大,且提取效果较索氏提取器差。

(6)制样时,试样量必须合适。试样量过多,制得的试样晶片太"厚",透光率差,导致收集到的谱图中强峰超出检测范围;试样量太少,制得的晶片太"薄",收集到的谱图信噪比差。

(7)红外光谱实验应在干燥的环境中进行,因为红外光谱仪中的一些透光部件是由溴化钾等易溶于水的物质制成,在潮湿的环境中极易损坏。另外,水本身能吸收红外光并产生强的吸收峰,干扰试样的谱图。

五、实验用品与时间安排

实验用品:茶叶、95%乙醇、生石灰。60 ml索氏提取器、蒸发皿、玻璃漏斗、蒸馏头、接收管、50 ml锥形瓶、直形冷凝管。红外光谱仪、红外干燥灯、不锈钢镊子、样品刮刀、玛瑙研钵、试样纸片、压模机、压片机、磁性样品架、无水乙醇浸泡的脱脂棉等。

时间安排:要求在9学时内完成。

六、思考题

(1)咖啡因与鞣酸溶液作用生成什么沉淀?

(2)咖啡因与碘-碘化钾试剂作用生成什么颜色的沉淀?咖啡因与过氧化氢等氧化剂作用的实验现象是什么?

(3)化合物的红外光谱是怎样产生的?它能提供哪些重要的结构信息?

(4)为什么甲基的伸缩振动出现在高频区?

(5)单靠红外光谱解析能否得到未知物的准确结构?为什么?

(6)含水的样品是否能直接用于测定其红外光谱?为什么?

实验四 延胡索生物碱的系统分离法

中药延胡索为罂粟科植物延胡索(*Corydalis yanhusuo* W. T. Wang)的干燥块茎(见图4-26),主产于河北、山东、江苏、浙江等地。延胡索具有活血、利气、止痛等作用,用于治疗胸胁、脘腹疼痛、经闭痛经、产后淤阻、跌打疼痛等。其主要化学成分是生物碱(其中叔胺类含量约为0.65%,季胺类含量约为0.3%),目前已分离出近20种生物碱。

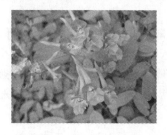
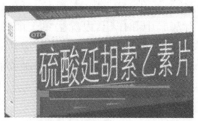

图4-26 延胡索及其制剂举例

一、实验目的

(1)了解生物碱的系统分离法的原理及应用。

(2)掌握生物碱的系统分离法的具体操作步骤。

二、实验原理

除水溶性生物碱外，大多数生物碱溶于有机溶剂却不溶于水，而生物碱的盐类能溶于乙醇及水，却难溶于有机溶剂。因此，生物碱盐的水溶液用醚萃取时，生物碱盐不能自水溶液中提出，必须加碱碱化使生物碱游离，游离的生物碱则可溶于有机溶剂而被分离出。常用的生物碱萃取溶剂为乙醚、氯仿。生物碱根据其结构可分为四种类型，由于生物碱的理化性质与其结构有关，根据其理化性质不同，可将各类型生物碱进行分离（见图 4-27）。

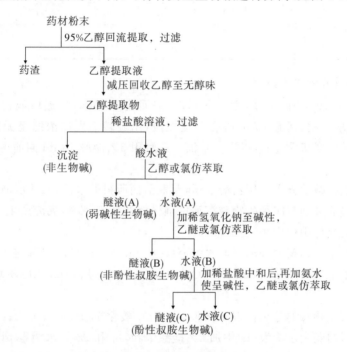

图 4-27　延胡索生物碱的系统分离流程图

（1）弱碱性生物碱。因其碱性极弱，与酸结合成盐不稳固，易从中性或酸性水溶液中转溶于有机溶剂，故在醚液 A 中可能出现。

（2）非酚性叔胺生物碱。一般碱性较强，其盐类在碱化后，生物碱游离，转溶于有机溶剂，故在醚液 B 中出现。

（3）酚性叔胺生物碱。酚性叔胺生物碱可与苛性碱（NaOH，KOH 或 Ca(OH)$_2$）生成钠盐、钾盐或钙盐，可溶于水而不溶于有机溶剂，酸化中和后再加碱（氨水或碳酸钠）则游离出生物碱，从而可溶于有机溶剂，故在醚液 C 中出现。

（4）水溶性生物碱。水溶性生物碱包括季铵生物碱、氮氧化物等，易溶于水，不溶于有机溶剂，故最终保留在水溶液中。

三、实验步骤

1. 预试验

按天然药物化学成分鉴别项下实验方法进行，结果填入表 4-4 中。

表 4-4 生物碱沉淀反应结果

试剂＼试液	预实验	醚 A	水 A	醚 B	水 B	醚 C	水 C
碘化汞钾试液							
碘化铋钾试液							
碘-碘化钾试液							
硅钨酸试液							

2. 生物碱的系统分离及鉴定

取延胡索粉末 10 g,加 95％乙醇 15 ml,水浴回流 30 min,将提取液转于圆底烧瓶中。药渣如前法再提取一次,回流 10 min,合并提取液,用旋转蒸发仪浓缩至无醇味。用 5％盐酸 30 ml 搅拌溶解,冷却后过滤,得澄清水液。残渣用 5％盐酸 15 ml 同前再操作一次,合并水液。

(1) 弱碱性生物碱的分离。用乙醚 8 ml 萃取前面所得酸水液,取醚层液 4 ml,再以稀酸水萃取,取酸水层液分别与四种生物碱沉淀试剂作沉淀反应,根据沉淀产生与否决定是否再萃取,直至沉淀反应呈阴性为止,得醚液(A)。

(2) 非酚性叔胺生物碱的分离。取水溶液(A) 2 ml,分为四份,作沉淀反应,若产生明显沉淀,则将其余水溶液(A)用 2 mol/L NaOH 调至 pH≥10,用 8 ml 乙醚萃取,同上法操作,得醚液(B)。

(3) 酚性叔胺生物碱的分离。取水溶液(B) 2 ml 酸化至 pH<3,分为四份作沉淀反应,若产生明显沉淀,向剩余水溶液(B)中加 2％盐酸中和,再用 5％氨水调至 pH＝9 左右,同上法操作,得醚液(C)。

(4) 水溶性生物碱的鉴定。取 2 ml 水溶液(C)用 2％盐酸化至 pH<3,分为四份作沉淀反应。若沉淀反应为阳性,则表明含水溶性生物碱。

3. 实验记录格式

各 pH 条件下的有机层和水层经生物碱沉淀试剂检查后,用"－"代表负反应,用"＋"、"＋＋"、"＋＋＋"代表正反应及强弱程度,记录于表 4-4,并推断含何种类型生物碱。

四、实验用品与时间安排

实验用品:延胡索、95％乙醇、盐酸、乙醚、NaOH、氨水、碘化铋钾、碘化汞钾、硅钨酸、碘-碘化钾、pH 试纸。旋转蒸发仪、圆底烧瓶、胶头滴管、试管、回流装置、分液漏斗、烧杯。

时间安排:要求在 6 学时内完成。

五、思考题

(1) 做生物碱沉淀反应,检查生物碱萃取是否完全时,能否用乙醚层直接检查?为什么?

(2) 以下四种成分用生物碱的系统分离法分离,它们将分别存在于醚液 A,B,C 或水液中的哪部分？

① 降氧化北美黄连次碱

② 去氢紫堇碱

③ 延胡索单酚碱

④ 四氢黄连碱

第五章 各类成分预试验

第一节 天然药物化学成分系统预试验

天然产物中所含的化学成分种类很多,在深入研究之前,应首先了解其中含有哪些类型的化学成分,如生物碱、皂苷、黄酮类等。这就需要进行各类化学成分的系统定性预试验,或根据研究的需要进行单项预试法来初步判断。利用各类成分的颜色反应和沉淀反应,对天然产物的提取液进行检查,可以初步判断其中的化学成分。由于提取液大多数颜色较深,影响对颜色变化的观察,可以使用薄层色谱(TLC)或纸色谱(PC)等方法对天然产物的提取液进行初步分离,再进一步检查。

一、实验目的

掌握未知成分的天然产物是怎样初步提取分离的,熟悉各主要成分的试管实验、沉淀反应和纸色谱、薄层色谱的方法,并根据试验结果判断含有什么类型的化学成分。

二、实验原理

利用试管实验、纸色谱和薄层色谱对多种天然药物化学成分进行系统试验,产生特定的颜色反应,初步判断其中的化学成分类型。

三、实验步骤

利用不同成分在各种溶剂中的溶解度的不同,一般可采用以下3种溶剂分别提取。

1. 水浸液

取中草药粗粉 5 g,加水 60 ml,在 50～60℃水浴上加热 1 h,过滤,用滤液做表 5-1 中试验。

表 5-1 水浸液预试验

检查项目	试剂名称	实验结果
糖	*1. 酚醛缩合反应	
	*2. 菲林试剂	
有机酸	△1. pH 试纸检查	
	△2. 溴甲酚绿试剂	
酚类	△1% $FeCl_3$ 试剂	

续表

检查项目	试剂名称	实验结果
鞣质	△1.1% FeCl₃ 试剂	
	*2.明胶试剂	
氨基酸	△茚三酮试剂	
蛋白质	*双缩脲反应	
苷类或多糖	*1.酚醛缩合反应	
	*2.加 6 mol/L HCl 酸化,加热煮沸数分钟,冷后仔细观察有无絮状沉淀	
	*3.菲林试剂,观察水解前后 Cu_2O 沉淀量有无增加	
皂苷	*泡沫试验	
生物碱	*1.碘化铋钾试剂	
	*2.硅钨酸试剂	

注:* 表示在试管中进行,△表示在滤纸或硅胶 CMC-Na 薄层板上进行,下同。

2. 乙醇提取液

取中草药粗粉 10 g,加 5～12 倍量 95% 乙醇,在水浴上加热回流提取 1 h,过滤。滤液留 2 ml 做表 5-2 所示试验,其余回收乙醇至无醇味,并浓缩成浸膏状。浸膏分为两部分:一部分加少量 2% HCl,振摇溶解过滤,分出酸液,做表 5-3 所示试验,附于滤纸上的部分再用少量乙醇溶解,其溶液做表 5-4 所示试验;另一部分浸膏用少量乙酸乙酯溶解,溶液置分液漏斗中,加适量 5% NaOH 振摇,使酚性物质及有机酸等转入下层氢氧化钠水溶液中,剩下的乙酸乙酯为中性部分,用蒸馏水洗去碱性即可备用。将乙酸乙酯 2～3 ml 在水浴上蒸干,用 1～2 ml 乙醇溶解,做表 5-5 中试验。

表 5-2　乙醇提取液预试验一

检查项目	酚类	鞣质	有机酸
试剂名称	△1% FeCl₃	△1% FeCl₃	△溴甲酚绿试剂
结果			

表 5-3　乙醇提取液预试验二

检查项目	试剂名称
生物碱	*1.碘化铋钾试剂
	*2.硅钨酸试剂
	*3.鞣酸试剂
	*4.苦味酸试剂
结果	

表 5-4　乙醇提取液预试验三

检查项目	黄酮	蒽醌
试剂名称	△1.1% AlCl₃ 试剂 *2.盐酸镁粉反应	△1.10% KOH 液 △2.0.5% Mg(Ac)₂ 试剂 △3.氨熏
结果		

表 5-5　乙醇提取液预试验四

检查项目	香豆素与萜类内酯	强心苷
试剂名称	*1. 开环与闭环反应 △2. 氨基安替比林－铁氰化钾呈色反应 △3. 羟胺反应	△1. Kedde 试剂 △2. 三氯乙酸试剂 *3. 苦味酸试剂
结果		

3. 石油醚提取液

取中草药粗粉 1 g，加 10 ml 石油醚（沸程 60～90℃），放置 2～3 h，过滤，滤液置表面皿上任其挥发，用残留物做表 5-6 中试验。

表 5-6　石油醚提取液预试验

检查项目	甾体或三萜类	挥发油和油脂
试剂名称	*1. 乙酸酐－浓硫酸试验 △2. 25％磷钼酸试剂	将石油醚提取液滴于滤纸片上，观察有无油斑并在加热后能否挥发
结果		

氰苷的检查：取中草药粗粉 0.2 g，置于试管中，加入 3～5 ml 5％硫酸溶液，摇匀混合。在试管口置一条浸泡过苦味酸钠盐溶液的滤纸条，然后塞紧试管口（滤纸不要接触溶液）。将试管置于沸水浴上加热十几分钟，如纸条呈红色，则表示有氰苷。

中草药化学成分的预试验，除上述颜色反应及沉淀反应外，如能配合色谱方法，不仅可以减少成分间的相互干扰，而且可以根据其极性及溶解性能（通过所用展开剂及 Rf 值判断）较为准确地判断中草药中所含的化学成分。

各类成分的色谱预试验条件大致见表 5-7，还可根据具体对象适当调整展开剂的比例。

表 5-7　中草药各类成分薄层色谱种类、展开条件和显色试剂

化合物类别	色谱种类	展开条件	显色试剂
酚类化合物	硅胶 TLC	氯仿－丙酮（8∶2）	1％三氯化铁乙醇液
有机酸	硅胶 TLC	氯仿－丙酮－甲醇－乙酸（7∶2∶1.5∶0.5）	溴甲酚绿
氨基酸	PC	正丁醇－乙酸－水（4∶1∶5，上层），酚以水饱和	茚三酮
生物碱	硅胶 TLC	氯仿－甲醇（9∶1），氨熏	改良碘化铋钾
强心苷	PC 滑石粉－TLC （甲酰胺为固定相）	氯仿－丙酮－甲醇－甲酰胺（8∶2∶0.5∶0.5）	呫吨氢醇
甾体，三萜	硅胶 TLC	氯仿－丙酮（8∶2）	硫酸－乙酸酐或 5％硫酸－乙醇
蒽醌	硅胶 TLC	环己烷－乙酸乙酯（7∶3）	氨熏
挥发油	硅胶 TLC	石油醚－乙酸乙酯（85∶15）	香草醛－浓硫酸
香豆素	硅胶 TLC	正丁醇－乙酸－水（4∶1∶1）	用 5％ KOH－甲醇喷后荧光观察
黄酮苷及苷元	PC	乙酸－水（15∶85），正丁醇－乙酸－水（4∶1∶1）	三氯化铝
糖	PC	正丁醇－乙酸－水（4∶1∶1），乙酸乙酯－吡啶－水（2∶1∶2）	苯胺－邻苯二甲酸

第二节 天然药物化学成分的鉴别方法

一、生物碱

样品制备：取药材的水溶液加 2％盐酸（或 1％乙酸）至酸性，或取药材的乙醇提取物加同上酸液至部分溶解，置小试管中，分别滴加下列生物碱沉淀剂 1～2 滴，观察并记录实验现象（沉淀、混浊、结晶、颜色）。本反应也可用毛细管取样品点于薄层板上，再滴加试剂观察变化（与空白对照）。

1. 沉淀试剂

（1）碘化铋（Dragendorff）试剂。出现橘红色或黄色沉淀。

（2）碘化汞钾（Mayer）试剂。出现白色或淡黄色沉淀。

（3）硅钨酸（Bertrand）试剂。出现淡黄色或灰白色沉淀，在薄层板上反应时，加热后出现黑色斑点。

（4）苦味酸（Hager）试剂。样品液需调至中性后加试剂，出现黄色晶形沉淀。

2. 记录形式举例

样品名称：

结果现象：

薄层分析：

3. 硅胶-CMC-Na 薄层举例

样品：黄连和延胡索提取液，巴马汀、小檗碱、药根碱和延胡索乙素的对照品。

展开剂：氯仿—甲醇（3∶1），展开前薄层板先在氨缸中饱和 5 min。

显色：先在紫外灯下观察荧光，然后再喷以改良碘化铋钾试液显色。

如果用中性或碱性氧化铝薄层，展开剂可用氯仿。

记录：薄层色谱图谱。

二、酚类、鞣质（用水或乙醇浸出液进行检查）

（1）1％三氯化铁水溶液或乙醇试剂：试液应为酸性，滴加试剂，出现蓝色、绿色或蓝紫色。也可以在滤纸片上进行检测。

（2）三氯化铁－铁氰化钾试剂：1％三氯化铁水溶液，1％铁氰化钾水溶液，临用时等体积混合。将试液点在滤纸上，滴加试剂，立即出现明显的蓝色斑点。但时间长后背景也渐呈蓝色。

（3）明胶试剂：0.5％明胶水溶液加等量的 10％氯化钠溶液。试液滴加试剂后产生沉淀，证明含有鞣质。

三、有机酸（用水或乙醇浸出液进行检查）

（1）pH 试纸检查。应呈酸性。

（2）溴甲酚绿试剂。1％溴甲酚绿乙醇（70％乙醇）溶液。将试液点于滤纸上，滴加试剂后,在蓝色的背景上立即显黄色斑点。若不明显,再喷洒氨水,然后暴露在盐酸气体中,背景逐渐由蓝色变为黄色,而有机酸盐的斑点仍为蓝色。

四、氨基酸、蛋白质、肽(用在60℃以下加热浸出的水溶液检查)

(1)茚三酮(Ninhydrin)试剂。0.2%茚三酮乙醇溶液。将试液滴于滤纸上,滴上试剂后在110℃左右的烘箱中放置2 min,如有氨基酸、肽,则应出现紫红色或蓝色斑点,少数出现黄色斑点。

(2)双缩脲反应(Biuret reaction)试剂。1%硫酸铜水溶液和40%氢氧化钠水溶液等量混合。取1 ml水浸液加入试剂1~2滴,振摇,冷时显紫红色说明可能有蛋白质或肽。

五、糖、多糖和苷(用水或稀醇溶液检查)

1. 酚醛缩合反应(α-萘酚试剂、Molisch 试剂)

将试液置试管内,加入10% α-萘酚乙醇溶液1~2滴,振摇后,倾斜试管,沿管壁加入浓硫酸数滴,在两液的接触面产生紫红色环即说明有还原糖。

2. 菲林氏反应(Fehling 试剂)

配制溶液Ⅰ:69.3 g 结晶硫酸铜溶于1000 ml水中;配制溶液Ⅱ:349 g 酒石酸钾钠及氢氧化钠100 g,溶于1000 ml水中。上述两种溶液如不够澄清,可滤过一次。临用前等体积混合。

操作:水试液加等量菲林氏液,摇匀,在沸水浴上加热2~3 min,如果产生砖红色氧化亚铜沉淀,证明水试液中含有还原糖。

若水试液中不含还原糖,可加6 mol/L HCl 酸化,加热煮沸数分钟至0.5 h,冷后仔细观察有无絮状沉淀。如果产生沉淀,表明可能含有苷或低聚糖。将滤液加碳酸钠中和至碱性,然后再加等量菲林氏液,摇匀,在沸水浴上加热2~3 min,如果产生氧化亚铜沉淀,证明苷或多糖已水解产生还原糖。此时氧化亚铜的沉淀比水解前增加。

3. 氨性硝酸银试剂(Tollens 试剂)

配制:将5%硝酸银溶液2 ml置洁净试管内,加入1滴10%氢氧化钠溶液。逐滴加入20%氨水,同时不断振摇,直到氧化银沉淀恰巧溶解为止。为制得灵敏试剂,氨的量不可过量。本试剂应在临用前配制,因为久放会分解,并会沉积出一种高度爆炸性的沉淀。

操作:将试液点在滤纸上,再滴上新鲜配制的试剂,于100℃加热5~10 min,如果试液呈深褐色,证明含有带醛基的还原糖。

4. 苯胺─邻苯二甲酸盐

配制:将0.93 g 苯胺、1.66 g 邻苯二甲酸溶于100 ml 水饱和的正丁醇中。

操作:将试液点于滤纸上,再滴加试液,在105℃加热10 min。还原糖呈桃红色,有时也呈棕色。呈红色说明还原糖为戊醛糖或2-己酮糖酸,呈棕色说明还原糖为己醛糖或5-己酮糖酸。

5. (碱式)乙酸铅水溶液

为了进一步确证是苷类,将试液加乙酸铅饱和水溶液,如果产生沉淀,则试液就可能含有有机酸、黏液质、鞣质、蛋白质和苷类。待沉淀完全后,滤去沉淀,滤液加碱式乙酸铅饱和水溶液,如果产生沉淀,就可能含有苷类。

6. 碘液或碘化钾—碘试液(wagner 试剂)

配制:5%碘的氯仿溶液。取 1 g 碘及 10 g 碘化钾,溶于 50 ml 水中,加热,加 2 ml 乙酸,再用水稀释至 100 ml。

操作:取试液的浓缩水溶液 1 ml,加 5 倍量的乙醇使其产生沉淀,加热过滤,并用少量热乙醇洗涤。将此沉淀溶于 3 ml 水中,进行多糖试验。取此试液 1 ml,加少量碘液或 Wagner 试剂。如试液呈褐色则为糊精,呈蓝黑色则为地衣糖。

7. 皂苷

(1)泡沫试验。取穿山龙的水浸出液 2 ml 置小试管中,用力振摇 1 min,如产生大量泡沫,放置 10 min,泡沫没有显著消失,即表明含有皂苷。另取试管 2 支,各加入穿山龙热水溶液 1 ml;一管加入 2 ml 0.1 mol/L 氢氧化钠溶液,另一管加入 2 ml 0.1 mol/L 盐酸溶液,将两管塞紧,用力振摇 1 min,观察两管出现泡沫的情况。如两管的泡沫高度相近,表明含有三萜皂苷,如含碱液管比含酸液管的泡沫多数倍,表明含有甾体皂苷。

(2)溶血试验。取清洁试管 2 支,其中一支试管加入蒸馏水 0.5 ml,另一支试管加入穿山龙的水浸出液0.5 ml,然后分别加入 0.5 ml 0.8% NaCl 水溶液,摇匀,再加 1 ml 2%红细胞悬浮液,充分摇匀,观察溶血现象。

根据下列标准判断实验结果:

全溶——试管中溶液透明,为鲜红色,管底无红色沉淀物。

不溶——试管中溶液透明,为无色,管底沉着大量红细胞,振摇立即发生浑浊。

8. 皂苷元

将所提取的薯蓣皂苷元用于下列试验。

(1)磷钼酸试剂(3%~10%乙醇液)。将薯蓣皂苷元重结晶的乙醇母液点于滤纸片或硅胶薄板上,点加磷钼酸试剂,略加热,颜色变蓝,与空白组对照。

(2)三氯乙酸试剂(Rosen-Heimer 反应)。将薯蓣皂苷元结晶少许置于干燥试管中,加等量固体三氯乙酸,放在 60~70℃恒温水浴中加热。数分钟后由红色变为紫色,说明为甾体皂苷。若加热至 100℃由红色变为紫色,应为三萜类皂苷。

(3)硫酸—乙酸酐试剂(Liedermann-Burchard 反应)。取薯蓣皂苷元结晶少许,置白瓷板上,加硫酸—乙酸酐试剂 2~3 滴,观察颜色由红色变为紫色再变为蓝色,放置后变为暗绿色。

(4)浓硫酸试剂。取薯蓣皂苷元结晶少许,置白瓷板上,加浓硫酸 2 滴,观察颜色变化,久置后由红紫色变为暗绿色。

薄层色谱:

薄层板:硅胶 CMC-Na 板。

样品:薯蓣皂苷元粗品、乙醇重结晶母液,薯蓣皂苷元精制品乙醇液。

对照品:薯蓣皂苷元标准品乙醇溶液。

展开剂:石油醚—乙酸乙酯(7:3)。

显色剂:5%磷钼酸乙醇液,喷雾后加热,显蓝色斑点。

六、黄酮类

1. 盐酸—镁粉反应

取样品(芦丁、槲皮素)1 mg 置于试管内,加 50%乙醇 2 ml,在水浴上加热溶解,滴加浓盐酸 2 滴,再加镁粉约 50 mg。溶液由黄色变为红色。

2. 氨熏

取水溶液试样滴于滤纸上,在浓氨水瓶上熏,立即置于紫外灯下观察,呈亮黄色荧光斑点。

3. 1%三氯化铝乙醇溶液

将水试液滴在滤纸上,再滴上试剂,呈黄色斑点。挥干后置于紫外灯下观察显亮黄色荧光斑点。

4. 硼氢化钾(钠)反应

专门还原二氢黄酮而使之呈现红色至紫色。取橙皮苷 5 滴溶于 50%乙醇,置于试管内,加硼氢化钾 1 粒(米粒大小),再滴加浓盐酸,观察颜色变化。

5. 乙酸镁反应

取样品(芦丁、橙皮苷)数毫克,溶于 50%乙醇中,倒入试管中或点样于滤纸上,加 1%乙酸镁甲醇液,黄酮类(芦丁)呈黄色荧光,二氢黄酮类(橙皮苷)呈天蓝色荧光。

6. 浓硫酸反应

取芦丁数毫克置于白色有孔瓷板上,滴加浓硫酸后生成锌盐,呈橙色,待加酸溶解后,加较多量水稀释后转为浅黄色,并析出芦丁黄色沉淀。

7. 锆盐—柠檬酸反应

取槲皮素、黄芩素各 0.1 mg,分别置于试管内,加甲醇于水浴上加热溶解,再分别加 2%二氯化锆 3~4 滴,凡有 C_3—OH 的黄酮即呈鲜黄色。然后分别加 2%柠檬酸甲醇溶液 3~4 滴,具有 C_3—OH 的黄酮黄色不褪,具有 C_5—OH 的黄酮黄色减褪。

8. 1%三氯化铁乙醇液

取试液滴于滤纸上,再滴试液,观察颜色(酚羟基反应)。

七、香豆素类

1. 荧光

秦皮的极稀溶液发生蓝色荧光,若加氨水后,呈明显黄色(成盐)。

2. 1%三氯化铁水溶液

秦皮的水溶液加 1%三氯化铁溶液数滴,呈蓝绿色,若再加入氨水,转为暗红色。

3. 异羟肟酸铁反应(羟胺反应)

取 1%香豆素甲醇液 1 ml,置于小试管中,加新鲜的 1 mol/L 盐酸羟胺甲醇液 0.5 ml,加 2 mol/L KOH 甲醇液 0.5 ml,使溶液呈碱性,在水浴上微热,冷却后加 1%$FeCl_3$ 的 1%盐酸液 1~2 滴,然后滴加 5%HCl,使溶液呈微酸性。若有紫红色出现,表明含有香豆素及其他内酯化合物和酯类化合物。

4. Gibb's 反应

反应条件：此反应必须有游离酚羟基，且酚羟基对位无取代者，才能呈阳性反应。本试剂在弱碱性条件下与酚羟基对位活性氢缩合成蓝色化合物。

试剂甲：0.5% 2,6-二氯苯醌-4-氯亚胺乙醇溶液。试剂乙：硼酸－氯化钾－氢氧化钠缓冲液（pH＝9.4）。用毛细管将 7,8-二羟基香豆素和 7-羟基香豆素乙醇液滴在滤纸上，吹干，再用毛细管滴加试剂甲，待干后再滴加试剂乙。该反应呈深蓝色或蓝色。

5. 4-氨基安替比林－铁氰化钾（Emerson）

配制溶液Ⅰ：2% 4-氨基安替比林乙醇溶液；溶液Ⅱ：8%铁氰化钾水溶液。或用 0.9% 4-氨基安替比林和 5.4%铁氰化钾水溶液。

操作：将试液滴于滤纸上，先喷洒溶液Ⅰ，再喷洒溶液Ⅱ，随即显色，或再放置于密闭缸内，缸内放 25%氢氧化铵，溶液即呈橙红色至深红色。

6. 内酯化合物的开环闭环反应

取 1 ml 乙醇浸出液，加 2 ml 1%氢氧化钠，于沸水浴中煮 3～4 min。液体在未加热前澄清，说明开环，若再加 2%盐酸使之酸化，液体变为混浊，说明闭环，有时产生沉淀。

八、强心苷类

1. 强心苷的检测

甲型强心苷在碱性溶液中能与活性次甲基试剂作用而呈色。

(1) 亚硝基铁氰化钠－氢氧化钠（Legal 试剂）。检查不饱和内酯、甲基酮或活性次甲基，常用于强心苷等。

喷洒剂：取 1 g 亚硝基铁氰化钠溶于 100 ml 2 mol/L 氢氧化钠－乙醇（1∶1）的水溶液。显红色或紫色斑点。

(2) 3,5-二硝基苯甲酸（Kedde 试剂）。检查强心苷，α、β-不饱和内酯。

喷洒剂：取 1 g 3,5-二硝基苯甲酸溶于 50 ml 甲醇，加入 1 mol/L 氢氧化钾 50 ml。强心苷呈紫红色斑点。

(3) Baljet 反应。取毛花洋地黄总苷的醇溶液滴于硅胶板上，加上新鲜配制的碱性甘味酸试剂（1%苦味酸乙醇溶液和 5%氢氧化钠水溶液等量混合）1 滴，呈现橙色或橙红色。此反应有时发生较慢，需放置 15 min 后才显色。须设置空白对照。

(4) 氯胺 T－三氯乙酸。检查强心苷。

喷洒剂Ⅰ：3%氯胺 T 水溶液，新鲜制备。喷洒剂Ⅱ：25%三氯乙酸乙醇溶液（能保存整天）。10 ml 喷洒剂Ⅰ加 40 ml 喷洒剂Ⅱ，用前混合。

喷洒后处理：110℃加热 7 min，紫外荧光分析下检示呈蓝色或黄色荧光。

2. 2,6-去氧糖的颜色反应

(1) Keller-Killani 反应。取毛花洋地黄总苷 1 mg 溶于 1 ml 冰乙酸中，加 1 滴 2%三氯化铁水溶液，置试管中，沿管壁注入 0.5 ml 浓硫酸，观察界面和乙酸层的颜色变化。如有 2,6-去氧糖存在，乙酸层渐呈蓝色。

(2)呫吨氢醇(xanthydrol)反应。取毛花洋地黄总苷的乙醇液滴在硅胶板上,再加呫吨氢醇试剂 1 滴,用电吹风加热 3 min,呈红色。

九、挥发油

香草醛－浓硫酸试剂:配制 5％香草醛浓硫酸乙醇液(0.5 g 香草醛溶解于 100 ml 硫酸和 25 ml 95％乙醇中),喷洒在薄层色谱上,在 105 ℃下加热,不同挥发油呈不同颜色。

实验 断血流化学成分预实验、提取和分离工艺设计

断血流为唇形科植物灯笼草(*Clinopodium polycephalum* (Vaniot) C. Y. Wu et Hsuan)或风轮菜(*C. chinensis* (Benth.) D. Kuntze)的干燥地上部分(见图 5-1),为安徽省的特色药材。断血流具有止血功能,可用于崩漏、尿血、鼻出血、创伤出血、子宫肌瘤出血等。断血流的化学成分复杂,其主要化学成分为皂苷和黄酮类化合物,用于临床的主要制剂有断血流片剂、断血流胶囊和断血流颗粒等。

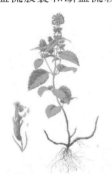
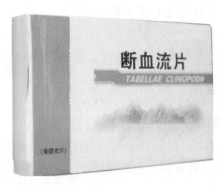

图 5-1 断血流及其制剂举例

一、实验目的

(1)掌握断血流中化学成分的预实验方法。
(2)熟悉断血流中主要化学成分的提取、分离方法及工艺流程设计方法。
(3)了解各提取、分离方法及工艺流程中常用的仪器、设备、试剂和试药。

二、实验步骤

(1)做预实验时设计不同方法,确定断血流可能含有的化学成分。
(2)查阅资料,设计提取、分离断血流中总皂苷和总黄酮成分的工艺流程。
(3)查阅资料,设计断血流皂苷 A 和香蜂草苷单体化合物的分离流程。
(4)选择一种提取、分离工艺用于实验,提取出断血流中总皂苷和总黄酮成分。

三、注意事项

(1)要求每组同学独立完成实验的设计、试剂的准备和实验操作过程,不得出现工艺流程重复现象。
(2)结合提取、分离产率,不同小组在实验结束后将设计路线的优缺点写出来,并对实验

过程进行讨论。

（3）通过实验，学生应主要掌握文献检索、实验设计、试剂准备、实验操作和报告撰写的方法，具备一定的科研训练能力。

四、思考题

根据实验设计、操作过程，计算断血流中总皂苷和总黄酮的初步提取率；思考如何根据现有条件，优化提取工艺，提高提取率。

附　录

附录一　实验思考题参考答案

第二章　色谱分离技术

实验一　四季青中酚性化合物（原儿茶酸、原儿茶醛）的提取和分离

1. 2,4-二硝基苯肼试剂与羰基反应的第一步是羰基的亲核加成，但加成产物不稳定，立即进行第二步反应，即分子内失去一分子水，结果 $R_2C=O$ 变成 $R_2C=N-$，生成2,4-二硝基苯腙。以上反应都是由碱性的氮原子进攻羰基显正电性的碳原子，故是亲核加成。2,4-二硝基苯肼又称为羰基试剂，但其亲核性不如 CN^-、R^- 强，所以加成反应一般需在酸的催化下进行。酸的作用是增加羰基的亲电性，有利于亲核试剂的进攻。反应生成物有固定的结晶形状和熔点，生成物在稀酸作用下，可水解得到原来的醛和酮，因此又可用于鉴定、分离、纯化醛和酮。

2. (1)薄层厚度：层厚小于 0.2 mm 时对 Rf 值的影响较大，层厚超过 0.2 mm 时则可以认为没有影响，但不能超过 0.35 mm。(2)展开距离：展开距离最好固定，展开距离加大时，有些物质的 Rf 值会稍有增大，而有些物质又稍有减小。(3)点样量：点样量过多时，会使斑点变大，甚至拖尾，Rf 值也会随之变化。(4)薄层含水量：特别是黏合薄层板，如干燥不均匀，或其他原因使薄层各部分含水量不一致，就会影响 Rf 值。(5)展开容器中展开剂蒸气的饱和度——边缘效应。最好用较小体积的展开缸或将薄层在缸内放置一段时间，待溶剂蒸气达到饱和后再展开；如在展开缸内壁贴上浸湿展开剂的滤纸条，效果也很好；如采用3 cm 以下的狭小薄板，只点 2～3 个点时，也会减小边缘效应。

实验二　红辣椒中色素的分离

1. 粗红色素的色素组分为辣椒红素二酯、辣椒玉红素、玉米黄质二酯和 β-胡萝卜素，各单体组分对温度均较为敏感，随着加热温度和时间的增加，辣椒色素损失加快，且加热温度对各色素的稳定性均有极显著影响。由于二氯甲烷的沸点较低，控制温度在50℃，既能保证粗红色素的稳定性和产率，又能保持溶剂的沸腾状态。

2. 硅胶吸附剂的颗粒大小一般应在100～200目，在柱子下端塞上脱脂棉防止硅胶流出柱子。脱脂棉对洗脱物质不影响，需注意的问题：(1)干装法要将吸附剂均匀地倒入柱内，中间不应间断。(2)柱装好后,剪一直径大小适合的滤纸放入吸附剂上面,防止倒入样品或洗脱剂时将吸附剂冲起,再打开下端活塞。(3)柱内必须没有气泡,如有气泡,可再加溶剂,并在柱的上端通入压缩空气,使气泡随溶剂由下端流出。(4)湿装法应注意"走柱",直到吸附剂的沉降不再变动,并且柱内没有气泡。如有气泡,会使液体的流动不规则,形成"沟流"现象,各部分快慢不一致,因而造成色带的变形,影响分离效果。

实验三　绿叶中色素的提取和分离

1. 选择鲜嫩、颜色浓绿的新鲜叶片,以保证含有较多的色素。二氧化硅能增加杵棒与研钵间的摩擦力,破坏细胞结构,使研磨充分;碳酸钙可防止研磨过程中色素被破坏。

2. 避免将滤液细线中的色素分子溶解到展开剂中。由于色素在展开剂中的溶解度不同、扩散速度不同,所以才能将其分离开。但是,滤纸会吸收展开剂,从而使色素在滤纸上分散开来。若滤液细线触及展开剂,那么滤纸上的色素就会溶于展开剂中,而得不到色素扩散图样。

第四章　各类成分的提取和分离实例

第一节　糖　类

实验一　香菇多糖的提取

1. 多糖溶于热水,不溶于60%以上乙醇,也不溶于氯仿－正丁醇,所以用热水提取,乙醇沉淀可除去部分醇溶性杂质;另外,热水也可以将蛋白质类物质提取出来,所以用氯仿－正丁醇萃取除去提取液中的蛋白质。

2. (1)料液比:当料液比在1:(10~25)之间,多糖提取率增长较快,继续提高料液比,多糖提取率仍有升高,但提高速率降低。对于料液比的选择,若加水太少,提取不彻底;加水太多,则降低了提取液的固形物含量,不利于以后的分离。(2)提取温度:随着提取温度的升高,粗多糖提取率逐渐升高。在80~95℃时,粗多糖提取率升高趋势明显,再提高温度时,粗多糖提取率升高趋势趋于平缓。高温提取会破坏多糖的结构,影响其生物活性。(3)提取时间:随着提取时间的延长,粗多糖提取率呈增加趋势,0.5~3 h之间增加趋势明显,继续延长提取时间,多糖提取率增加趋势逐渐趋于平缓。(4)乙醇添加倍数:随着乙醇添加倍数的逐渐提高,多糖提取率逐渐升高,3倍之后再继续提高乙醇添加倍数,对粗多糖提取率的影响趋于减弱。(5)提取次数:多糖的提取率随着提取次数的增加而增加,但提取次数超过2次后,多糖的提取率增加缓慢,趋于平缓。

实验二　麻黄多糖的提取

1. 乙醇沉淀麻黄提取液的主要原理是,通过降低溶液的介电常数,使多糖脱水,从而产生沉淀来分离多糖,由于多糖的相对分子质量都比较大,具有较高的黏度,利用乙醇沉淀麻黄提取液时,多糖聚集在一起易成黏稠的沉淀,使多糖脱水困难,搅拌则有利于沉淀完全。

2. 超声提取法、微波辅助提取法。

第二节 苯丙素类

实验一 秦皮中七叶苷、七叶内酯的提取、分离与鉴定

1. 硅胶 G 薄层色谱分离原理为物理吸附,且硅胶为极性吸附剂,对极性大的化合物吸附力强,七叶苷的极性比七叶内酯大,所以七叶苷的 Rf 值比七叶内酯小,即在薄层色谱图中,Rf 值大者为七叶内酯,Rf 值小者为七叶苷。

2. (1)荧光:香豆素母体本身无荧光,羟基香豆素在紫外灯下大多能显出蓝色荧光,在碱溶液中(或加碱后)荧光大都增强。(2)异羟肟酸铁反应(显色反应):香豆素类具有内酯环,在碱性条件下可开环,与盐酸羟胺缩合成异羟肟酸,然后于酸性条件下与三价铁离子络合成盐而显红色。

实验二 丹皮酚的提取、分离和鉴定

1. 挥发性。
2. 购买中成药中药材的对照品,提取、纯化后,进行薄层色谱或高效液相色谱对照鉴别。

第三节 醌 类

实验一 大黄中蒽醌类化合物的提取和分离

1. 酸性大小顺序为:大黄酸>大黄素>芦荟大黄素>大黄素甲醚>大黄酚。因为大黄酸有羧基,酸性最强;大黄素有 β-OH,酸性次之;芦荟大黄素与大黄素甲醚比较,均含有吸电子氧原子,且前者没有供电子基团(CH_3),故前者吸电子作用强;大黄酚没有 OCH_3 或 CH_2OH,酸性最弱。

2. 应用萃取法,根据强酸首先与弱碱反应,先用最弱碱与强酸反应,再依次增加碱性,依次萃取出不同的酸性物质。本实验依据大黄中大黄酸、大黄素、芦荟大黄素、大黄素甲醚和大黄酚的酸性不同,依次用 5% $NaHCO_3$、5% Na_2CO_3、2.5% NaOH、5% NaOH 进行梯度萃取分离。

实验二 虎杖中大黄素的提取、分离和鉴定

1. 苯醌和萘醌多以游离态存在,易溶于乙醇、乙醚、苯、三氯甲烷等有机溶剂,基本上不溶于水。而蒽醌一般结合糖成苷,易溶于甲醇、乙醇、热水,但在冷水中溶解度较低,几乎不溶于苯、乙醚、三氯甲烷等极性小的溶剂。本实验采用酸水解和脂溶性试剂同时提取的方法,再用硅胶柱色谱和 pH 梯度萃取法进行分离。

2.

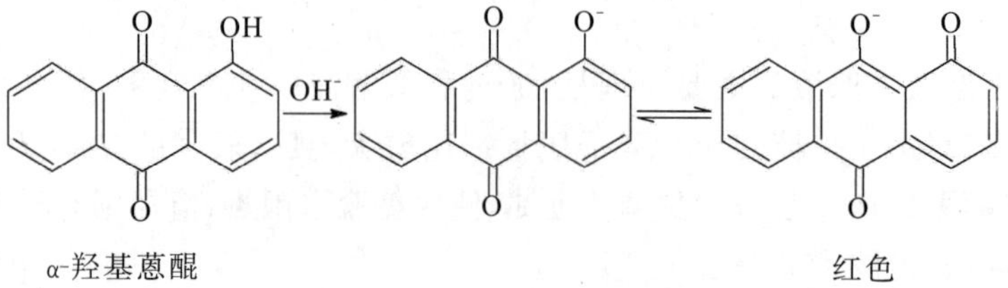

α-羟基蒽醌 　　　　　　　　　　　　　　　红色

β-羟基蒽醌　　　　　　　　　　　红色

第四节　黄酮类

实验　芦丁的提取、分离和鉴定

1. 鉴别芦丁结构中的双糖，即葡萄糖和鼠李糖，仅能说明该物质结构中含有糖类成分。
2. 不一定，因为显色反应仅能判定是否为某一类成分，或者判定该类成分可能有哪些基团，不能用来完全确认结构。
3. 水解不完全会在抽滤时全部进入滤液，而无小针状结晶。水解的产物是槲皮素和糖。
4. 注意碱和酸的浓度，即 pH，它是影响产量和质量的关键因素。加入硼砂可对芦丁酚羟基起保护作用。

第五节　萜类和挥发油

实验一　橙皮中柠檬烯的提取

加两分子氢的产物是 1-异丙基-4-甲基环己烷；这个物质没有光学活性，因为它具有对称中心。

实验二　穿心莲中穿心莲内酯的提取、分离和鉴定

1.（1）石油醚萃取。（2）粗提物可用丙酮溶解后，拌样于 3 倍量的聚酰胺，然后以 1∶1 的比例上一根短柱，先用 80% 乙醇－水洗脱，然后用 90% 乙醇－水洗脱，去除叶绿素。如果样品量不大，将提取物通过装有 C_{18} 硅胶的短柱，可把所含的叶绿素方便地除去。缺点是反相 C_{18} 较为昂贵，有时会吸附在色谱柱上难以清除。（3）MCI GEL 系列由日本三菱公司生产，MCI GEL 系列反相分离填料是在三菱化学 Diaion 和 Sepabeads 大孔吸附树脂基础上设计的，因为基于现代的 HPLC 高压液相色谱分离技术，较小的颗粒有更高的色谱分离性能，因此广泛地用于天然产物和发酵产物的分离。MCI GEL 脱叶绿素的效果非常好，石油醚浸膏、乙酸乙酯浸膏都可以使用（石油醚浸膏用得多一些，色素重）。MCI 用水装柱，样品最好用水溶解（低极性的可用一定比例甲醇水溶解）上样，用甲醇水洗脱，也可用不同比例的甲醇水洗脱分段，流出液不含色素，色素留在 MCI 柱上。用无水甲醇和丙酮可将色素洗下，MCI GEL 可以反复使用。一般情况下，可以将快报废的 MCI GEL 专用于脱除叶绿素。（4）也可以使用大孔吸附树脂去除叶绿素，某些特定的树脂，如 Amberlite™ FP 系列就具有脱除色素的功能。如果到了后期的纯化阶段，样品有 5~200 mg，但是还带有一点颜色，感觉不太纯时，可用 TSK Toyopearl HW-40 凝胶，上一根短柱，稍微粗一点，即可分开，效果较好。也可以使用 Sephadex LH-20，与 Toyopearl HW-40 类似。

2.(1)采用高速逆流色谱(HSCCC),在流速为 2.0 ml/min 的正己烷、乙酸乙酯、乙醇和水(体积比为 1∶4∶2.3∶2.7)的两相溶剂系统分离。HSCCC 为可逆吸附,回收率高,操作简便,进样量较大,最多可达数克,分离能力强,分离时间短。但分辨率较低,分离时间较长,溶剂用量大。(2)大孔吸附树脂色谱法,用 40%乙醇水溶液洗去杂质后,45%乙醇洗脱液中富含穿心莲内酯,55%乙醇洗脱液中富含脱水穿心莲内酯。该法具有操作简便、成本低等特点,但是分离耗损较大。

3. Legal 反应机制可能是:亚硝酰铁氰化钠试剂中的亚硝基和活性次甲基反应生成肟基衍生物而留在络合阴离子内,Fe^{3+} 被还原成 Fe^{2+}。Kedde 反应机制是五元不饱和内酯与 Kedde 试剂在碱性条件下,双键移位,形成了活性亚甲基和 3,5 二硝基苯甲酸,形成大共轭体系,显红紫色。一般只有具有不饱和内酯环结构的化合物才能呈现阳性反应。

实验三 八角茴香挥发油的提取和鉴定

1. 提取采用水蒸气蒸馏法,分离采用冷冻法。
2. 点滴试验是一种微量化学分析方法。只用一滴试液,在滤纸或点滴板上,即可进行分析,常能用一滴试液检出 1 微克(μg)以下的物质。特点是迅速、经济、可靠,不用复杂仪器,对无机物和有机物都适用。20 世纪 20 年代,F·法伊格尔系统地研究了利用灵敏的有机试剂检出金属离子的试验,奠定了点滴试验的基础。
3. 要考虑到如果是正相硅胶板,先用极性大的展开剂将小极性物质充分分开,推到一定高度,再用极性小的溶剂展开。但是,如果是反相色谱,则应先用极性小的展开剂。

实验四 栀子中京尼平苷的提取、分离和纯化

1. 分子筛和物理吸附作用。
2. 因为京尼平苷为含糖类结构,极性较大,在水中有一定溶解度。
3. 利用物理吸附原理,与京尼平苷产生吸附作用,再选择适宜的洗脱剂洗脱。

第六节 三萜苷类

实验一 甘草酸的提取和鉴定

1. 甘草酸具羧基,具有酸性,所以水提液加 H_2SO_4 后可沉淀析出。
2. 甘草酸为三萜皂苷类化合物,常见的三萜类的显色反应有醋酐-浓硫酸反应、五氯化锑反应、三氯乙酸反应、氯仿-浓硫酸反应、冰乙酸-乙酰氯反应。

实验二 齐墩果酸的提取、分离和鉴定

1. 果皮中齐墩果酸含量比全果实的齐墩果酸含量高,所以采用果皮作原料更容易提取出齐墩果酸。
2. 两相溶剂水解又称双相水解,即在水解液中加入与水不互溶的有机溶剂,使水解后的苷元立即进入有机相,避免苷元长时间与酸接触。
3. 齐墩果酸具羧基,可与氢氧化钠发生皂化反应,利用这一性质可以用于齐墩果酸的纯化,与其他杂质分开。

4. 齐墩果酸的20位碳连了2个甲基,为齐墩果烷型的骨架,熊果酸的20位碳上只有1个甲基,还有1个甲基在19位碳上,为乌苏烷型的骨架。二者为同分异构体,极性差异很小,利用薄层色谱基本上分不开,宜采用分离效果更好的HPLC进行分离。

第七节　甾体类

实验　薯蓣皂苷元的提取和鉴定

1. 可用 Liebermann-Burchard 反应、Salkowski 反应、Rosen-Heimer 反应和三氯化锑(五氯化锑)反应。

2.
穿山龙粗粉
↓加2倍水润湿12 h,于40℃预发酵16 h
酸性药渣
↓加6%硫酸,用量为原料量的6倍,于高压灭菌锅中水解5 h,过滤,药渣用水洗涤3次
水解后药渣
↓用饱和碳酸钠溶液中和至pH=7,抽滤,洗涤,干燥
干燥药渣
↓置索氏提取器中,以石油醚(60~90℃)为溶剂,回流提取6 h
石油醚提取液
↓浓缩后析晶,抽滤,固体用少量新鲜石油醚洗涤2次,抽滤
粗品薯蓣皂苷元
↓95%乙醇重结晶(色深时可加1%~2%活性炭脱色)
薯蓣皂苷元

提取时先酶解,再用弱酸水解,最后用脂溶性溶剂进行提取。分离主要采用重结晶法。

3. 石油醚有30~60℃沸点,也有60~90℃和90~120℃沸点,应根据待提取物的性质、浓缩的需求来选择不同沸程的石油醚。在使用石油醚时,不能有明火,尤其挥散时不要达到闪点,否则会引起爆炸。石油醚的蒸气或雾对眼睛、黏膜和呼吸道有刺激性。中毒表现有烧灼感、咳嗽、喘息、喉炎、气短、头痛、恶心和呕吐,可引起周围神经炎,对皮肤有强烈刺激性。

处理方法:①皮肤接触,应立即脱去被污染的衣服,用肥皂水和清水彻底冲洗皮肤。②眼睛接触:立即提起眼睑,用大量流动清水或生理盐水彻底冲洗至少15 min。就医。③吸入:迅速脱离现场至空气新鲜处,保持呼吸道通畅。如呼吸困难,给输氧;如呼吸停止,立即进行人工呼吸。就医。④食入:误服者用水漱口,给饮牛奶或蛋清。就医。

第八节　生物碱类

实验一　氧化苦参碱的提取、分离和鉴定

1. 生物碱与酸结合成盐,可用酸水提取出来,酸提取后的生物碱呈阳离子状态而被阳离

子交换树脂所交换,再用氨水碱化后使生物碱游离,再用有机溶剂回流提取可得生物碱。

2.(1)通过生物碱沉淀反应判断。取 1 ml 渗漉液,滴加 1~2 滴碘-碘化钾试剂、碘化汞钾试剂、碘化铋钾试剂或硅钨酸试剂,若有沉淀产生或产生明显浑浊,表明渗漉液中含有生物碱。或将溶液滴在滤纸上,再喷雾碘化铋钾试剂,若有橙红色斑点,说明溶液中含生物碱。(2)①检查离子交换树脂柱流出液的 pH 变化,流出液的 pH 低于上柱前的 pH 说明生物碱交换到树脂柱上。②用碘化铋钾等生物碱检识试剂检查树脂柱流出液,如果呈阴性,说明生物碱交换到树脂柱上。(3)①检查离子交换树脂柱流出液的 pH 变化,若 pH 同上柱前,说明树脂柱已饱和。②用碘化铋钾等检识试剂检查流出液,若呈阳性,说明树脂柱已经饱和。

3.索氏提取器提取是利用溶剂回流及虹吸原理,使固体物质连续不断地被纯溶剂萃取,具有节约溶剂、萃取效率高等特点。索氏提取器由提取瓶、提取管和冷凝器三部分组成,提取管两侧分别有虹吸管和连接管。提取时,将待测样品包在脱脂滤纸包内,放入提取管内,提取瓶内加入溶剂,加热提取瓶,溶剂气化,由连接管上升进入冷凝器,凝成液体滴入提取管内,浸提样品中的脂类物质。待提取管内溶剂液面达到一定高度,溶有粗脂肪的溶剂经虹吸管流入提取瓶,流入提取瓶内的溶剂继续被加热气化、上升、冷凝、滴入提取管内,如此循环往复,直到提取完全为止。

4.闪柱是闪式柱色谱的简称,闪柱色谱的最大特点是分离相当迅速。完成一个重量为 0.01~10 g 的混合物样品的分离,从装柱、上样到洗脱分离,整个过程只需要 15~60 min。

5.制备性薄层色谱是指使用薄层色谱板进行制备分离,从混合物中提取所需要的单体。与常用的柱色谱相比,具有简单、快速、节省溶剂与人力等优点。

6.酸水提取,离子交换树脂法分离得氧化苦参碱粗品,进一步使用制备性薄层色谱或闪柱色谱纯化得氧化苦参碱纯品。氧化苦参碱的波谱数据:UV:202 nm;IR:3470 cm^{-1}, 2940 cm^{-1}, 1615 cm^{-1}, 1470 cm^{-1}, 1440 cm^{-1}, 1420 cm^{-1};^{13}C-NMR:68.7(C-2), 17.0(C-3), 25.9(C-4), 34.3(C-5), 66.6(C-6), 42.4(C-7), 24.4(C-8), 17.0(C-9), 69.1(C-10), 52.8(C-11), 28.3(C-12), 18.5(C-13), 32.7(C-14), 169.8(C-15), 41.6(C-17)。

实验二 黄柏中小檗碱的提取、分离和鉴定

1.可用熔点测定仪测定所得产品的熔点,观察熔距的大小,熔距越小,纯度越高;用 TLC 方法检测,若在三种展开系统中均呈现单一斑点,可确认为单一化合物;通过高效液相色谱法检测,观察其是否为单一对称的峰。

2.TLC 与标准品对照;HPLC 与标准品的色谱峰对照;还可通过测定其紫外光谱、红外光谱、核磁共振谱、质谱来鉴定(可与标准品的光谱作对照)。

3.小檗碱为水溶性生物碱,可溶于碱水,盐酸小檗碱难溶于水,所以先用碱水自黄柏中提出小檗碱(加入氯化钠盐析),再加盐酸使其转化为盐酸小檗碱,使其沉淀析出;黄柏中富含黏液质,加石灰乳可以沉淀黏液质。

4.分离碱性物质,多数情况下是以氧化铝为吸附剂。用薄层色谱法检识盐酸小檗碱时,若选用氧化铝为吸附剂,则要选用中性溶剂为展开剂,如氯仿-乙醇(9:1);若采用硅胶为吸附剂,则以选用碱性展开剂为宜,如展开剂为苯-乙酸乙酯-异丙醇-甲醇-氨水(6:3:1.5:1.5:0.3,氨蒸汽饱和)、乙酸乙酯-三氯甲烷-甲醇-二乙胺(8:2:2:1)。

实验三 茶叶中咖啡因的提取及其红外光谱测定

1. 咖啡因属于嘌呤衍生物，可与鞣酸生成白色沉淀。

2. 红褐色的沉淀。咖啡因可被过氧化氢、氯酸钾等氧化剂氧化，生成 1,3,7,8-四甲基黄嘌呤，将其用水浴蒸干，呈玫瑰色，后者与氨作用即生成紫色。

3. 当分子吸收红外光子，引起分子内振动和转动能级跃迁，所产生的吸收光谱即为红外光谱，从谱中可得知某些特殊键或官能团是否存在。

4. 化学键的力常数越大，原子折合质量越小，则振动频率越高，吸收峰将出现在高波数区，C—H 的伸缩振动主要出现在高频区，2800～3000 cm^{-1} 为甲基。

5. 红外吸收光谱只能提供特征官能团的吸收峰，因而单靠红外光谱解析得不到未知物的准确结构。

6. 含水的样品不能直接测定其红外光谱，因为红外光谱实验应在干燥的环境中进行。红外光谱仪中的一些透光部件是由溴化钾等易溶于水的物质制成，在潮湿的环境中极易损坏。另外，水本身能吸收红外光产生强的吸收峰，干扰试样的谱图。

实验四 延胡索生物碱的系统分离法

1. 检查生物碱萃取是否完全时，不能用乙醚层直接检查或用含有醚层的酸水检查，必须要经过处理除去干扰成分，避免得到假阳性结果。

2. 红褐色的沉淀。咖啡因可被过氧化氢、氯酸钾等氧化剂氧化，如与盐酸、氯酸钾在水浴上加热蒸干，所得残渣遇氨即生成紫色的四甲基紫脲酸铵，再加氢氧化钠，紫色即消失。此反应即紫脲酸铵反应，是黄嘌呤类生物碱的特征鉴别反应。其反应式如下：

附录二 常用溶剂性质及精制方法

在我们的实验中,常常需要应用很多的有机溶剂,这些溶剂用过以后就会混入许多有机及无机物质,并带进了很多水分。除去这些杂质和水分后,这些溶剂又可以重新使用。因此,使用再生溶剂也是贯彻增产节约方针的具体表现。在分析和色谱实验中,对溶剂的纯度要求更高。一般重蒸的溶剂或市售工业品均不能直接应用,必须进一步精制,否则将影响实验结果。下面分别介绍各种溶剂的再生和精制方法。

一、石油醚

石油醚是石油馏分之一,主要是饱和脂肪烃的混合物,极性很低,不溶于水,不能和甲醇、乙醇等溶剂无限制地混合。实验室中常用的石油馏分根据沸点不同有下列数种,其再生方法大致相同。

	沸 点	比 重
轻石油醚	35～60℃	0.59～0.62
重石油醚	60～80℃	0.64～0.66
汽油	80～120℃	0.67～0.72
汽油	120～150℃	0.72～0.75

再生方法:用过的石油醚,如含有少量低分子醇、丙酮或乙醚,则置分液漏斗中用水洗数次,用氯化钙脱水、重蒸,收集一定沸点范围内的部分;如含有少量氯仿,在分液漏斗中先用稀碱液洗涤,再用水洗脱数次,氯化钙脱水后重蒸。

精制方法:工业规格的石油醚用浓硫酸精制,每千克加 50～100 g 浓硫酸,振摇后放置 1 h,分去下层硫酸液,可以溶去不饱和烃类,根据硫酸层的颜色深浅,酌情用硫酸振摇萃取 2～3 次。上层石油醚再用 5% 稀碱液洗一次,然后用水洗数次,氯化钙脱水后重蒸。如需绝对无水,再加金属钠丝或五氯化二磷脱水干燥。

二、环己烷

环己烷沸点为 81℃,性质与石油醚相似,再生时先用稀碱洗涤,再用水洗,脱水重蒸。精制方法为:将工业规格的环己烷加浓硫酸及少量硝酸钾放置数小时后,分去硫酸层,再用水洗,重蒸。如需绝对无水,再用金属钠丝脱水干燥。

三、苯

苯沸点为 80℃,比重为 0.879,不溶于水,可与乙醚、氯仿、丙酮等在各种比例下混溶。

再生方法:用稀碱水和水洗涤后,用氯化钙脱水重蒸。

精制方法:工业规格的苯常含有噻吩、吡啶和高沸点同系物,如甲苯等。可将苯 1000 ml 在室温下用浓硫酸振摇数次,每次 80 ml,至硫酸层呈色较浅时为止,再经水洗,用氯化钙脱水重蒸,收集 79～81℃ 馏分。对于甲苯等高沸点同系物,则用二次冷却结晶法除去。苯在

54℃固化成为结晶,可以冷却到0℃,滤取结晶,杂质留在液体中。

四、氯仿

氯仿沸点为61℃,比重为1.488,不溶于水,易与乙醚、乙醇等混溶,在日光下易氧化分解成Cl_2、HCl、CO_2及光气($COCl_2$)。后者有毒,故应贮在棕色瓶中。氯仿在稀碱水作用下易分解产生甲酸盐,在浓碱水作用下则生成碳酸盐。

再生及精制方法:医用氯仿含有1%酒精(作为安定剂,以防止其分解),可用水洗涤,氯化钙脱水重蒸,收集61℃馏分,贮于棕色瓶中。

五、四氯化碳

四氯化碳沸点为77℃,比重为1.589,极性很小,不溶于水。工业规格的四氯化碳中常含有2%~3%二硫化碳,其除去方法为:取1000 ml四氯化碳加5% KOH乙醇溶液100 ml,60℃加热30 min,冷却后,用水洗涤(氯化钙或固体),分去水层;再用少量浓硫酸振摇多次,直至硫酸不变色;最后用水洗涤,用氯化钙或固体氢氧化钠脱水,加液状石蜡少许后蒸馏,可得精制品。

注意:氯仿和四氯化碳脱水干燥时,切忌用金属钠,否则将发生爆炸事故。

六、二硫化碳

二硫化碳沸点为46℃,性质与四氯化碳相似。纯的二硫化碳为无色液体,味香,有毒性。市售工业规格的二硫化碳常含硫化氢、硫氢化碳等分解产物,因而其味难闻。二硫化碳久置色变黄。精制时先用金属汞振摇,再用饱和氯化汞冷溶液振摇,最后用高锰酸钾液洗涤后蒸馏而得。

七、乙醚

乙醚沸点为35℃,比重为0.714,在水中的溶解度为8.11%。用过的乙醚常含有水及醇,如用水洗涤损失很大,可用饱和氯化钙水液洗涤,同时又可去除乙醇,再用无水氯化钙脱水干燥,重蒸即得。

乙醚久置于空气中,尤其是暴露于日光下,会逐渐氧化成醛、酸及过氧化物。当过氧化物含量达到万分之几时,蒸馏时有发生爆炸的危险。过氧化物可以通过用碘化钾溶液与少量乙醚共振摇生成游离碘而检出,其除去方法为:可用稀碱液、高锰酸钾液、亚硫酸钠液顺次洗涤,再用水洗,干燥,重蒸而得。贮存时,加少量表面洁净的铁丝或铜,以防止氧化。

其他除法:少量醇类可在乙醚中加少量高锰酸钾粉末和氢氧化钠2块,放置数小时后,在氢氧化钠表面如有棕色的醛缩合树脂生成,则重复这一操作,直至氢氧化钠表面不生棕色物为止。然后将乙醚倒入另一瓶内,加无水氯化钙脱水,重蒸而得。如需绝对无水,再将金属钠压成钠丝加入,将瓶塞打孔,附一氯化钙管。为了减少蒸发,在氯化钙管上安装一根一端拉成毛细管的玻璃管,与外界相通。

八、丙酮

丙酮沸点为56℃,比重为0.792,与水、醇能以任意比混溶。

再生方法：丙酮中如含有大量的水时，可加食盐或固体碳酸钾等盐类，盐析成二层，分去下层盐水层，上层丙酮液蒸馏收集54～57℃馏分，再用无水氧化钙脱水干燥、重蒸。

精制方法：

1. 一般工业用丙酮常含有甲醇、醛和有机酸等杂质，精制时加高锰酸钾粉末回流，所加的量应使丙酮一直保持紫色，如不加热，放置3～4天也可。加热后冷却，滤去沉淀，加无水碳酸钾或氯化钙脱水干燥，蒸馏收集。

2. 如丙酮中混有少量乙醇、乙醚、氯仿等溶剂，精制时加2倍量的饱和亚硫酸氢钠溶液振摇，生成亚硫酸氢钠丙酮加成体，再在其中加等量的酒精，析出结晶，过滤收集，顺次用酒精、乙醚洗涤，干燥。将此结晶与少量水相混合，加入10%碳酸钠或10%盐酸，使加成物分解，滤液分级蒸馏，取丙酮的馏分，再加无水氯化钙或碳酸钾脱水干燥，重蒸而得。

注意：丙酮不宜用金属钠或五氧化二磷脱水。

九、乙醇

乙醇沸点为78℃，比重为0.79，与水能以任意比混溶，蒸馏时与水共沸，共沸点78.1℃，共沸混合液含水4.43%（即95%乙醇）。

再生方法：先在用过的乙醇中加生石灰（氧化钙），每升加25～50 g，加热回流脱水后，分级蒸馏，收集76～81℃馏分，含醇80%～90%。再置圆底烧瓶中，加比计算量多1倍的生碳，回流5 h，再蒸馏收集76～78℃馏分，含醇98.5%～99.5%。如需绝对无水，可用下列方法之一。

1. 99.5%乙醇1000 ml，加27.5 g苯二甲酸二乙酯和7 g金属钠，放置后蒸馏得无水乙醇。

$$C_6H_4(COOC_2H_5)_2+2C_2H_5ONa+2H_2O \rightarrow C_6H_4(COONa)_2+4C_2H_5OH$$

2. 98%以上的乙醇60 ml，置于2 L圆底烧瓶中，加入5 g金属镁、0.5 g碘，使其发生反应，促进镁溶解成醇镁，再加900 ml乙醇，回流加热5 h，蒸馏可得100%乙醇。

$$(C_2H_5O)_2Mg+2H_2O \rightarrow 2C_2H_5OH+Mg(OH)_2$$

如乙醇用于紫外光谱分析，则对纯度要求较高。普通发酵乙醇常混有少量醛和酮，无水乙醇用苯共沸蒸馏后常含有苯、甲苯，均不宜用于光谱分析。其精制法如下：95%普通乙醇1000 ml，加入25 ml$(NH_4)_2SO_4$，在水浴上回流加热数小时，以除去苯及甲苯等杂质。蒸馏，除去初馏分50 ml及残馏分100 ml。主馏分中加硝酸银8 g，加热使其溶解，再加入粒状氢氧化钾15 g。回流加热1 h，此时溶液从黏土色的AgOH悬浊液变为黑色的还原银粒凝集沉淀下来。此反应需20～30 min。如果黑色沉淀生成很早，则表示能被氧化的物质含量较多。蒸馏后的溶液再加入少量硝酸银和氢氧化钾（1:2）（W/W），重复上述操作，直至没有黑色沉淀生成为止。再继续加热30 min，蒸馏，除去初馏分约50 ml及残馏分约100 ml。收集主馏分，但有可能带入微量的碱和银离子，会促进乙醇的氧化。应重蒸馏一次，用此法制得的乙醇含水3%～6%，在206 nm处透明，在200 nm处有末端吸收。

十、甲醇

甲醇沸点为65℃，比重为0.79，能与水、乙醇、乙醚、氯仿等以任意比例混溶，不与水共沸，利用分馏法可得99.8%的浓度。绝对无水的甲醇，可用镁和碘等制得（同乙醇项下）。甲醇有毒,对视神经有损伤,应用和操作时应注意。

精制方法:工业规格的甲醇主要含丙酮和甲醛等杂质,可用硫酸汞酸性溶液与甲醇一起加热,使丙酮生成络合物析出。或与碘的碱性溶液共热,使醛或酮氧化成碘仿,然后再分馏精制。

注意:甲醇不能用生石灰脱水,因 CaO 能吸收 20% 甲醇,CaO、CH_3OH、H_2O 会处于某一平衡状态,完全脱水不可能。

十一、乙酸乙酯

乙酸乙酯沸点为 77℃,比重为 0.90。含水的乙酸乙酯在日光下会逐渐水解为乙酸和乙醇,精制时用 5% 碳酸钠(或碳酸钾)溶液、饱和氯化钙溶液分别洗去乙酸和醇。再以水洗、分级蒸馏,取乙酸乙酯馏分,经无水氯化钙脱水干燥后重蒸一次,或在乙酸乙酯中加少量水。每 500 g 加 2 g 水,蒸馏,水和乙醇在第一馏分中被蒸出。

十二、乙酸

乙酸沸点为 118℃,冰点为 16.5℃,比重为 1.06。纯的乙酸(99%~100%)在较低温度时结成固体,故又称冰乙酸。其精制可用冰冻法,即冷却至 0~10℃,乙酸结成结晶,分去液体,结晶加热重复熔化,再经冷冻一次,可得冰乙酸。乙酸中如含有乙醇和醛等杂质,可在乙酸中加 2% 左右的重铬酸钾(或钠)后进行分馏,若含有少量水分,则加适量的乙酸酐后进行分馏,收集 117~118℃ 的馏分。

十三、吡啶

吡啶沸点为 116℃,比重为 0.98,能与水、乙醇、乙醚等混溶,和水共沸,共沸点为 92~93℃。吡啶中的水分可加适量的固体氢氧化钠放置,分去析出水层后,再加固体氢氧化钠至无水层分出为止,蒸馏,收集 116℃ 馏分,即得无水吡啶。

十四、二甲基甲酰胺(DMF)

二甲基甲酰胺沸点为 153℃,比重为 0.95,能与水、乙醇、乙醚等许多有机溶剂任意混溶。二甲基甲酰胺与水形成共沸混合物,故含有水分的二甲基甲酰胺不能用分馏法除去,可加无水碳酸钾干燥后,蒸馏精制而得。

附录三　常用干燥剂性能

化学干燥剂可分两类,一类能与水生成水合物,如硫酸、氯化钙、硫酸铜、硫酸钠、硫酸镁和氯化镁等;另一类与水反应后能生成其他化合物,如五氧化二磷、氧化钙、金属钠、金属镁、金属钙和碳酸钙等。必须注意的是,有些化学干燥剂是酸或与水作用后变为酸的物质,有一些化学干燥剂是碱或与水作用后变为碱的物质。在用这些干燥剂时,应考虑到被干燥物的酸碱性质。应用中性盐类作干燥剂时,如氯化钙,它能与多种有机物形成分子复合物,也要加以考虑。因此在选择干燥剂时,首先应了解干燥剂和被干燥物的化学性质是否相容。下面介绍一些实验室常用的干燥剂的性能。

一、无水氯化钙

无水氯化钙对固体、液体和气体的干燥均可使用。有干燥能力的是含 2 分子结晶水的氯化钙($CaCl_2 \cdot 2H_2O$),潮解吸水后成为含 6 分子结晶水的氯化钙($CaCl_2 \cdot 6H_2O$),加热至 30℃ 时成 $CaCl_2 \cdot 4H_2O$,加热至 200℃ 恢复为 $CaCl_2 \cdot 2H_2O$,如加热至 800℃,则水分完全失去,成为熔融的氯化钙。可以用氯化钙脱水的化合物有烃类、卤代烃类、醚类。对于沸点较高的溶剂,干燥后重蒸溶剂时,应将干燥剂滤出,不可一起加热蒸馏,以免被吸去的水分在加热时再度放出。它的缺点是脱水能力不强,并且能和多种有机物生成复合物,如醇、酚、胺、氨基酸、脂肪酸等,因此不可作为醇等溶剂的脱水干燥剂。对结构不明的化合物溶液,不宜使用氯化钙来干燥。

二、无水硫酸钠

无水硫酸钠可用作中性、酸性和碱性物质的脱水干燥剂,与有机物没有反应,可以广泛应用,吸水后成为带有 10 分子结晶水的硫酸钠($Na_2SO_4 \cdot 10H_2O$)。但无水硫酸钠的脱水能力弱,而且作用慢,不能用加热来促使其脱水,因为含水的硫酸钠在 33℃ 以上又失去结晶水;对于含水量较多的醇类不宜用作脱水干燥剂;适用于醚、苯、氯仿等溶剂,新买来的应加热焙干后使用。

三、无水硫酸镁

无水硫酸镁的性质同无水硫酸钠,其吸水效力强一些,与水生成的水合物含 7 分子结晶水。

四、无水硫酸铜

无水硫酸铜常用于制备无水醇,是干燥能力相当弱的干燥剂。无水硫酸铜呈浅绿色,生成水合物质后变蓝($CuSO_4 \cdot 5H_2O$),根据颜色变化说明发生吸水过程,故可用来检验溶剂的含水多少。$CuSO_4 \cdot 5H_2O$ 加热至 100℃ 失去 4 分子结晶水,从而再生。加热时温度不宜超过 220~230℃,否则就生成碱性盐类而失去水合的效力。

五、无水硫酸钙

无水硫酸钙是由石膏加热至 160~180℃ 而得，而在 500~700℃ 灼烧所得的无水硫酸钙，几乎不能与水结合。它是强烈干燥剂之一，但吸水量不大，只能达到自身重量的 6.6%，吸水后形成相当稳定的水合物 $2CaSO_4 \cdot H_2O$。它和其他形成水合物的盐类不同，不需要把它与被干燥的有机液体事先分开，可以放在一起蒸馏。甲醇、乙醇、乙醚、丙酮、甲酸和乙酸用无水硫酸钙脱水可获得良好的效果。

六、苛性碱

苛性钠（NaOH）和苛性钾（KOH）是碱性干燥剂，适用于干燥有机碱类，如氨气、胺类、吡啶、重氮甲烷、生物碱等。作为干燥器内的干燥剂，用来排除被干燥物质中挥发出来的酸性杂质时，应用更多，苛性钾的效力较苛性钠大 60 倍，对于酸性物或酮、醛等均不适用。

七、无水碳酸钾

无水碳酸钾的碱性比苛性碱弱，应用范围较广一些，除适用于碱性物质外，对醇类也适用。

八、氧化钙

氧化钙俗称"生石灰"，是一种碱性干燥剂，常用来在实验室里制造无水乙醇，因为来源方便，生成的氢氧化钙不溶于乙醇，要得到绝对无水的乙醇，需要用过量的氧化钙，吸收 1 g 水大约要 5 g 块状氧化钙（理论量是 3.11 g）。氧化钙也适用于干燥有机碱液体，但不适用于干燥甲醇，因 CaO、H_2O、CH_3OH 与形成的复合物成一平衡，不能完全脱水，而且要吸收 20% 的甲醇。

九、金属钠

金属钠有很强的脱水作用，被广泛应用于各种惰性有机溶剂的最后干燥，如用于乙醚、苯、甲苯、石油醚等。由于金属钠有可工塑性，脱水时可将钠块周围的杂质切去，用压钠机压成条状，置入装有溶剂的容器内，这样使金属钠与液体接触的表面大大增加，不至于因金属钠含有的杂质在钠块表面形成一层薄膜，妨碍钠进一步与水作用。必须注意，对于 $CHCl_3$、CCl_4 及其他含有 $-OH$、$>C=O$ 等反应性强的官能团的溶剂，都不能用金属钠脱水，含水量多的溶剂也不能用钠脱水，因为钠遇水发生爆炸，易引起危险事故。

十、浓硫酸

浓硫酸是一种酸性干燥剂，由于它对许多有机化合物具有腐蚀性，限制了它在干燥上的应用，因此浓硫酸多半应用于无机物的干燥或作为干燥器内的干燥剂。对于气体，并不是所有中性和酸性气体对浓硫酸都不起作用，硫酸除了有酸的作用外，还有氧化作用，例如，溴化氢遇到硫酸将大部分被氧化成溴。干燥器内以硫酸为干燥剂的应用很广，但是真空干燥器内应用硫酸应十分小心，因为它在 1 毫米汞柱的压力下有一部分要挥发，它的蒸气与干燥物质就能起作用。放在干燥器内的硫酸不需要特别纯，在硫酸中可加 1% 硫酸钡（18 g 硫酸钡加在 1 L 硫酸内,比重 1.84)。当硫酸吸水后浓度降低至 93% 时,即析出 $BaSO_4 \cdot 2H_2SO_4 \cdot H_2O$ 的针状结晶;当硫酸浓度降低至 84% 时,$H_2SO_4 \cdot H_2O$ 变成很细的结晶。如果发现有细小的硫酸钡结晶出现时,就应该更换硫酸。

十一、五氧化二磷

五氧化二磷即磷酸酐,吸水后生成磷酸。它的脱水反应是不可逆的,在酸性干燥剂中,它的脱水效力最高,可用于一般固体、气体和惰性液体的脱水。碱性物质或有羟基的化合物不宜用五氧化二磷来脱水。它的最大缺点是吸水后表面生成一层很黏的磷酸,妨碍它的进一步干燥。需要注意的是,五氧化二磷中常含有少量的三氧化二磷,此物大量地与热水作用,可生成剧毒的磷化氢。

$$2P_2O_3 + 6H_2O \rightarrow PH_3 + 3H_3PO_4$$

十二、硅胶

二氧化硅与少量水(2%~10%)结合形成的胶状硅胶($SiO_2 \cdot xH_2O$),称为硅胶,呈无色透明玻璃块状,其中有无数细孔,可吸收湿气,发挥干燥作用,常用作气体干燥剂。吸水硅胶外观无变化,为了便于观察,可加 $CoCl_2$ 盐,干燥时呈蓝色,吸水后呈淡黄色($CoCl_2$ 用量少时则褪色)。蓝色硅胶由于含有少量的氯化钴(有毒),应避免和食品接触或吸入口中,如发生中毒事件,应立即就医。

硅胶再生时,将其铺在器皿中成一薄层,放入烘箱,在 150~180℃ 加热,小心温度勿超过 200℃。

十三、分子筛

结晶的铝硅酸盐中,主要由硅铝通过氧桥连接组成空旷的骨架结构,在结构中有很多孔径均匀的孔道和排列整齐、内表面积很大的空穴,此外还含有电价较低而离子半径较大的金属离子和化合态水。由于水分子在加热后连续失去,但晶体骨架结构不变,形成了许多大小相同的空腔,空腔又有许多直径相同的微孔相连,比孔道直径小的物质分子吸附在空腔内部,而把比孔道大的分子排斥在外,因而称作分子筛。分子筛适用于各类有机化合物的干燥。例如:

3A 型分子筛,化学式:$2/3K_2O \cdot 1/3Na_2O \cdot Al_2O_3 \cdot 2SiO_2 \cdot 9/2H_2O$。主要用途:液体(如乙醇)的干燥;中空玻璃中的空气干燥;氮氢混合气体的干燥;制冷剂的干燥。

4A 型分子筛,化学式:$Na_2O \cdot Al_2O_3 \cdot 2SiO_2 \cdot 9/2H_2O$。主要用途:空气、天然气、烷烃、制冷剂等气体和液体的深度干燥;氩气的制取和净化;易受潮变质物质的静态干燥;在油漆、聚酯类、染料、涂料中作脱水剂。

5A 型分子筛,化学式:$3/4CaO \cdot 1/4Na_2O \cdot Al_2O_3 \cdot 2SiO_2 \cdot 9/2H_2O$。主要用途:脱硫、脱二氧化碳;氮氧分离、氮氢分离,制取氧、氮和氢;石油脱蜡,从支烃、环烃中分离正构烃。

13X 分子筛,化学式:$Na_2O \cdot Al_2O_3 \cdot (2.8 \pm 0.2)SiO_2 \cdot (6 \sim 7)H_2O$,硅铝比:$SiO_2/Al_2O_3 \approx 2.6 \sim 3.0$。分子筛能承受 600~700℃ 的短暂高温,在 350~400℃ 可活化 4~6 小时。

十四、活性氧化铝

活性氧化铝吸水量大、干燥速度快,适用于烃、胺、酯、甲酰胺等,能再生(110~300℃烘烤)。高强度的 x-ρ 型氧化铝对水有较强的亲和力,是一种微量水深度干燥用的干燥剂。活性氧化铝具有在使用介质中用水浸泡不变软、不膨胀、不粉化等特点。活性氧化铝具有许多毛细孔道,表面积大,可作为吸附剂、干燥剂及催化剂使用。活性氧化铝对水、氧化物、乙酸、碱等极性物质具有较强的亲和力,除氟时类似于阴离子交换树脂,但对氟离子的选择性比阴离子树脂大。

附录四　常用试剂配制及显色方法

一、通用显色剂

1. 重铬酸钾-硫酸:一般有机物均能显色,不同化合物显示不同颜色。
喷洒剂:5 g 重铬酸钾溶于 100 ml 40%硫酸中。喷洒后加热至 150℃斑点出现。
2. 碘:检查杂原子、双键、芳环等基团。
碘蒸气:在一个密闭玻璃皿中先放入碘片,使缸内空气被碘蒸气饱和,将薄层或纸层放入缸内数分钟即显色。有时在缸内放一只盛水的小杯,增加缸内的湿度,可提高显色的灵敏度。
3. 5%碘的氯仿溶液:取出挥发过量的碘,再喷 1%淀粉的水溶液,斑点转成蓝色。
4. 碘-碘化钾溶液:检查普通有机物,很多有机物呈黄色(配法见后)。
5. 5%磷钼酸乙醇溶液:检查还原性化合物、类脂体、生物碱、甾体。喷后在 120℃下烘烤,还原性物质显蓝色,再用氨气熏,则背景变为无色。
6. 20%磷酸乙醇溶液:喷后在 120℃下烤,还原性物质显蓝色。
7. 碱性高锰酸钾试剂:检测含有双键、三键的不饱和化合物。还原性物质在淡红色背景上显黄色。溶液Ⅰ:1%高锰酸钾溶液。溶液Ⅱ:5%碳酸钠溶液。溶液Ⅰ和溶液Ⅱ等量混合使用。
8. 中性 0.5%高锰酸钾溶液:检查含有双键、三键的不饱和化合物。易还原性物质在淡红色背景上显黄色。
9. 硝酸银-氢氧化铵(Tollen's-zoffaronl)试剂:喷后在 105℃下烤 5~10 min,还原性物质显黑色。溶液Ⅰ:0.1 mol/L 硝酸银溶液。溶液Ⅱ:氢氧化铵溶液。临用前将溶液Ⅰ和溶液Ⅱ以 1:5 混合。注意:久放易生成爆炸性的叠氮化银。
10. 硝酸银-高锰酸钾试剂:还原性物质在蓝绿色背景上立即显黄色。溶液Ⅰ:0.1 mol/L 硝酸银溶液、2 mol/L 氢氧化铵溶液和 2 mol/L 氢氧化钠溶液(1:1:2),临用前配制。溶液Ⅱ:高锰酸钾 0.5 g,碳酸钠 1 g,加水配成 100 ml 溶液。临用前将溶液Ⅰ和溶液Ⅱ等量混合。
11. 四唑蓝试剂:还原性物质在室温或微加热时显紫色。溶液Ⅰ:0.5%四唑蓝甲醇溶液。溶液Ⅱ:6 mol/L 氢氧化钠溶液。临用前将溶液Ⅰ和溶液Ⅱ等量混合。
12. 铁氰化钾-三氯化铁试剂:还原性物质显蓝色,再喷 2 mol/L 盐酸溶液,则蓝色加深。溶液Ⅰ:1%铁氰化钾溶液。溶液Ⅱ:2%三氯化铁溶液。临用前将溶液Ⅰ和溶液Ⅱ等量混合。
13. 浓硫酸-甲醇(1:1)溶液,或 5%硫酸的乙醇溶液:喷后在 100℃下烤 15 min,不同物质显不同颜色。
14. 荧光显色剂溶液:试喷以下某一种溶液,不同的物质在荧光背景上可能显黑色或其他荧光斑点。
A:0.2% 2,7-二氯荧光素乙醇溶液

B:0.01%荧光素乙醇溶液

C:0.1%桑色素乙醇溶液

D:0.05%罗丹明B乙醇溶液

15.荧光素-溴试液:溶液Ⅰ:0.1%荧光素乙醇溶液。溶液Ⅱ:5%溴的CCl_4溶液。喷洒溶液Ⅰ以后,置于含溶液Ⅱ的缸内,可在UV光下检查荧光,荧光素与溴化合成曙红(无荧光),而光饱和化合物则与溴加成,保留了原来的荧光;若点样量较多,则成黄色斑点,底板成红色。

16.碱式乙酸铅试剂(可做喷洒或沉淀试剂,与多种有机化合物均反应):取PbO 14 g置乳钵内,加蒸馏水10 ml,研成糊状后,倾入玻璃瓶中,乳钵用10 ml蒸馏水洗净,洗液并入瓶中,加乙酸铅溶液(取乙酸铅22 g,加蒸馏水70 ml制成)70 ml,用力振摇,放置7天,滤过,并向滤器中添加适量新沸过的冷蒸馏水,配制成100 ml溶液即得。

二、生物碱类显色剂

1.改良碘化铋钾(Dragendorff)试剂:生物碱和某些含氯化合物显橙红色。溶液Ⅰ:碱式硝酸铋0.85 g,溶于冰乙酸10 ml和40 ml。溶液Ⅱ:碘化钾0.8 g溶于水20 ml。

储存液:溶液Ⅰ和溶液Ⅱ等量混合(置棕色瓶中可长期保存)。显色剂:储存液1 ml与冰乙酸2 ml和水10 ml混合,用前配制。

2.碘化铂钾(碘铂酸)试剂:不同的生物碱显不同的颜色。10%六氯化铂酸溶液3 ml和水97 ml混合,加6%碘化钾溶液100 ml,混合均匀,临用前配制。

3.碘-碘化钾(Wagner)试剂:生物碱显棕褐色。碘1 g和碘化钾10 g溶于50 ml水中,加热,加冰乙酸2 ml,用水稀释到100 ml。

4.碘化铋钾。溶液Ⅰ:碱式硝酸铋0.85 g,加入蒸馏水40 ml和冰乙酸10 ml,充分搅匀。溶液Ⅱ:碘化钾8 g溶于20 ml蒸馏水中。临用时取溶液Ⅰ、Ⅱ各5 ml,加入20 ml冰乙酸及60 ml蒸馏水混合,用棕色瓶保存。

5.硫酸铈-硫酸试剂(改良Sonnenschein试剂):喷后在110℃下烤几分钟,不同的生物碱显不同的颜色。将硫酸铈0.1 g悬浮于4 ml水中,加三氯化乙酸1 g,加热煮沸,放冷,逐滴加入浓硫酸,直到混浊消失为止。

6.碘化汞钾(Mayer)试剂(沉淀试剂):取$HgCl_2$ 1.35 g加蒸馏水60 ml,溶解后,量取碘化钾5 g,加蒸馏水10 ml使其溶解,将两液混合,加蒸馏水稀释至100 ml即得。

7.硅钨酸(Bertrand)试剂(沉淀试剂):取5 g硅钨酸溶于100 ml蒸馏水中,加稀盐酸使呈酸性即得。阳性结果为产生灰白色或浅黄色沉淀。

8.氢氧化钠试液:取氢氧化钠4.3 g,加水溶解,配成100 ml溶液即得。

三、强心苷类显色剂

1.碱性3,5-二硝基苯甲酸试剂(Kedde试剂):强心苷显紫红色,几分钟后褪色。配制2% 3,5-二硝基苯甲酸甲醇溶液与2 mol/L氢氧化钾溶液,用前按1:1混合。

2.碱性三硝基苯:在浅橙色背景上显橙红色。溶液Ⅰ:取间三硝基苯100 mg,溶于二甲基甲酰胺40 ml,加浓盐酸3~4滴,加水至100 ml,避光能长期保存。溶液Ⅱ:5%碳酸钠溶液。先喷溶液Ⅰ,再喷溶液Ⅱ,喷后在90~103℃下烤5 min。

3. 三氯乙酸试剂：喷后在110℃下烤7～10 min，紫外光下观察荧光。试剂Ⅰ：25％三氯乙酸的乙醇或氯仿溶液，配制后可放置数日。或用试剂Ⅱ：上述乙醇溶液用前每10 ml加过氧化氢溶液4滴，或新配3％氯铵T水溶液按4∶1混合。

4. 三氯化锑试剂：喷后在100℃下烤5 min，日光下或紫外光下观察。配制25％或饱和的三氯化锑氯仿溶液。

5. 磷酸—溴试剂：溶液Ⅰ：10％磷酸溶液。溶液Ⅱ：溴化钾饱和溶液、溴酸钾饱和溶液及25％盐酸溶液按1∶1∶1混合。薄层用溶液Ⅰ喷洒后，在125℃下烤12 min（薄层太湿时，烤的时间可适当延长），在紫外光下观察一次，将薄层再烤热，趁热喷溶液Ⅱ，再在紫外光下观察。

6. Keller-Kiliani试剂：检测α-去氧糖。试液：100 ml冰乙酸和$FeCl_3$试液0.5 ml混匀，试样1 ml混匀。试样1 ml加试液2 ml溶解后，沿试管壁滴入浓硫酸2 ml，接触面即显棕色，渐变为浅绿色、蓝色，最后冰乙酸层全部呈蓝色。

四、黄酮类显色剂

黄酮类成分在紫外光下大多显出不同颜色，用氨熏，喷三氯化铝溶液或喷氢氧化钠等碱性溶液，则颜色变深或变色。

1. 氨气。

2. 10％氢氧化钠或氢氧化钾溶液。

3. 1％或5％碳酸钠溶液。

4. 1％或5％三氯化铝乙醇溶液。

5. 2％乙酸镁甲醇溶液。

6. 饱和三氯化锑的氯仿溶液，在100℃下烤5 min。

在使用以上6种试剂前后，将薄层分别置于日光与紫外光下观察。

7. 1％～2％三氯化铁乙醇溶液。

8. 1％中性乙酸铅或碱式乙酸铅溶液。

9. 0.1 mol/L硝酸银溶液。

10. 铁氰化钾—三氯化铁试剂。溶液Ⅰ：2％铁氰化钾溶液。溶液Ⅱ：2％三氯化铁溶液。临用前将溶液Ⅰ与溶液Ⅱ等量混合。

11. 硼氢化钾试剂。二氢黄酮化合物显红色或橙红色。溶液Ⅰ：1％～2％硼氢化钾异丙醇溶液，必须新鲜配制。溶液Ⅱ：浓盐酸。先喷溶液Ⅰ，5 min后放入盐酸蒸气槽内。

12. Shinoda试剂。在混有锌粉的硅胶薄层上喷盐酸，黄酮醇显红紫色。制备硅胶薄层时，加入2％（W/W）锌粉并混合。薄层展开后喷盐酸溶液，如展开剂为酸性，可在展开后先喷锌—丙酮混悬液，再喷盐酸溶液。

13. 罗丹明—氨试剂。溶液Ⅰ：0.1％罗丹明B的4％盐酸溶液。溶液Ⅱ：浓氨溶液。先喷溶液Ⅰ，然后再将薄层放入氨气槽内。

14. 对氨基苯磺酸试剂。溶液Ⅰ：将对氨基苯磺酸0.3 g，加入8％盐酸溶液100 ml中溶解。溶液Ⅱ：5％亚硝酸钠溶液。取溶液Ⅰ 25 ml用冰冷却，加预冷的溶液Ⅱ 1.5 ml。

15. 硼酸—柠檬酸试剂。溶液Ⅰ：饱和硼酸的丙酮溶液。溶液Ⅱ：柠檬酸丙酮溶液。先喷溶液Ⅰ，再喷溶液Ⅱ。

16. 福林试剂(Folin-Ciocalteu's reagent)。取钨酸钠 10 g 和钼酸钠 2.5 g 溶于 70 ml 水中,再缓缓加 85% 磷酸 5 ml 和浓盐酸 10 ml,将混合液回流煮沸 10 h,然后加硫酸锂 15 g,水 5 ml 及溴 1 滴,再回流煮沸 15 min。所得溶液冷却后移至 100 ml 溶量瓶中,并用水稀释到刻度(贮备液),溶液应不显绿色。溶液Ⅰ:20% 碳酸钠溶液。溶液Ⅱ:临用前将上述贮备液 1 份用水 3 份稀释。先喷溶液Ⅰ,稍干后再喷溶液Ⅱ。

17. 苯胺一邻苯二甲酸试液配制。取 0.93 g 苯胺、1.66 g 邻苯二甲酸,溶于 100 ml 水饱和的正丁醇。

18. 三氯化铝试剂:1% 三氯化铝乙醇液。

19. 斐林试剂。溶液甲:取 1.93 g 硫酸铜溶于 100 ml 水中。溶液乙:取 34.6 g 酒石酸钾钠及 10 g 氢氧化钠溶于 100 ml 水中。临用前,将甲、乙二液等体积混合,如甲或乙不透明,可先过滤再混合。

五、三萜、甾体类显色剂

1. 25% 磷钼酸乙醇溶液。喷后在 140℃下加热 5~10 min,呈深蓝色。
2. 三氯化锑浓盐酸或氯仿溶液。三氯化锑 1 ml 加氯仿 4 ml,溶解。喷后在 90℃下烤 10 min(应在通风橱中进行),不同的皂苷元在可见光或紫外光下显出各种颜色。
3. 硫酸一甲醇(1:2)溶液。喷后加热,不同的皂苷元可显红褐色、紫色、黄色或黑色,所显颜色与温度无关。
4. 氟磺酸一乙酸(1:1)溶液。喷后在 130℃下加热 5 min。可显天蓝色、紫色、粉红色或淡棕色,在紫外光下也显不同荧光。
5. 碘蒸气。将薄层置于碘蒸气筒中,皂苷元皆显棕黄色斑点。
6. 三氯乙酸一乙酸(1:2)溶液。喷后在 100℃下加热 20 min,皆显黄色。
7. 2% 血球生理盐水混悬液(溶血试验、检测皂苷)。取新鲜兔血(由心脏或静脉取血)适量,用洁净小毛刷迅速搅拌除去纤维蛋白,并用生理盐水反复离心洗涤至上清液无色后,量取沉降红细胞,用生理盐水配成 2% 混悬液,贮冰箱内备用(贮存期 2~3 天)。

六、蒽醌类显色剂

蒽醌及其苷在日光下显黄色,在紫外光下显黄色或红橙色荧光。在薄层上用氨熏或喷氢氧化钾与碱溶液,则颜色变深或变色。

1. 氨气。
2. 10% 氢氧化钾甲醇溶液。
3. 3% 氢氧化钠溶液或碳酸钠溶液。
4. 50% 哌啶的苯溶液。
5. 饱和硼酸锂溶液。
6. 饱和硼砂溶液。
7. 0.5% 乙酸镁甲醇溶液,喷后在 90℃下烤 5 min。
8. 0.5% 乙酸铝溶液,喷后在紫外光下观察荧光。
9. 0.5% 牢固兰 B 试剂。喷本试剂后,原来氢氧化钠、氢氧化锂、氢氧化钾等碱溶液显荧光,此时在可见光下显棕色、紫色或绿色。也可先喷本试剂,再喷稀氢氧化钠溶液而显色。

也用于酚类及芳香胺的显色。溶液Ⅰ：新配的0.5%牢固兰B盐的水溶液。溶液Ⅱ：0.1 mol/L氢氧化钠溶液。

七、香豆素显色剂

1. 0.5%碘的碘化钾溶液。香豆精显各种颜色，也可用于其他类型的化合显色。
2. 重氮化氨基苯磺酸试剂。香豆精显黄、橙、红、棕、紫等颜色。取对氨基苯磺酸0.9 g，加热溶于12 mol/L盐酸9 ml，用水稀释到100 ml，取此溶液10 ml用冰冷却，加冰冷的4.5%亚硝酸钠溶液10 ml，0℃放15 min（在0℃可保存3天），用前加等体积1%碳酸钠溶液。
3. 重氮化对硝基苯胺试剂。香豆精显黄、红、棕、紫等颜色，也可用于酚类的显色。

取对硝基苯胺0.7 g，溶于12 mol/L盐酸9 ml，用水稀释到100 ml，将此溶液逐渐滴加到冰冷的1%亚硝酸钠溶液，再用冰冷的水稀释到100 ml，需临用时新配。

4. 4-氨基安替比林－铁氰化钾试剂。香豆素和酚类显橙红色至深红色。溶液Ⅰ：2%4-氨基安替比林乙醇溶液。溶液Ⅱ：8%铁氰化钾溶液。先喷溶液Ⅰ，再喷溶液Ⅱ，最后用氨气熏。
5. 稀氢氧化钠溶液。喷前喷后在短波长的紫外光下观察薄层的荧光。

八、挥发油显色剂

1. 茴香醛－浓硫酸试剂：喷后在150℃下烤。挥发油中各成分显不同颜色。取浓硫酸1 ml加到冰乙酸50 ml中，冷却后加茴香醛0.5 ml，必须临用时配制。
2. 荧光素－溴试剂：检测含乙烯的化合物（配法及使用见前）。
3. 碘化钾－冰乙酸－淀粉试剂：斑点显蓝色则为过氧化物。溶液Ⅰ：4%碘化钾溶液10 ml与冰乙酸40 ml混合，再加锌粉一小勺过滤。溶液Ⅱ：新制的1%淀粉溶液。先喷溶液Ⅰ，5 min后喷大量溶液Ⅱ，喷到薄层透明为止。
4. 对二甲氨基苯甲醛试剂：检出菌与菌前体在室温或80℃下烤10 min显深蓝色。取对二甲氨基苯甲醛0.25 g，溶于冰乙酸50 g、85%磷酸5 g和水20 ml的混合液中，此试剂储于棕色瓶中能稳定数月。
5. 异羟肟酸铁试剂：斑点显淡红色，可能是酯和内酯。溶液Ⅰ：取盐酸羟胺5 g溶于水12 ml，用乙醇稀释到50 ml，储于冷处。溶液Ⅱ：取氢氧化钾10 g溶于少量水，再用乙醇稀释到50 ml，储于冷处。溶液Ⅲ：溶液Ⅰ和溶液Ⅱ以1∶2混合，滤去氯化钾沉淀，所得滤液必须放入冰箱中，可稳定2星期。溶液Ⅳ：取三氯化铁（$FeCl_3 \cdot 6H_2O$）10 g溶于36%盐酸20 ml，与乙醚200 ml振摇，得均匀的溶液，密塞储存可长久使用。先喷溶液Ⅲ，在室温中干燥后，再喷溶液Ⅳ。
6. 2,4-二硝基苯肼试剂。醛和酮化合物显黄色。取36%盐酸10 ml和2,4-二硝基苯肼试剂1 g，加到乙醇1000 ml中。
7. 0.3%邻联二茴香胺冰乙酸溶液：醛和酮化合物显各种颜色。
8. 三氯化铁试剂：酚性物质显蓝绿色。配制1%～5%三氯化铁的0.5 mol/L盐酸溶液。
9. 4-氨基安替比林－铁氰化钾试剂：酚性物质显橙红色至深红色。溶液Ⅰ：2% 4-氨基安替比林乙醇溶液。溶液Ⅱ：8%铁氰化钾溶液。先喷溶液Ⅰ，再喷溶液Ⅱ，最后用氨气熏。
10. 硝酸铈试剂：醇在黄色背景下显棕色。取硝酸铈铵6 g溶于4 mol/L硝酸溶液100 ml。

11. 钒酸铵(钠)8-羟基喹啉试剂：醇在蓝灰色背景下显淡红色，有时需加热。取1%钒酸铵(钠)溶液1 ml和25% 8-羟基喹啉的6%乙醇溶液1 ml，加苯30 ml，振摇，分出蓝灰色的苯溶液使用。

12. 溴甲酚绿试剂：有机酸显黄色。取双甲酮30 mg溶于乙醇90 ml，慢慢加入85%磷酸10 ml，配制后的试剂放置于冷处能用几个星期，但新配的效果较好。

13. 酚—硫酸试剂：喷后在110℃下烤10～15 min，糖显棕色，取酚3 g及浓硫酸5 ml溶于乙酸95 ml。

14. 3,5-二氨基苯甲酸—硫酸试剂：喷后在100℃下烤15 min，2-去氧糖在日光下显红棕色，在紫外光下显黄绿色荧光。取甲基红1 g及溴酚蓝3 g溶于95%乙醇1000 ml。

15. 溴酚蓝指示剂：显黄色。配制0.04 mol/L溴酚蓝乙醇溶液，用氢氧化钠溶液调至微碱性。

16. 溴甲酚绿指示剂：如展开剂中含乙酸，则喷前薄层在120℃下烘烤除去乙酸，在蓝色背景上显黄色。取溴甲酚绿0.04 g溶于乙醇100 ml，加0.1 mol/L氢氧化钠溶液至蓝色刚刚出现。

17. 溴甲酚紫指示剂：喷前薄层在100℃下烤10 min，冷却到室温后，喷显色剂。在蓝色背景上显黄色。取溴甲酚紫0.04 g溶于50%乙醇100 ml，用0.1 mol/L氢氧化钠溶液调至pH为10.0。

18. 溴甲酚紫柠檬酸试剂：取溴甲酚紫25 ml及柠檬酸100 mg，溶于丙酮—水(9:1)混合液100 ml。

19. 百里酚酞碱溶液：在灰色或蓝色背景上显红色或白色。取0.1 g百里酚酞溶于乙醇，用乙醇稀释至100 ml。

20. 二氯靛酚试剂：喷后加热片刻，在天蓝色背景上显粉红色，如加热时间延长，则钼酸转变为白色，故可识别酮酸。2,6-二氯靛酚0.1 g溶于95%乙醇100 ml。

21. 芳香胺—还原糖试剂：取芳香胺(如苯胺5 g)和还有糖(如木糖5 g)溶于95%乙醇。

22. 碘化物淀粉试剂：在白色或浅蓝色背景上显深蓝色，灵敏度为2μg。取8%碘化钾溶液、2%碘酸钾溶液及1%淀粉溶液等量混合，用前新鲜配制。

23. 硝酸铈铵—吲哚乙醇溶液：溶液Ⅰ：10%硝酸铈铵溶液。溶液Ⅱ：吲哚乙醇溶液。

24. 联苯胺—亚硝酸钠试剂：喷后在254nm紫外光下观察荧光。溶液Ⅰ：取联苯胺2.5 g溶于浓盐酸7 ml及水500 ml。溶液Ⅱ：10%亚硝酸溶液。临用前将3份溶液Ⅰ和2份溶液Ⅱ混合。

九、氨基酸显色剂

1. 茚三酮试剂：用于氨基酸、氨及氨基糖检测。试剂Ⅰ：取茚三酮0.3 g溶于正丁醇100 ml中，加乙醇3 ml。试剂Ⅱ：取茚三酮0.2 g溶于乙醇100 ml中。试剂Ⅲ：饱和硝酸铜溶液1 ml与10%硝酸银溶液0.2 ml、乙醇100 ml混合。方法：在色谱上喷洒试剂Ⅰ或试剂Ⅱ，喷后在110℃下加热至显出颜色，或可继续喷洒试剂Ⅲ，斑点由蓝紫色转成红色。

2. 吲哚醌试剂：将1 g吲哚醌溶于100 ml乙醇中，加冰乙酸10 ml，混合均匀。

3. 茚三酮—硝酸铜试剂(Moffatt-Lytle反应)：试剂Ⅰ：取0.2 g茚三酮，用100 ml乙醇溶解。试剂Ⅱ：分别取1 ml饱和硝酸铜溶液、0.2 ml 10%硝酸银溶液、100 ml乙醇，混合均匀。试剂Ⅰ和试剂Ⅱ等量混合。在色谱上喷洒显色剂,然后在110℃下加热,直至斑点刚刚显色,颜色在日光中逐渐加深,不同氨基酸的显色速度不同。

4. 1,2-萘醌-4-磺酸钠试剂(Folin 试剂):喷后在室温干燥,不同的氨基产生不同的颜色。取 1,2-萘醌-4-磺酸钠 0.02 g 溶于 5%碳酸钠溶液 100 ml 中(需新鲜配制)。

5. 氯气－联甲苯胺试剂:将薄层放在氯气中,假如氯气从气筒中得到,则放置 5～10 min;假如由 1.5%高锰酸钾溶液及 10%盐酸(1:1)的混合物制得,则需放置 5～20 min。然后将薄层置空气中数分钟,以除去过量的氯气,再喷试剂。试剂配制:取邻联甲苯胺160 mg 溶于乙醇酸 30 ml 中,溶液用蒸馏水 500 ml 稀释,然后加碘化钾 1 g。

十、糖显色剂

1. 茴香醛－硫酸试剂:喷后在 100～105℃下烤,各种糖显不同颜色,取浓硫酸 1 ml 加到含茴香醛的乙醇溶液 50 ml 中,需临用前配制。

2. 1,3-二羟基苯萘酚－硫酸试剂:在 110℃预热的薄层上喷试剂,几分钟后在白色背景上显不同颜色,再加热,颜色加深,背景也变深。

3. 苯胺－二苯胺－磷酸试剂:喷后在 85℃下烤 10 min,各种糖显不同颜色。取二苯胺 4 g、苯胺 4 ml 及 85%磷酸 20 ml 溶于丙酮 200 ml 中。

4. 苯胺－邻苯二甲酸试剂:取苯胺 0.93 g 和邻苯二甲酸 1.66 g,溶于 100 ml 用水饱和的正丁醇中。喷后在 105～110℃下烤 10 min,糖显红棕色。

5. α-萘酚－硫酸试剂:喷后在 100℃下烤 3～6 min,多数糖显蓝色,鼠李糖显橙色,所显颜色于室温稳定 2～3 天。将 15% α-萘酚乙醇溶液 21 ml、浓硫酸 13 ml、乙醇 87 ml 及水 8 ml 混匀后使用。

6. 1,3-二羟基萘酚－磷酸试剂:喷后在 105℃烤 5～10 min,酮糖显红色,醛糖显淡蓝色。将 0.2% 1,3-二羟基萘酚乙醇溶液 100 ml 与 85%磷酸溶液 10 ml 混合。

7. 双甲酮－磷酸试剂:喷后在 110℃烤 15～20 min,仅酮显暗绿灰色。

8. Keller-Kiliani 试剂:检查 α-去氧糖。配法及使用见强心苷项下。

9. 3,5-二氨基苯甲酸－磷酸试剂:取 3,5-二氨基苯甲酸 1 g 溶于 80%磷酸 25 ml,加水稀释至 60 ml。喷后在 100℃烤 10～15 min,糖显棕色,在紫外光下显黄绿色荧光。

10. 苯酚－硫酸试剂:将苯酚 3 g 及浓硫酸 5 ml 溶于乙醇 95 ml。喷后在 100℃烤 10～15 min,糖显棕色。

11. 对硝基苯胺－过碘酸试剂。溶液Ⅰ:饱和过碘酸 1 份加水 2 份稀释。溶液Ⅱ:1%对硝基苯胺乙醇溶液 4 份与盐酸 1 份混合。先喷溶液Ⅰ,放置 10 min,再喷溶液Ⅱ。去氧糖显黄色,紫外光下显强荧光,再喷 5%氢氧化钠醇溶液,颜色转为绿色,乙二醇同样显色。

十一、鞣质显色剂

1. 氯化钠明胶试剂:取明胶 1 g 溶于 50 ml 水中,加 10 g NaCl 使其溶解,然后加水稀释至 100 ml 即得。保存期为 2～3 个月。

2. 铁铵明矾试液:取硫酸铁铵结晶 1 g 加蒸馏水溶解后,稀释至 100 ml 即得。

3. 新鲜石灰水:新鲜石灰水上清液。滴加新鲜石灰水,鞣质产生青灰色或棕红色沉淀。

参考文献

[1] 李嘉蓉.天然药物化学实验[M],第1版.北京:中国医药科技出版社,2004.
[2] 黄涛.有机化学实验[M],第2版.北京:高等教育出版社,1998.
[3] 成都中医药大学内部教材.中药化学实验.2003.
[4] 吴立军.天然药物化学实验指导[M],第3版.北京:人民卫生出版社,2011.

Experimental Code for Chemistry of Natural Products

1. Experimental Requirement

(1) Before the experiment, you should prepare lessons which includes preparing the preliminary note, understanding the purpose of the experiment, knowing the principle of experiment, and comprehending the experimental steps.

(2) Students should abide by the laboratory system, operate conscientious, use the various instruments properly, record faithfully the observed phenomenon and results such as the weight, volume and temperature or other data, and develop such good habits.

(3) During the course of the experiment, keep quiet and clean, avoid loud noise and no smoking should be obeyed. In addition, students should not be late to the class or leave the lab before the class is over. On the contrary, students should observe the experimental reactions and phenomenon carefully, make preparation for the next step, and always keep the experimental table, apparatus, sink and floor clean. Throwing the discarded waste or filter paper into the sewer must be forbidden.

(4) After finishing the experiment, students should wrap the product and tag the bottles. Furthermore, analyzing the test phenomenon carefully, drawing a reasonable conclusion and writing out experimental report should be done in time.

(5) When the experiment was finished, students on duty should arrange the public apparatus, clean the experimental table and floor, clear the waste tank, check the water faucet and electric switch, and close the door and window.

(6) Please handle the apparatus with care, don't use expensive instrument without the permission of the teacher, then report and replace the damaged equipment in time.

(7) Don't use the wrong bottle stopper of public drugs in order to protect them from cross contamination.

2. Experimental Safety

(1) The circuit should always be open to the atmosphere and the pipe shouldn't be blocked before reflux or distillation.

(2) Don't heat anything with open fire during the course of refluxing or distilling inflammable solvent. Water bath, oil bath, or electric heating-jacket can be chosen according to the boiling point of the solvent. Before heating, you should add some zeolites into solvent in order to prevent bumping. If forget to put zeolites or activated carbon into solvent, you can redo it when the solvent cools to room temperature.

(3) When you refluxing or distilling the inflammable, volatile or toxic solvents, you must pay attention to the gas leakage of apparatus and guide the residual gas to outdoor or sink with rubber pipe.

(4) Pressure relief system should be equipped with a safety bottle. When using compression column, you should pay attention to the mechanical property of chromatography column and storage tanks, and control the pressure to avoid glass cracking.

(5) When using the inflammable solvent, you should keep away from sources of ignition and avoid ventilation. When unsealing the bottle cap of volatile solvent, please take care of your face.

(6) Assure safekeeping of the toxic or caustic drugs, wash your hands after using them, and don't touch your face or wound.

(7) Before using electrical equipments or analytical instruments, you should learn the operating rules and do not touch the power with wet hand.

(8) Before inserting the glass tube into rubber stopper, you should apply some water or glycerol to the plug hole, wrap the glass tube with cloth and screw it into rubber stopper and avoid breaking the glass.

(9) Once fire accident happens in the lab, you should keep calm and take appropriate measures. You should cut off the electricity supply and take away the inflammable solvents. Small fire can be quenched by a wet cloth, yellow sand or a fire extinguisher.

3. Injury Rescue

(1) Wound: Sterilize the wound with hydrogen peroxide or apply pharmaceutical mercurochrome to it.

(2) Scald or burn injury: Apply scald drugs, glycerol or boric acid vaseline to it.

(3) Acid-base corrosive injury: Wash the wound at first, then use 5% sodium bicarbonate solution or dilute ammonia solution if wounded by acid corrosive reagents, or use 1% acetate solution if wounded by alkaline corrosive reagents, and flush with water at last.

If acid or alkali splashes into the eyes, wash the wound at first, then flush with 1% sodium bicarbonate solution if wounded by acid corrosive reagents, or use 1% boric acid if wounded by alkaline corrosive reagents, and flush with water at last.

(4) In case students eat toxic drugs by accident, the teacher should weigh 0.3~0.5 g copper sulfate and dissolve it in 150~250 ml warm water for the student to drink, or let the student insert a finger into throat to vomit.

(5) The wounded should be sent to the hospital if it is severe.

4. How to Wash the Apparatus

Common washing method is as follows.

(1) Brushing with water: It can draw off soluble impurity, dust, and insoluble substance, except oil pollution or organic compounds.

(2) Brushing with synthetic detergent or abstergent: The dirty apparatuses should be moistened at first. Then you can add the proper synthetic detergent or abstergent to brush it, flush and wash it to cleanliness at last.

(3) Brushing by washing solution: As for stubborn stains or residues, they can be washed away by washing solution. The most commonly used washing solution is composed of concentrated sulfuric acid and isovolumetric saturated potassium bichromate solution.

The standard of clean apparatus is that insoluble substance, oil pollution or obvious bead should be not found; the water only leaves a thin layer of membrane on the glass surface when you turn it upside down.

5. How to Dry the Apparatus

(1) Heat-drying: The emergency apparatus can be dried in the oven at 105℃. Or invert them in the glass drying apparatus.

(2) Drying in the air or blow-drying: Non-emergency apparatus can be kept in a dry place. For glass containers with scale, add a little volatile solvent in it and rotate up and down, and they can be dried in the air or dried at low temperature after dumping the solvent.

6. Experimental Report

Experimental report should be well organized and has recognizable handwriting. The format of experimental report can be adjusted based on test contents. Besides the information of major, class, name, experiment teams and date, it should also include the following items.

(1) Title.

(2) Purposes and requirements.

(3) Basic principle: It should involve basic principle of extraction, isolation or identification.

(4) Operation: It should be presented by flow chart briefly. The phenomenon should be recorded correctly.

(5) Identification: It should include chemical reagent, phenomenon, result, conclusion etc.

(6) Products: It should include color, crystal form, weight, melting point and yield.

(7) Discussion: It should include notice, key step, the reasons for success or failure and comments.

(8) Questions: According to the teacher's requests, you should answer some questions in the report.

Chapter 1
Common Technology of Extraction and Separation

Natural pharmaceutical chemistry is the subject that mainly studies effective components of natural medicines. Because the complex components contain effective components, ineffective compositions and impurities, we should extract effective components in order to lay the foundation of structure identification and pharmacological research. The essence of extraction is the process of extract chemical components from the medicine by proper method, obviously, it can be viewed as the pretreatment task of drug production.

1. Basic Principle of Solvent Extraction

According to the different solubility properties of multiple components of natural drugs, it is beneficial to choose the solvent with high solubility for active components and low solubility for unwanted compositions. When the solvent is added to Chinese herbal medicine, it enters plant cell through the cell wall because of the mechanism of diffusion and permeation, and makes the soluble substance dissolve. It causes concentration difference between internal and external plant cell, and accelerates the process of diffusion and permeation. Repetition goes on until the concentration of internal and external plant cell reaches dynamic equilibrium. After filtering the saturated solution and adding the same solvent once more, the needed components can be extracted as much as possible.

2. Factors of Influencing the Extraction Effect

The key to solvent extraction is to select appropriate solvent and measure, such as grinding degree of medicinal materials, temperature and time etc.

2.1 Grinding Degree

Solvent extraction includes many complex procedures, such as saturation, dissolution, and diffusion etc. Generally, the finer powder of medicinal materials, the greater its surface area and the higher its extraction efficiency. If the powder is too fine, it will lead to increasement of powder particle surface area, enhancement of adsorption, and influence of diffusion. At the same time, the fine powder containing compositions of proteins or polysaccharides makes the extract very sticky, which will effect the extraction and separation of the effective components. Therefore, when extracted with water, materials should be made into middlings or flake.

2.2 Temperature

Higher temperature can speed up molecular motion and enhance the diffusion and permeation. So hot-extraction has better efficiency than cold-extraction. Because over high temperature will destroy some components of drugs and increase the dissolution of impurities, the extraction temperature should be between 60℃ and 100℃.

2.3 Time

The extraction efficiency increases with the passage of time until the concentration of internal and external plant cells reaches the dynamic equilibrium. So there is no need for extending extraction time. The time for water extraction is 0.5～1 h, while the time for alcohol extraction is 1～2 h.

3. Selection of Solvents

Selection of appropriate solvents is the key of extraction, which needs to pay attention to the following three points: High solubility for active components and low solubility for unwanted compositions; no chemical reaction with active compositions; it should be economical, available and safe.

Common extraction solvent can be divided into three types as follows.

3.1 Water

Water is a kind of strong polar solvent which can dissolve lots of compositions such as inorganic salts, small molecular polysaccharides, tannins, amino acids, proteins, organic acid salts, alkaloid salts, and glycosides. In order to improve the solubility, acid or basic water usually can be used as extraction solvent. The former can dissolve alkaloids; the latter can dissolve organic acid, flavonoids, anthraquinones, lactones, coumarin and phenols etc. Disadvantages: Water extraction will cause mildew and deterioration easily, which lead to the difficulty in filtering, especially for some Chinese herbal medicine containing pectin and mucilage; extracting with hot or boiling water will produce starch gelatinization and increase the difficulty of filtering. Therefore, traditional Chinese drug decoction pieces are directly boiled; water extract could produce a large amount of foam, which makes the concentration and isolation difficult, especially for some components of saponin or mucilage. Installation of gas-liquid seperation glass ball on a distilling apparatus in a lab or membrane concentration in industry can prevent the generation of foam.

3.2 Hydrophilic Solvents

Hydrophilic solvents are miscible with water, such as ethanol, methanol, acetone and so on. The most commonly used hydrophilic solvent is ethanol. Its advantages are as follows: Good solubility and good penetrating power, which enable it to dissolve lots of components except protein, mucilage, pectin, starch and some polysaccharides; low dosage, short extraction time, and few water soluble impurities; low boiling point, low toxicity, low price, wild source, easily recyclable and mildew-proof. Its disadvantage is being combustible.

The characteristics of methanol and ethanol are similar, but the boiling point of methanol is lower (64.5℃). What's more, it is toxic to optic nerve.

3.3 Lipophilic Solvents

Lipophilic solvents are not miscible with water, such as petroleum ether, benzene, chloroform, ether, ethyl acetate, dichloroethane, etc. Good selectivity and hardly extracting water soluble impurities are its advantages. Its disadvantages are as follows: highly volatile, mostly combustible except chloroform, mostly toxic and expensive; weakly penetrating power makes the extraction need more extraction time; if crude drugs contain too much water, it's difficult to extract the active components with lipophilic solvent. So there are some limitations in extraction of a large number of Chinese herbal medicines with lipoplilic solvents.

Section 1 Common Extraction Technology

1. Impregnation

1.1 Cold Impregnation

The crude drugs are weighed at first and put into suitable and airtight container. Add a certain amount of solvent, such as water, acid water, basic water or alcohol. Stir and shake them from time to time, impregnate $1 \sim 2$ d at room temperature, and then filter out the active components. Add appropriate solvent once more and impregnate the rest of components for $2 \sim 3$ times, filter it, and combine the filtrate with the former. The mixed extraction was concentrated to get the total extracts.

1.2 Hot impregnation

Its operation is on the whole the same as cold impregnation, but its temperature range is $40 \sim 60$ ℃. Because of the higher temperature, its extract efficiency is better. It is essential to filter the sediment and then concentrate the filtrate.

2. Percolation

2.1 Device

Common percolation device is usually cylindrical or conical percolator (see fig. 1-1). The length of percolator is $2 \sim 4$ times the diameter of it. The cylindrical and conical percolator is suitable respectively for low and high expansion of Chinese herbal medicines.

2.2 Operation

Put coarse powder of medicinal materials into the container with a cover, add the extraction solvent which is the volume of $60\% \sim 70\%$ coarse powder, moisten it evenly and keep it closed, stand a while for 15 minutes to several hours, and make the medicine fully expanded. Take some adsorbent cotton and moisten with the extraction solvents, pave it at the bottom of the barrel, and then put the expansion materials into percolator. After adding the medicine, you should flatten it uniformly. The degree of tightness is decided by the characteristic of materials and extraction solvent. The solvent containing water or alcohol should be pressed respectively loose or compact. After loading the powder, use filter paper or gauze to cover the medicine, and add some glass beads or broken tiles into it in order to prevent the powder from being washed away. Then slowly add the solvent, and open the piston of the percolator to exhaust the air. After the solution flows from the bottom,

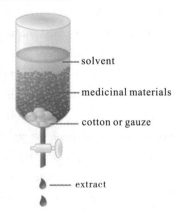

Fig. 1-1 Percolation device

pour it into the percolator once again and close the piston, continue to add the solvent until its height is several centimeters higher than the powder, and stand a while for 24~48 h to make the solvent fully permeated and diffused. If the weight of medicinal materials is 1000 g, its flow rate should be approximately 1~5 ml/min. It is essential to supply the solvent in time. The ratio of the medicinal powder to solvent is 1 : (4~8).

2.3 Notice

(1) The medicine powder should not be too thin, so as not to clog the pore and prevent the solvents from flowing into it. Generally, when percolating a large number of medicinal materials, they should be sliced about 0.5 cm long; when percolating a small amount of medicinal materials, they should be ground to a meal. If fine powder has existed, you can mix it with the meal evenly so as not to clog the percolator.

(2) Before putting the powder into the percolator, it must be moistened for some time in order to avoid clogging because of expansion and causing an incomplete extraction.

(3) Compactness and uniformity have an important influence on leaching effects. If the powder is packed too tight, it will block the solvent outlet and stop the percolation. On the contrary, if the powder is packed too loose, the solvent will go through the powder fast and cause incomplete leaching. Flattening off the powder surface with a mallet layer by layer is a correct way.

(4) The powder should not be excessive and its dosage is two-thirds volume of percolator. Some space is left for storage of solvents.

(5) After the powder is filled enough, you should first open the piston of the percolator, and then add the solvent. If the order of installment is opposite, there will be many bubbles. During the course of percolation, the height of the solvent must be higher than that of the powder, otherwise cracking of the powder will happen soon. Continuous percolation device (see fig. 1-2) can prevent it happening.

3. Decoction

Take the medicine tablet or the meal, put it in the suitable vessel (non-iron ware), and add enough water into it. After the solution boils, keep decocting and filter the solution at last. The time of decoction is decided by the weight and characteristic of raw materials. Generally speaking, it may boil 20~30 minutes at the first time according to the quantity and texture of medicines. Hard texture or large quantity of Chinese medicine should be extracted for 1~2 hours. Time may be reduced according to the actual situation.

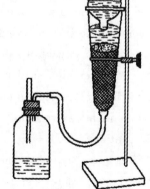

Fig. 1-2 Continuous percolation device

4. Reflux

Load the meal of medicinal materials in a round flask, and add the solvent until its liquid level is 1~2 cm higher than that of the powder. It is noteworthy that total dosage of the solvent and meal should be 1/2~2/3 the volume of flask. Condenser tube is connected to upper side of the flask, meanwhile, put the bottom of flask in a water bath within stipulated time, filter it, add the residue in the solvent and go on extracting 2~3 times, and then combine all the extracts (see fig. 1-3).

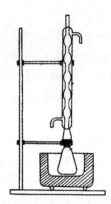

Fig. 1-3　Reflux device

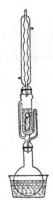

Fig. 1-4　Soxhlet extractor

5. Soxhlet Extraction

5.1　Device

Soxhlet extractor consists of three parts. There are a condenser pipe, an extraction tube with the siphon, and a round flask on the upper, middle and lower parts respectively. The three parts connect with each other tightly with ground glass joints (see fig. 1-4).

5.2　Operation

Put the powder into filter paper cylinder, and then put into the extraction tube and connect all apparatuses. After installing them completely, heat them in the water bath. When the solvent boils, steam reaches condenser pipe through the side tube, which is condensed into liquid and dropped into the extraction tube. When liquid level reaches the highest point of the siphon, the extract solution will flow into the siphon rapidly because of siphon effect. The solvent of solution will evaporate by heating and ascend through the side tube into condenser pipe until it flows into the middle extraction tube once more, which leads to producing new siphon effect. So keeping the continuous extracting will make most soluble components extracted. Generally, it spends several hours.

5.3　Notice

(1) Filter paper cylinder can be strapped or folded and its liquid level should exceed 1~2 cm of Soxhlet extractor's siphon. Internal diameter of filter paper cylinder should be less than that of extraction tube.

(2) It is right that height of the loaded powder is lower than that of the siphon. The powder should not be dropped onto filter paper cylinder lest it blocks the siphon during experiment.

(3) Before heating, zeolites should be added in the flask to prevent bumping.

6. Distillation

6.1 Device and Installation

The most commonly used atmospheric distillation device (see fig. 1-5) is consisted of distilling flask, distilling head, thermometer, condenser pipe, horn tube, and conical flask.

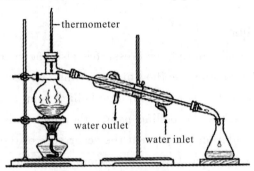

Fig. 1-5 Distillation device

Choose an appropriate flask, adjust the position of thermometer's mercury bulb and make its lower part stand in the same horizontal line with the upper part of distilling flask's branch pipe. Its installation starts generally from the heat source at first, then follows the order of bottom-to-top and left-to-right. When you install condenser pipes, condenser pipe tongs should clamp its center of gravity position. Keep condenser pipes in a straight line with distilling flask's branch pipe, and then connect with the flask uniformly in a straight line so as not to break pipes. Condenser tube tongs should not clamp too tight or loose and the tube should be able to rotate freely. The center line of installed devices should be in a straight line viewed from the front and the side.

6.2 Operation

(1) Feeding: Add the solution into flask with a long neck funnel; prevent the liquid from flowing into branch pipe. Next, add enough zeolites, install the thermometer, and check if the connection is tight and if there is air leak.

(2) Heating: Add the cold water into condenser pipe and begin heating. When steam reaches the mercury bulb of the thermometer, the temperature rises dramatically. You should control the temperature, and adjust the distillation speed to $1 \sim 2$ drops per second usually.

(3) Collecting: Because different distillation components have different boiling points, prepare enough flasks and collect low boiling point liquid in time. If maintaining temperature doesn't produce new distillation liquid, you should stop heating at first, then shut off the tap and remove the instruments.

6.3 Notice

(1) The solvent volume should be $1/3 \sim 2/3$ the volume of the flask.

(2) When distilling volatile and flammable liquids, avoid using open fire. It is better to use water bath as heat source.

(3) Don't forget to add zeolites before heating. If you forget to add zeolites, you must redo it when the solvent cools to room temperature, otherwise it will produce large quantities of steam which can spout out of the flask. It could injure you and cause fire or burn accidents. Before heating again, we should add new zeolites if we stop distillation half way for some reasons.

7. Vacuum Distillation

Distillation under normal atmospheric pressure is also known as common distillation or simple distillation. It is a common method of separating, extracting or purifying organic compounds. Because some compositions with high boiling point often decompose or oxidize before the temperature reaches the boiling point, they cannot be distilled under normal atmospheric. Vacuum distillation can prevent the occurrence of this phenomenon. Vacuum distillation device which is connected to vacuum pump will reduce the system pressure and cut down the boiling point of organic compounds.

7.1 Device

Vacuum distillation can be divided into three parts (see fig. 1-6): distillation system, vacuum system and pressure-measuring device.

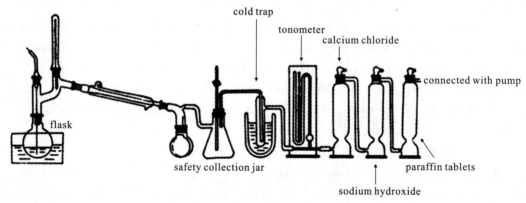

Fig. 1-6 Device of vacuum distillation

Device of vacuum distillation is consisted of flask, Claisen distilling flask, straight condenser pipe, vacuum tube, receiving bottle, safety collection jar, tonometer and vacuum pump (oil vacuum pump or circulating water vacuum pump), as shown in fig. 1-7 to fig. 1-9. You cannot use flat bottom instrument as distilling flask and receiving bottle, such as Erlenmeyer flask, flat bottom flask, and thin-wall or damaged instrument, because the external pressure can cause an

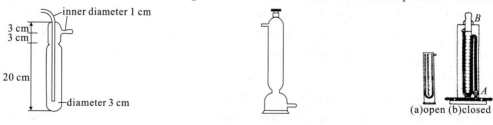

Fig. 1-7 Cold trap   Fig. 1-8 Adsorption tower   Fig. 1-9 Tonometer

explosion. Before installing the equipments, smear a little special grease on the surface of ground glass in order to ensure the sealing of device and lubricate the join.

Insert a capillary to the bottom of Claisen distilling flask and ensure the steam can pass through the capillary. Capillary plays the role of stirring and gasification center which can prevent the liquid bumping. However, zeolites don't play the role of gasification center in the reduced pressure condition. Insert a thin copper wire on the top of capillary tube, clamp it with a spiral clip and adjust air inflow.

Vacuum receiving pipe connects with a safety collection jar, which not only prevents oil or water from entering the receiving bottle in order to avoid mutual contamination, but also prevents materials from entering the reduced pressure system. The safety collection jar connects with a pump and tonometer.

7.2 Operation

The volume of the distillates should not exceed 1/2 the volume of the flask. When the pressure is stable, some continuous and stable minute bubbles will pass through the capillary. If the bubbles are very big and rush into the branch pipe of Claisen distilling flask, there may be two kinds of cases: the first is that air inflow is too strong, and the second is that vacuum degree is too low. At this moment, adjusting the spiral clip of the capillary should be done slowly. Most of liquid can evaporate at low temperature and low pressure, therefore, the heating is not too fast. When the distillation is finished, rotate the vacuum tube and begin to receive fractions. Adjust the distillation speed to $1 \sim 2$ drops per second. When the pressure is stable and the compound is pure, boiling range should be controlled in $1 \sim 2\,^\circ\!C$.

7.3 Notice

Move the heater at the end of the experiment and open the spiral clip. After cooling down, slowly open air release valve of the safety collection jar, make the tonometer return to zero position, and shut off the pump. Otherwise, oil or water will enter the cold trap or the safety collection jar because of low pressure.

With the continuous development of modern instrument technology, traditional vacuum distillation device has been gradually replaced by rotary evaporator due to its complex installment and low security during the course of concentration (see fig. 1-10).

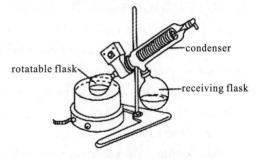

Fig. 1-10 Rotary evaporator

8. Steam Distillation

8.1 Device

Simple device of steam distillation is commonly used in laboratory (see fig. 1-11), which is consisted of steam generator, distiller, condenser and receiving flask.

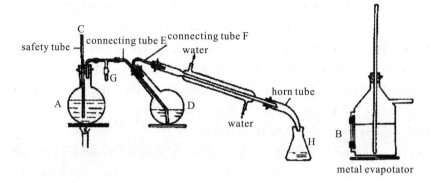

Fig. 1-11 Steam distillation device

A is a steam generator which is generally made of metal (it could be replaced by large short-neck round flasks). Glass tube B is the water level gauge which can help to observe the height of the water. C is a safety tube (the glass tube is 1 cm long and its internal diameter is 5 mm). Insert safety tube near the bottom of steam generator. When the pressure of steam generator is too high, water ascends along the safety pipe, which adjusts the internal pressure. If distillation system is clogged up, water will spout out of the safety tube, thus you should check the distillation flask and assure if the steam pipe has been blocked.

Distillation device is usually a 500 ml long-neck and round-bottom flask. In order to prevent boiling liquid in the flask from jumping and splashing into condenser pipe, the angle between the flask and the steam generator is 45 degrees. The volume of liquid should not exceed one-third the volume of the flask. The end of vapor pipe E should be tortuous and inserted vertically near the bottom of the bottle. Internal diameter of steam outlet tube F (bending angle is about 30°) should be slightly larger than that of pipe E. Insert one end of tube F in the diplopore stopper of round-bottom flask with leakage of 5 mm long, and the other end is connected with condenser pipe. Distillate flows into receiving flask H. If necessary, cold water bath can be used to cool the liquid.

A T-tube connected with rubber pipe and spiral clamp G should be equipped between round-bottom flask and steam generator. On the one hand, T-tube can remove condensate water. On the other hand, T-tube can be immediately opened in order to ensure safety when abnormal operation or emergency situation occurs.

8.2 Operation

Add distillate (miscible liquid or solid mixed with a small amount of water) in device D. At the same time, add hot water of three-quarters the volume of the steam generator and zeolites. After examining air tightness of the entire device, open spiral clamp G and heat steam generator right away. Close spiral clamp G when large quantities of steam rushes out of the T-tube. Steam will enter the round-bottom flask. In the process of distillation, condensate water will make the volume of distillate increase constantly. Once the liquid volume exceeds two-thirds the volume of distillation flask, and the distillation speed is low, the flask could be directly heated above asbestos wire gauze. During the course of heating, care should be taken to prevent the occurrence of jumping phenomenon. Distillation speed should be controlled within 2～3 drops per second. In the process of distillation, check the water level of safety tube; observe whether distillation liquid in round-bottom flask splashes acutely. Once there is an abnormal phenomenon, immediately open spiral clamp G, discharge water vapor, and then remove the heater and the devices to check the blocked point. When the distillation is finished, open spiral clamp G at first, and then stop heating, or else distillate will be reversely adsorbed into the steam generator.

8.3 Notice

(1) If volatile material has high melting point which produces solid precipitate because of condensation effect, you should cut down the velocity of condensate water to make the material maintain in liquid state. If the condenser pipe has some solid materials which can block the flow of distillate, the condensate water can be switched off or discharged temporarily in order to increase the temperature of condenser pipe. Distillate will melt into liquid and flow into the receiving flask. Adding cold water into the condenser pipe once more should be done slowly and carefully in order to avoid breaking the condenser pipe because of shock cooling. If the condenser pipe has been blocked, you should stop the distillation immediately, and try to dredge. you can use a glass rod to clear up the crystal or pour hot water into condenser pipe to make the crystal melt into liquid and flow out, and then continue the distillation.

(2) If the volume of distillation solution is small, Kjeldahl's flask should be used to replace round-bottom flask.

9. Supercritical Fluid Extraction

Supercritical fluid extraction (SFE) is a new fleetly developmental technology and is widely used in many fields. Traditional extracting methods such as steam distillation, vacuum distillation, solvent extraction and so on, have complex process and low purity, and cause residue of harmful substances. Fluid in supercritical state has the character of high density, low viscosity, and high diffusion co-efficiency. It has some advantages such as high extraction yield, high product purity, simple production process, and low energy consumption.

9.1 The Concept of SFE

What is SFE? Any kind of substance has three phases: gas, liquid, and solid. Three-phase point is the point at which three phases coexist in equilibrium state. Critical point is the point at which liquid phase and gas phase are in equilibrium. Temperature and pressure at the critical point are called critical temperature and critical pressure respectively. Different materials have different critical temperature and critical pressure. Supercritical fluid (SCF) is any substance at a temperature and pressure above its critical point. State close to the critical point is called supercritical state (see tab. 1-1).

Tab. 1-1 Physical property comparison of SCF, gas, and liquid

phase	density (g/ml)	diffusion coefficient (cm^2/s)	viscosity (g/cms)
gas(G)	10^{-3}	10^{-1}	10^{-4}
supercritical fluid(SCF)	0.3~0.9	$10^{-4} \sim 10^{-3}$	$10^{-4} \sim 10^{-3}$
liquid(L)	1	10^{-5}	10^{-2}

9.2 The Principle of SFE

SFE is the process of separating one component from another using supercritical fluid as the extrating solvent. In supercritical conditions, SCF has good flowability and permeability which can separate different ingredients according to different polarity, boiling point and molecular weight. Because the extract separated at different pressures isn't a monomeric compound, we can get the best proportion of mixture by controlling the conditions. Then change the supercritical fluid into ordinary gas with the help of reduced pressure or high temperature. Effective constituents are extracted completely so as to achieve the process of purification. The process of SFE is consisted of extraction and separation (see fig. 1-12).

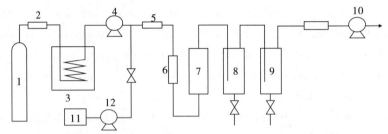

1. steel cylinder of CO_2 2. filter 3. refrigeration compressor 4. high pressure metering pump 5. mixer 6. preheater 7. extractor 8. separator Ⅰ 9. separator Ⅱ 10. flow quantity recorder 11. entrainer 12. centrifugal pump

Fig. 1-12 Device of SFE

The major influencing factors of SFE are as follows:

(1) Density: Solvent strength is relevant to the density of SCF. When the temperature is constant, strength and solubility of solvent increase with increasing density and pressure.

(2) Entrainer: Most fluids applied to SFE have low polarity which is beneficial to selective extraction, but restricts application of some components with high polarity. So we can add a little entrainer (such as ethanol) to change the polarity of the solvent and greatly improve the yield.

(3) Size: The diffusion of solvents from sample particles can be described by Fick's second law. The size of the particles can influence extraction yield. Generally speaking, small particles are beneficial to SFE-CO_2 extraction.

(4) Fluid volume: Increasing fluid volume can improve the recovery because extract solubility is relevant to the volume of SCF.

10. Ultrasonic Extraction

10.1 Brief Introduction

Ultrasonic Extraction (UE) technology is applied to Chinese herbal medicines in recent years and becomes an effective and new method of extraction and separation of ingredients. Ultrasonic is the electromagnetic wave with the 20~50 MHz frequency range. It is a kind of mechanical wave and propagates in energy carrier and medium. During the course of propagation, ultrasound has alternating cycle of the positive and negative pressure. In positive phase medium molecules are extruded, and the medium density is increased; in negative phase medium molecules become sparse and discrete and the medium density is decreased. In other words, ultrasonic cannot make sample molecules polarize, but can produce sonic wave cavitation between solvent and sample, which leads to the formation, growth and blasting compression of bubbles in the solvent. Thus it makes solid sample scattered, increases the contact area between extraction solvent and sample, and improves mass transfer rate of transferring target from solid phase to liquid phase.

The principle of UE: Extraction superiority of UE is based on the special physical properties of ultrasonic. It mainly reduces the force between target extraction and sample matrix through fast mechanical vibration wave generated by a piezoelectric transducer so as to accomplish the solid-fluid extraction or separation. The basic processes are as follows:

(1) Ultrasonic is able to speed up motion of the effective particles, and make ultrasonic energy act on the particles of medicinal ingredients. The particles will obtain huge acceleration and kinetic energy, and escape rapidly from the medicine.

(2) Ultrasonic propagating in liquid produces special cavitation effect, which makes the compositions of Chinese herbal medicine escape, produces constant exfoliation of matrixes, and accelerates leaching extraction of effective ingredients which do not belong to plant structure.

(3) Uniform vibration of ultrasonic makes the whole sample extraction more effective.

To sum up, active substances of natural drugs in ultrasonic field not only get great accelerated speed and kinetic energy as a particle, but also get the strong external shocks by cavitation effect, which gets high efficiency of isolation (see fig. 1-13).

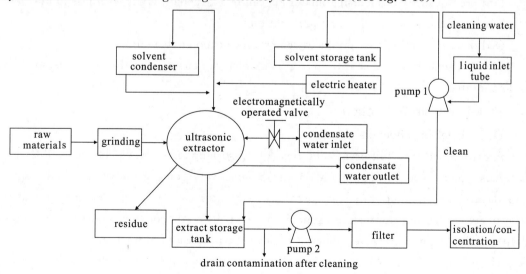

Fig. 1-13 Industrial ultrasonic extractor

10.2 Characteristics of UE

UE is applicable to extract effective ingredients of Chinese traditional medicines, and is a new method and new technique of changing completely the extraction method of traditional water-extracting and alcohol-precipitating. Compared with traditional extraction, ultrasonic extraction has the following prominent characteristics.

(1) No need for high temperature: UE does not destroy chemical ingredients of easy hydrolysis or oxidation in water at 40~50℃. UE can break the plant cell wall and improve the curative effect of Chinese traditional medicine.

(2) Atmospheric extraction, safe, simple in operation and convenient in maintenance.

(3) High extraction efficiency: UE wins the best extraction yield in the extraction time of 20~40 minutes. Extraction time is one third of water-extracting and alcohol-precipitating time or less. Extraction yield is twice the yield of traditional methods. According to statistics, ultrasonic extraction efficiency is very high at 65~70℃. Effective ingredients in Chinese herbal medicine will not be destroyed at temperature below 65℃. Extraction time is about 40 minutes when UE is used at 65℃. While decoction methods usually cost two to three hours which is triple the time of UE methods. Extract three times and then you can extract basically more than 90% effective ingredients of traditional Chinese medicine.

(4) Wide application: With wide serviceability, the majority of Chinese herbal medicines can be extracted by UE.

(5) It can be used with different ultrasonic extraction solvents. Therefore, there are many kinds of extraction solvents and extraction targets to be chosen.

(6) Lower energy consumption: UE is used without heating, its extracting temperature is low and extracting time is short at the same time, thus it greatly reduces energy consumption.

(7) Large quantity of medicinal materials can be extracted by UE with less impurities, which is beneficial to separation and purification.

(8) Lower extraction cost produces remarkable economic benefits.

(9) Ultrasonic has certain antiseptic effect which can ensure that the extract is not easy to deteriorate.

11. Microwave Extraction

11.1 Brief Introduction

According to the different abilities of absorbing microwave between different materials, microwave extraction (ME) heats selectively some areas of matrix or some components in extraction system so that extracted materials are separated from the matrix or system, and go into extraction agent with lower dielectric constant and relatively poor ability of absorbing microwave, so as to achieve the purpose of extraction.

The principle of ME: Microwave is a kind of electromagnetic wave in the frequency range 300 MHz to 300 000 MHz. It has four basic characteristics: wave property, high frequency, thermal characteristic and non-thermal characteristic. Microwave frequency commonly used is

2 450 MHz. Microwave heating is a method that heated polar molecules (such as H_2O, CH_2Cl_2) rotate fastly and orient in microwave electromagnetic field, which generates heat according to the effect of laceration and mutual friction. Microwave heating makes its energy have direct effect on the heated substances. Air and containers don't absorb or reflect microwave basically, which ensures that the energy transfers rapidly and is utilized fully.

11.2 Characteristics of ME

(1) Good selectivity, only heating polar molecule and producing selective dissolution.

(2) ME greatly reduces the extraction time. Traditional extraction methods need a few hours, UE also needs half an hour to an hour, but ME only needs a few seconds to a few minutes. Therefore, the extraction rate increases dozens or hundreds, even thousands of time.

(3) ME is less limited by solvent affinity, so there is a wider selection of the solvents, and ME reduces the dosage of the solvent.

ME is generally suitable for materials with thermal stability. Heat sensitive components extracted by ME can become deformed and inactive. Therefore, raw materials should have good water absorption, otherwise the cells can not absorb enough microwave and break itself. It is difficult to make the product release, because ME has a poor selectivity of components. With the development of modern technology, continuous microwave extraction has entered the stage of industrialization (see fig. 1-14).

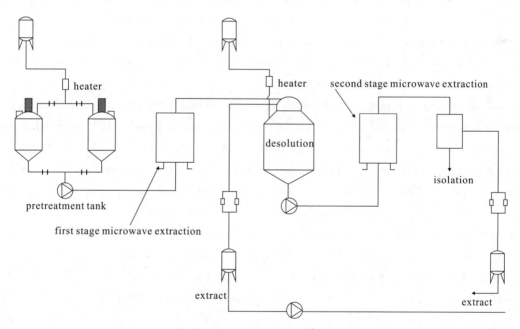

Fig. 1-14 Device of industrial continuous extraction microwave

12. Enzymatic Extraction and Bionic Extraction

12.1 Enzymatic Extraction

Enzymatic extraction is a new technology. In recent years, cellulose enzymes are widely used in various fields; especially its industrial application in Chinese herbal medicine extraction has entered the early development stage. Most of cell walls which wrap effective components of Chinese herbal medicine are composed of cellulose. Cellulose is composed of β-D-glucose which is connected with the chain of 1,4-β-glucoside. Cellulose enzyme can destroy the bond of β-D-glucose, which is beneficial to extract effective components. Traditional extraction methods such as decoction and reflux demand high extraction temperature, large quantities of ethanol and high cost with low efficiency and poor security. Appropriate enzyme can decompose plant tissues through gentle enzyme reaction, and accelerate the release of the effective components. Remove the residues of influencing liquid clarity such as starch, protein, pectin, and promote changing liposoluble constituents with low polarity into soluble glucoside.

Influencing factors of enzymatic extraction are as follows:

(1) Pretreatment of medicinal materials is beneficial to enzyme solution. For example, when using ball mill to pretreat raw materials, the finer powder, the easier to suspend in the enzyme solution. Furthermore, with the increase of effective contact area, materials are hydrolyzed more easily by the enzyme and the hydrolysis speed increases.

(2) pH, temperature and enzymolysis time are influencing factors of the extraction, which should be optimized based on the experimental data. At the same time, they are chosen according to the species of Chinese herbal medicines and enzymes.

Enzymatic extraction has great application potential, but it also has some restrictions such as the narrow choice of extraction enzymes and complexity in extraction process.

12.2 Semi-bionic Extraction (SBE)

SBE is a new extraction method which integrates overall drug research with molecular medicine research, imitates the principle of oral administration and gastrointestinal drug transport from a biopharmaceutical point of view, and lays the foundations for the design of digestive drug simultaneously. The process is as follows: extract respectively 2~3 times with acid and alkaline water which is similar to acidity and basicity in stomach and intestinal environments. It not only uses active mixed compositions, but also uses monomer composition to control its pharmaceutical quality. But its shortcoming is the necessity of decoction in high temperature which will destroy some effective ingredients.

12.3 Bionic Extraction (BE)

BE is mainly aimed at extraction of oral medicines. It imitates human stomach and intestinal environments, overcomes the weakness of SBE which needs high temperature decoction that easily destroys effective components, and shows advantages of enzymolysis. Most components are weak organic acids or weak organic alkalis in molecular or ionic form in body fluids. According to the physiology characteristic of alimentary canal, biological membrane between digestive tube and vessel is lipid membrane which only allows liposoluble substances to pass through, so molecular form of drug is adsorbed more easily.

Chapter 1　Common Technology of Extraction and Separation

New Words and Phrases

grind [graɪnd]　*v.* 磨碎,磨成(粉末)
melicera [melɪˈsərə]　*adj.* 黏稠的,糖浆状的
mesh [meʃ]　*n.* 网孔,网状物
　　　　　　vt. & vi. (使)吻合;用网捕
carbohydrate [ˌkɑːbəʊˈhaɪdreɪt]　*n.* 碳水化合物,糖类
polysaccharide [ˌpɒlɪˈsækəraɪd]　*n.* 多糖,多聚糖
alkaloid [ˈælkəlɒɪd]　*n.* 生物碱
mildew [ˈmɪlduː]　*n.* 霉,霉病
　　　　　　vt. & vi. (使)发霉,(使)长霉
deterioration [dɪˌtɪəˈreɪʃən]　*n.* 恶化;变坏;退化;堕落
mucilage [ˈmjuːsɪlɪdʒ]　*n.* 黏液,胶水
hydrophilic [ˌhaɪdrəʊˈfɪlɪk]　*adj.* 亲水的(等于 hydrophilous)
lipophilic [ˌlɪpəˈfɪlɪk]　*adj.* 亲脂性的
miscible [ˈmɪsɪbl]　*adj.* 易混合的
petroleum ether　石油醚
benzene [ˈbenˌziːn]　*n.* 苯
chloroform [ˈklɔːrəˌfɔːm]　*n.* 氯仿
ethyl acetate　乙酸乙酯
dichloromethane [daɪˌklɔːrəˈeθeɪn]　*n.* 二氯甲烷
impregnation [ˌɪmpregˈneɪʃən]　*n.* 浸渍,饱和作用
impregnate [ɪmˈpregneɪt]　*v.* 充满,浸渍
percolation [ˌpɜːkəˈleɪʃn]　*n.* 过滤,渗滤
conical [ˈkɒnɪkəl]　*adj.* 圆锥(形)的
cylindrical [səˈlɪndrɪkəl]　*adj.* 圆柱形的,圆筒状的
decoction [dɪˈkɒkʃən]　*n.* 煎煮,熬出物
noteworthy [ˈnəʊtˌwɜːðiː]　*adj.* 值得注意的,显著的
condenser tube　冷凝管
flask [flæsk]　*n.* 长颈瓶;烧瓶
round flask　圆底烧瓶
distillation [ˌdɪstəˈleɪʃən]　*n.* 蒸馏(过程);蒸馏物
tong [tɒŋ]　*n.* 钳;煤钳
evaporator [ɪˈvæpəˌreɪtə]　*n.* 蒸发器,脱水器
rotary evaporator　旋转蒸发仪
stopper [ˈstɒpə]　*n.* 阻塞物,(尤指)瓶塞
　　　　　　vt. (用瓶塞)塞住
perforated [ˈpɜːfəˌreɪtɪd]　*v.* 穿孔于,在……上打眼(perforate 的过去式和过去分词)
diplopore [dɪˈplɒpɔː]　*n.* 双孔

supercritical [ˌsjuːpəˈkrɪtɪkəl] adj. 超临界的
viscosity [vɪˈskɒsɪtɪ] n. 黏稠；黏性；黏质
ultrasonic [ˌʌltrəˈsɒnɪk] adj. 超声的，超音速的
　　　　　　　　　　　　　　n. 超声波
bionic [baɪˈɒnɪk] adj. 仿生学的；利用仿生学的
enzymatic [ˌenzaɪˈmætɪk] adj. 酶的；酶催化
zeolite [ˈziːəlaɪt] n. 沸石
thermometer [θəˈmɒmɪtə] n. 温度计
siphon [ˈsaɪfən] n. 虹吸管
　　　　　　　　vt. 用虹吸管吸或输送（液体）
　　　　　　　　vi. 通过虹吸管
filter paper　滤纸
gauze [ɡɔːz] n. 纱布（包扎伤口用）；纱网
ethanol [ˈeθənɔːl] n. 乙醇
methanol [ˈmeθənɒl] n. 甲醇
distilling head　蒸馏头
horn tube　尾接管
Soxhlet extractor　索氏提取器
rubber pipette bulb　吸耳球
screw clamp　螺旋夹
reducing bush　大变小转换接头

Section 2　Common Separation Technology

The extract is still a mixture which needs removing impurities and monomer should be acquired through separation and refinement. Separation is a process that uses certain method to make the constituents separate completely according to the difference of physical or chemical properties in the mixture. Refinement is a kind of separation process which can separate compounds with a certain purity and remove residual impurities in order to achieve the process of purification. The process of separation can be roughly divided into three stages: coarse separation, components separation and monomer separation. These three stages have no clear boundaries and should be chosen according to different chemical compositions of herbs. The commonly used methods of separation and refinement are systematic solvent separation, two-phase solvent extraction, precipitation, salting, dialysis, fractionation, recrystallization, liquid-liquid extraction, coinstanteneous distillation/extraction, solid-phase extraction and solid-phase microextraction.

1. Systematic Solvent Separation

Systematic solvent separation is a process that uses three or four kinds of solvents with different polarities to extract the total extracts according to the polarity from low to high, which will separate various ingredients dissolving in different solvents with different polarities. On the basis of pharmacology, we can determine the effective parts and separate them. Most extracts are jellies which are hard to disperse evenly in low polarity solvents or to be extracted fully. A way to solve the problem is to mix the extracts with inert bulking agent such as soil silicate and cellulose powder. Next, dry the mixture at low temperature, make it become powder, and extract with solvent in turn. Commonly used solvents are petroleum ether, ethyl ether, chloroform, ethyl acetate, ethanol, water, etc. If the chemical composition is not stable, you should avoid the following factors: high temperature, long heating, strong acid, strong alkali which can accelerate the decomposition and isomerization of effective ingredients.

2. Two-Phase Solvent Extraction

2.1 Simple Extraction

Simple extraction is a separation method which is based on the following principle: ingredients of mixture have different distribution coefficient in two immiscible liquids. The greater partition coefficient is in the two immiscible liquids, the higher the separation efficiency is. If effective ingredients of water extract are liposoluble, extraction solvents (such as benzene, chloroform, ethyl ether) are generally used for two-phase extraction; if effective components are slightly hydrophilic, they need solvents such as ethyl acetate, butanol, etc. Adding appropriate amount of ethanol or methanol in chloroform or ether can also increase the hydrophilicity. For extracting flavonoids ingredients, ethyl acetate and water are used as solvents. For extracting hydrophilic saponins, we usually choose n-butyl alcohol, isoamyl alcohol and water as two-phase solvents.

(1) Device: The most commonly used extraction device in laboratory is separating funnel (see fig. 1-15).

(2) Operation: Choose separating funnels whose volume is twice the volume of the separated liquid, dry the lower piston, smear a thin layer of grease onto the surface, insert the plug, and rotate the piston several times. Make the grease distribute evenly, and then put it in the circle of iron support stand. Close the lower piston, add separation solution and extraction solvent (usually 1/3 the volume of solution) into the top of separating funnel successively. Close the upper plug (do not smear grease), and rotate it tightly to prevent leakage of fluid. Take down the separating funnel, press your right palm against the plug, and hold the neck of funnel or the whole with your fingers. Hold the piston with your left hand, press the piston handle with your thumb and index finger, place middle finger under the plug to prevent the piston from slipping, and vibrate the funnel at a slanting angle. Vibrate the funnel several times slowly, make the mouth of

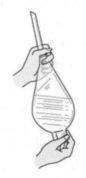

Fig. 1-15 **Separating funnel**

funnel face a safety place, and give off volatile gases from the piston to balance internal and external pressure. Repeat the process 2~3 times, and then vibrate it for some times to make two immiscible liquids contact completely, which will improve the extraction rate.

Put separating funnel into the iron ring, and it should stand a while until the solution is divided into two layers. Open the upper plug, unscrew the piston slowly to make the lower liquid and floccule discharge from the funnel, and separate the liquid as far as possible. Pour out supernatant liquid from the upper of the funnel so as to avoid crossed contamination. Extraction times depend on the distribution coefficient, generally 3~5 times.

(3) Notice.

①Put the solution in a small test tube, vibrate it vigorously for 1 minute and observe the layering effect. If emulsification phenomenon appears easily, the operation should avoid vigorous vibration and prolong the extraction time. If emulsification phenomenon arises, you should separate the emulsified layer, and add new solvent to extract it again. Alternatively, stand a while for a long time and rotate it once in a while. Continuous countercurrent extraction of two-phase solvents can be used when serious emulsification appears.

②Specific gravity of water extract should be 1.1~1.2, because dilute liquid needs large quantities of extraction solvents which will affect the operation.

③Maintain a certain proportion between solvent and water. At the first time you should add more solvent which is generally 1/3 the volume of water extract, and 1/4~1/6 the volume of water extract next time.

④Generally, extracting 3~4 times can be enough. Under the condition that water-soluble ingredient is not easy to dissolve in organic solvent layer, we must increase extraction times or change extraction solvent.

Extraction in industrial production is usually done in airtight container. Stir for a certain time with the blender to make the two liquids mix completely. Then, stand a while for some time until it divides into two layers; sometimes, mix the two-phase solution by spray in order to increase contact area and improve the efficiency of extraction. Alternatively, countercurrent continuous extraction equipment of two-phase solvent may be used.

⑤Alkaline solution often has emulsification phenomenon.

2.2 Countercurrent Continuous Extraction (CCE)

CCE is a continuous extraction of two-phase solvent. The device contains several or more extraction tubes which are filled with small porcelain circle or small stainless steel wire circle to increase contact area of two-phase solvent. For example, extracting the toosendanin from impregnated water extract of Melia toosendan bark with chloroform has the following process (see fig. 1-16): Add chloroform in tube, concentrate water extract whose specific gravity is less than that of chloroform stored in higher containers, and then open the piston. The extract at high pressure goes into extraction tube, hits porcelain circle and disperses into fine particles because of collision of small porcelain circle, which makes contact area increase and has complete extraction. If impregnated water extract of a

Chinese herbal medicine needs to extract with benzene and ethyl acetate that is lighter than water, the extract should be put in the tube, and benzene and ethyl acetate are stored in higher container. The method of thin layer chromatography, paper chromatography, color reaction and precipitation reaction can be used to check whether the extraction is complete or not.

2.3 Countercurrent Distribution (CCD)

The principle of CCD and CCE are the same, but the sample dosage of CCD is constant. It is a separation method that the extract and two-phase solvent undergo many shifts, distribution and extraction to achieve the purpose of separation. This apparatus is composed of several or even hundreds of pipes. If this instrument is unavailable, it can be replaced by glass funnel for low-dose extraction. Choose two-phase immiscible solvents with great difference in distribution coefficient. According to behavior analysis of chromatography test, measure the extraction times. CCD can often obtain good effect in separating the similar qualitative mixture. Its application is subject to long operation time, damages of extraction tube because of mechanical oscillation, and more solvent consumption.

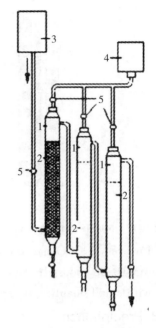

1. extraction tube   2. filler layer
3. higher container of water extract
4. solvent reservoir   5. control valve

Fig. 1-16 Device of countercurrent continuous extraction

2.4 Droplet Countercurrent Chromatography

Droplet flow distribution method is also known as droplet countercurrent chromatography (DCCC). DCCC is a modified method of two-phase solvent extraction based on CCD. The present application of instrument is as follows: connect 25 tubes (2.4 mm inner diameter and 60 cm height) on a plate, and use 12 plates (total 300 tubes) to form a continuous distribution extraction tube. The solvent system of DCCC and CCD are the same, but the solvent should be separated into two phases in a short time and produce valid droplet (see fig. 1-17 and fig. 1-18). Because of droplet formation of mobile phase, contact and increasement of friction with stationary phase effectively in fine extraction tubes will form a new surface that promotes the solute to distribute in the two-phase solvent. So the separation effect of DCCC is usually better than that of CCD and won't have emulsification phenomenon. Driving mobile phase with nitrogen pressure doesn't make separated material oxidized easily in the atmosphere. DCCC can effectively separate trace elements such as saikosaponin, quaternary ammonium base of protoberberine type etc.

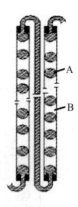
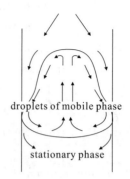

(A: mobile phase　B: stationary phase)

Fig. 1-17 Mobile phase and stationary phase of DCCC

Fig. 1-18 Distribution between droplets of mobile phase and stationary phase

However, DCCC has the following disadvantages: solvent systems which generate droplet must be choosed; the effect of separating polymer compounds is not good; it only deals with small quantity of samples less than 1 g, and needs certain equipments.

3. Precipitation

Precipitation is a method that add some reagent in the extract of Chinese herbal medicine to produce precipitation and remove the impurities.

3.1　Precipitation with Lead Salt

Precipitation with lead salt is a classic separation method of Chinese herbal medicine. Lead acetate and lead subacetate in water and alcohol solution can be integrated with various compositions of Chinese herbal medicine, such as organic acid, amino acid, protein, mucoid substance, tannic acid, resin, acidic saponins and part of flavonoids, and then generate lead salts or complex salt precipitation. Usually we add water or alcohol extract of Chinese herbal medicine into concentrated solution of lead acetate. Stand a while, filter out precipitation, combine the precipitation lotion and filtrate, and then add saturated solution of lead subacetate in the filtrate until the precipitation don't appear. In this way, lead acetate sediment, lead subacetate sediment and mother liquor can be gotten together. Suspend the sediment in a new solvent, pump hydrogen sulfide gas, and then make it decompose and turn to insoluble lead sulfide precipitation. Mother liquor containing lead salt should be treated by such deleading method. Then refine and purify it. Deleading with hydrogen sulfide is complete, but the solution might have redundant hydrogen sulfide. In order to avoid unwanted chemical reaction, pump air or carbon dioxide to remove excess hydrogen sulfide. New lead sulfide precipitation can adsorb some effective compositions and should be recycled with solvent.

Deleading can also use salts such as sulfuric acid, phosphoric acid, sodium sulfate, sodium, etc, while lead sulfate and lead orthophosphate in water still have certain solubility and lead salt can't be removed completely. Eliminating lead with cation exchange resin is fast and complete, but some effective components may be exchanged and resin regeneration is very difficult. In addition, the acidity of the solution increases after deleading, which sometimes need to be neutralized. Therefore, lead acetate and lead subacetate usually can be replaced by freshly prepared salts such as lead hydrate, calmogastrin, cupric hydroxide, lead carbonate, alums etc. For example, when adding alum solution in water extract of *Scutellaria baicalensis* Georgi, baicalin and aluminum salt generate insoluble complex in water which can be used directly for medicine after rinsing it with water.

3.2 Reagent Precipitation

When adding some alkaloid precipitation reagent in alkaloid salt solution, insoluble double salts are formed and can be separated. It is difficult to separate water soluble alkaloids with simple extraction method. Usually adding ammonium tetrathiocyanodiaminochromate can cement out alkaloid Reinecke's salt. When adding acid, alkaloid can be converted into precipitation such as hesperidin, rutin, baicalin, glycyrrhizin which are soluble in alkaline solution. Otherwise, changing the pH value of some protein solutions according to minimal solubility in isoelectric point can produce precipitation. In addition, use gelatin and protein solution to precipitate tannins; use cholesterol to precipitate digitonin.

4. Salt Fractionation

Its principle is as follows: Adding inorganic salt into water extract of Chinese herbal medicine to certain concentration or saturation to reduce solubility can make some ingredients generate precipitation and separate from water-soluble impurities. Commonly used inorganic salt for salting out includes sodium chloride, sodium sulfate, magnesium sulfate, ammonium sulfate, etc. For example, when adding magnesium sulfate into water extract of *Panax notoginseng* (Burk.) to saturation, saponins will precipitate. In addition, add sodium chloride or ammonia sulfate into extract to form salt fractionation in the production of berberine extracted from *Berberis julianae* Schneid or palmatine extracted from *Fibraurea recisa* Pierre. After adding enough salt in extract, some ingredients such as protoanemonin, ephedrine, matrine which has higher water solubility should be extracted by organic solvent.

5. Dialysis

Its principle is as follows: Small molecules in solution can pass through a semipermeable membrane, otherwise macromolecule can't pass through that membrane, which can achieve the purpose of separation. When separating and purifying the materials such as saponins, proteins, polypeptides, polysaccharides, etc, you can remove impurities, such as inorganic salts, monosaccharides and disaccharides with the method of dialysis. Conversely, macromolecular impurities can also be kept in a semipermeable membrane and refined when small molecular materials pass through the semipermeable membrane into the outer membrane solution (see fig. 1-19).

Add sample solution carefully in the dialysis bag, and then suspend the dialysis in a container which should be added into water. Change the water regularly to increase concentration difference of internal and external solution of dialysis membrane. Heating and stirring will be used to accelerate the speed of dialysis if necessary. You can also use electric dialysis method: place two electrodes at either end of pure solvents close to a semipermeable membrane, and then close an electric circuit. The components with a positive charge such as inorganic cations and alkaloids will move toward the cathode; the components with a negative charge such as inorganic anions and organic acids will move toward the anode; but neutral compounds and polymer compounds will be remained in dialysis membrane. Identifying the solution in dialysis membrane can check whether the dialysis is complete.

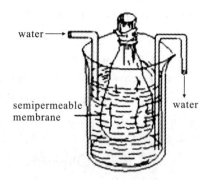

Fig. 1-19 Dialysis method

The completion of dialysis is closely related to the specification of dialysis membrane. Dialysis membrane includes animal membrane, collodion membrane, parchment membrane (sulfuric-paper membrane), protein membrane, cellophane paper membrane, etc. The sold cellophane or animal semipermeable membrane is usually bundled up like a pouch and protected with nylon bag outside. Dialysis membrane also can be prepared by yourself as following steps: use semipermeable membrane from animals such as bladder membrane from pig or cattle, rinse it with water, and defat with ether at last. Parchment membrane can be immersed in 50% sulfuric acid for 15~60 minutes, take it out and spread on the board, and flush it with water at last. The size of membrane hole is relative to concentration of sulphuric acid, soaking time and rinsing speed with water. The process of producing collodion membrane is as follows: dissolve collodion in ether and absolute ethyl alcohol, smear its solution on board, and dry in air. The size of membrane hole is relative to different solvents and volatilization speed of the solvent. At the same time, adding appropriate water can enlarge the hole size. Otherwise, adding a little acetic acid can reduce the size. The method of pretreating protein membrane (gelatin membrane) is as follows: smear 20% gelatin on fine cloth, place it in water after drying in air, add formaldehyde to make the membrane solid, and rinse it with water at last.

6. Fractionation

It is a kind of method which is used to separate liquid mixture according to the difference of boiling point among the components of liquid mixture after repeated distillation in the fractional distillation column. In the study of natural medicine chemistry, it usually can be used to separate volatile oil or some liquid alkaloids.

Each component in liquid mixture has their own fixed boiling point and certain saturated steam pressure at a certain temperature. The lower the boiling point is, the higher the steam pressure is. It means highly volatile. When the solution is vaporized, it gradually achieves the equilibrium between gas phase and liquid phase. Low boiling point component has high partial pressure, which leads to higher content in gas phase than in liquid phase. It means more ingredients with low boiling point are reserved in gas phase, and more ingredients with high boiling point are reserved in liquid phase. After an ideal distillation, the content of components with low boiling point increases, and the content of components with high boiling point decreases. After multiple distillations, various ingredients in the mixture can be separated basically. The process that repeated distillation makes the mixture separate is known as fractionation.

Fractionation is done in a fractional column which can finish the complex operation for many times (see fig. 1-20). In a fractional column, steam in the column is condensed into liquid because of air cooling. Heat exchange happens when ascending steam encounters descending liquor, and the gas-liquid equilibrium is achieved. If steam contains several components, the composition with high boiling point is more easily condensed. Compositions with high boiling

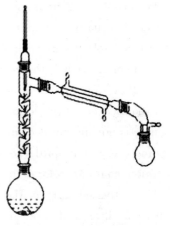

Fig. 1-20 Device of fractionation

point are on decrease because large quantities of steam ascend constantly. Pure components with low boiling point can be got at a certain height. Glass tubes or glass beads are often put in fractional column to increase the two-phase contact surface and reach balance faster.

If boiling point of separated components has a difference above 100℃, fractional column cann't be used; Otherwise, it can be used if boiling point has a difference below 25℃. Generally speaking, smaller difference of boiling point demands finer fractionation device. If liquid mixture can generate azeotropic mixture, and the components of liquid and steam are the same in the balance, it can't be separated by fractionation and must be done by chemical method.

Separating volatile oil by fractionation needs to operate under reduced pressure because ingredients have higher boiling point which leads to chemical reaction. Fractionation is hard to get monomer composition because volatile compositions are very complex and different boiling points are similar. But fractionation can get monomer components when cooperating with other methods such as chromatography.

7. Recrystallization

7.1 Operation

(1) Choice of solvent: Basic requirements of recrystallization solvents are that crystalline substances have high solubility in hot solvent and low solubility in cold solvent. The test of chosing solvent is as follows: put 0.1 g solid powder in a test tube, add the solvent with dropper and oscillate constantly, and heat it carefully until it boils after adding 1 ml solvent. If the substance is dissolved in 1 ml hot or cold solvent, the solvent can't be

used. If the substance is insoluble in boiling solvent, add 0.5 ml to 3 ml every time and heat up to boiling. If the material is still insoluble during the course of adding the solvent or it is soluble within 3 ml boiling solvent but doesn't form precipitation after cooling, the solvent can't be used. If the substance is soluble within 3 ml boiling solvent and it generates many crystalline substances after cooling, this solution can be applicable. If it is hard to choose a suitable solvent, mixed solvents can often be taken into account. Mixed solvent is usually composed of two solvents which are miscible in a proportion. Commonly used mixed solvents are ethanol and water, ethanol and ethyl ether, ethanol and acetone, ethanol and chloroform, ethyl ether and petroleum ether, etc.

(2) Dissolution and filtration: Add sample in a Erlenmeyer flask, add solvent less than the required quantity (according to solubility data), and then heat up to boiling. If the sample is not dissolved completely, you should add the solvent several times, heat up to boiling every time until the sample is dissolved completely, and filter while hot. If the solution contains colored materials, it can be decolorized by activated carbon. Before adding activated carbon, the solution should be appropriate cooling, then boil for 5~10 min, and filter while hot. In order to speed up the filtration, glass funnel with short and large neck can be used. Before filtration, keep the funnel hot in an oven, put folded filter paper in the funnel, and moisten it with a little hot solvent which can avoid crystallization and blocking the filter paper pores. A little crystal in the paper can be rinsed with a little hot solvent or abandoned. Too much crystal must be scratched away from the paper by a scraper and add a little solvent to dissolve it. After filtration, stand a while for crystal formation.

(3) Crystallization: Stirring the filtrate constantly during cooling can get tiny crystal which contains fewer impurities because of large surface, and more impurities are adsorbed on the surface. Placing the filtrate at room temperature and cooling slowly can get larger crystal. If the filtrate still has no crystal after cooling, use a glass rod to rub the container wall in order to form a rough surface which makes solute molecules form directional alignment, and use crystal seed to speed up crystal formation (if there is no crystal seed of this material, use a glass rod to dip a little solution and rub the container wall).

(4) Filtration under reduced pressure: Use Buchner funnel for filtration under reduced pressure in order to accelerate the filtration (see fig. 1-21). A thick rubber which can withstand gas pressure connects the side tube of suction flask to a safety bottle, and then connects with a vacuum pump. Put the plug in suction flask to avoid air leakage. The hole in Buchner funnel bottom should face the side tube of suction flask. The size of filter paper in Buchner funnel is slightly smaller than inside diameter of the funnel, but it should be able to cover all small holes.

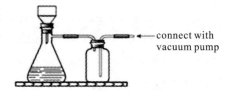

Fig. 1-21 Device of suction filtration

Before filtration, moisten the filter paper with the same solvent of recrystallization, then open the vacuum pump, and suck the filter paper tightly to prevent the crystal from being inhaled into buchner funnel from the gap of the filter paper. Add liquid and crystal into buchner funnel and begin to filter. After exhausting all solution, rinsing the crystal adhering to the vessel wall with a little filtrate can reduce the losses. Before rinsing crystal, stop the vacuum pump temporarily, add a little solvent on crystal, and scrape it with a scraper or stir carefully with a glass rod to make the crystal wet (don't make filter paper loose). Stand a while and begin to leach. At the same time, pressing the crystal surface with a clean glass stopper can make solvent and crystal separate easily. Generally, recrystallization operation is repeated $1 \sim 2$ times. Open the stopper of safety bottle at first when stopping the equipment, and then close the vacuum pump. Finally, take out the crystal, place it on a glass dish, and dry in the air or at the temperature below melting point of the crystal.

7.2 Notice

(1) Activated carbon can adsorb colored impurities, resin materials and homodisperse materials. Pay attention to the following points.

①Avoid excessive dosage which may adsorb samples. The dosage is decided by the color of impurities, generally $1\% \sim 5\%$ weight of dry coarse crystal. If the operation can't make the solution decolorized completely, repeat it with activated carbon.

②Forbid adding activated carbon in boiling solution in order to avoid the solution bumping.

③Decolorizing effect of activated carbon is good in water solution and bad in nonpolar solvent.

(2) If crystal grows too fast or the filtrate is too much during the filtration course, it should use hot filtration device (see fig. 1-22). A glass funnel is put in the metal funnel containing hot water. The benefit of the filtration method is that the preservation of hot water can decrease crystallization due to the drop in temperature in the process of filtration. When filtering flammable organic solvent, we must put out the flame around.

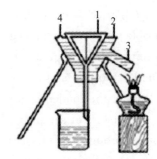

1. glass funnel 2. steel jacket 3. cupreous branch pipe 4. water injection hole

Fig. 1-22 Hot filtration device

(3) When using folded filter paper (also called filter paper of chrysanthemum type, see fig. 1-23), folded lines should not fold to the center of filter paper, otherwise, the central part of filter paper is easy to break during the course of filtration. Folded paper should be kept in order and put into the funnel, which can avoid contamination of filtrate.

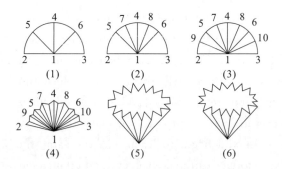

Fig. 1-23 Folding sequence of chrysanthemum type filter paper

8. Liquid-Liquid Extraction, Coinstantaneous Distillation/Extraction, Solid-Phase Extraction and Solid-Phase Microextraction

8.1 Liquid-Liquid Extraction

Liquid-liquid extraction is a most commonly used extraction method. Generally, the simplest equipment is separating funnel if you use multiple-low-dose method. If possible, automatic rotating continuous liquid-liquid extraction apparatus can also be used. The latter equipment costs more money and longer extraction time than separating funnel, but has higher extraction efficiency and saves the manpower. It is suitable for samples in water or water-soluble samples and has high magnification. Its weakness is that polar compounds have low recovery and easy emulsification, probably because oxidation produces new substances. When encountering emulsification, you can take the following measures: adding salts (light solvent) such as NaCl and Na_2SO_4, centrifugation, ultrasonic separation (non-flammable solvent), prolonging standing time, rotating slowly, and heating properly.

A continuous liquid-liquid extraction apparatus is shown in fig. 1-24. Add samples and water in the left bottle, and add extraction solvent in the right flask. After heating, the solvent will enter the condenser pipe, and the cooled solvent will go into the sample bottle. After the components of samples are extracted by the solvent extraction, it will return to solvent bottle through the phase separation. Repeat it several times until the components of samples are shifted to the solvent.

8.2 Coinstantaneous Distillation/Extraction

Advantages: It is suitable for samples in water, such as water-soluble sample, protein and oil; easily operating; cheap equipment; good reproducibility; high magnification.

Disadvantages: Polar compounds have low recovery rate because heating makes the sample decompose and produce new materials, such as furfural generated from saccharide, low carbon

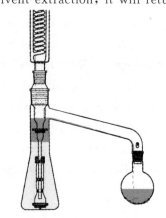

Fig. 1-24 Continuous liquid-liquid extraction apparatus

aldehyde generated from oil.

Common extraction solvents are ether, n-pentane, methylene chloride and so on. Diagrammatic sketch of coinstantaneous distillation/extraction instrument is shown in fig. 1-25. Add samples and water in the left bottle, and add extraction solvent in the right flask. After heating both flasks, volatile components are taken to the middle blending region between steam and solvent along with steam, exchange constantly with solvent and then have to be extracted and separated. The solvent with components of samples goes into the solvent flask once again, and then water returns to the sample bottle. Repeat it several times, so that volatile components of samples go into the solvent bottle.

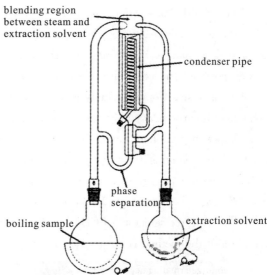

Fig. 1-25　Coinstantaneous distillation/extraction device

8.3　Solid-Phase Extraction (SPE)

SPE is a sample pretreatment technology with the development and combination of liquid-solid extraction and liquid column chromatography in recent years, and it is mainly used for separation, purification and concentration. Compared with traditional liquid-liquid extraction method, SPE can improve recovery rate of analysis ingredients, separate analyte and interfering components more efficiently, reduce pretreatment processes of the sample with simple operation, short extraction time and low energy consumption. SPE is a physical extraction process including liquid phase and solid phase. In the process of SPE, solid phase adheres to analyte more tightly than mother liquor. When the sample passes through a solid-phase extraction column, the analyte is adsorbed on the solid surface, and the other ingredients flow through the column along with mother liquor. Finally, the analyte is eluted with appropriate solvent.

Operation steps of SPE are as follows:

(1) Pretreatment of the column: In order to obtain high recovery rate and good reproducibility, solid-phase extraction column must be pretreated with appropriate solvent before it is used, which can remove impurities and deal with the packing to improve the reproducibility.

(2) Add the sample: After pretreated, sample solution is added and passes through the column at a certain flow rate. In this step, the analyte is held in adsorbent.

(3) Elution of the column: Select appropriate solvent to elute interfering components of sample and keep the analyte on the column.

(4) Elution of the analyte: Elute the analyte with the solvent, collect the eluent in collecting pipes, dry the analyte with nitrogen gas and dissolve it in a little solvent in order

to improve concentration of the analyte or analyze impurities in the solvent.

8.4 Solid-Phase Microextraction (SPME)

SPME is a new technology of sample pretreatment in 1990s, which has characteristics such as rapid development, environment-friendly extraction, and simple operation. The technology uses an portable and convenient extractor, which makes it suitable for indoor use and outdoor sampling analysis. Common analysis with many samples or shorter operation time can use the technology because it not only saves time, but also improves accuracy and reproducibility. This technology can complete sampling, extraction and enrichment in a simple process, which is beneficial to separating trace organic pollutants in liquid samples. SPME can separate materials combined with gas chromatography and liquid chromatography. The applicable detector are probably mass spectrometry (MS), FID detector (FID), flame photometric detector (FPD), electronic capture detector (ECD), atomic emission detector (AED), etc. The detectable limitation of the method is $ng(10^{-9}g)$ or even $pg(10^{-12}g)$.

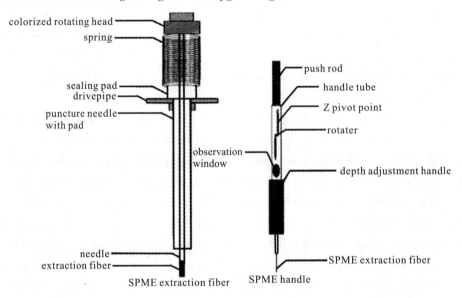

Fig. 1-26 Solid-phase microextraction device

SPME has two kinds of extraction methods. The first is that extraction fibers expose in samples which is suitable for analysing the sample containing gas organic compounds. The second is that extraction fibers expose in headspace of samples which is suitable for the analysis of volatile solids and semi-volatile organic compounds. Needles are coated with special adsorbent which can adsorb the gas composition in vapor-liquid equilibrium and can be desorbed in inlet of gas chromatography at high temperature. This method is suitable for qualitative and quantitative MS analysis(see fig. 1-26).

New Words and Phrases

  monomer [ˈmɒnəmə] *n.* 单体

  dialysis [daɪˈælɪsɪs] *n.* 透析,分离

Chapter 1　Common Technology of Extraction and Separation

isomerization [aɪˌsɒməraɪˈzeɪʃən]　n. 异构化(作用)
n-butyl　正丁基
isoamyl [ˌaɪsəʊˈæmɪl]　n. 异戊基
separating funnel　分液漏斗
plug [plʌɡ]　n. 塞子；插头
　　　　　　vt. 以(塞子)塞住；插入
vibrate [vaɪˈbreɪt]　vt. & vi. (使)振动，(使)颤动
test tube　试管
emulsification [ɪˌmʌlsɪfɪˈkeɪʃən]　n. 乳化(作用)
floccules [ˈflɒkjuːl]　n. 絮状物，絮凝粒
specific gravity　比重
countercurrent [ˈkaʊntəˌkʌrənt]　n. 逆流
cortex [ˈkɔː(r)teks]　n. 皮质；树皮
droplet [ˈdrɒplɪt]　n. 小滴，微滴
mobile phase　流动相
stationary phase　固定相；静止期
precipitation [prɪˌsɪpɪˈteɪʃən]　n. 匆促；沉淀
subacetaten [sʌbˈæsɪteɪt]　n. 碱式乙酸盐
hydrogen [ˈhaɪdrədʒən]　n. 氢
sulfide [ˈsʌlˌfaɪd]　n. 硫化物
Chinese herbal medicine　中草药
concentrate [ˈkɒnsəntreɪt]　vt. (使)浓缩
　　　　　　　　　　　　n. 浓缩物
delead [dɪˈled]　vi. 脱铅
carbonate [ˈkɑːbəneɪt]　n. 碳酸盐
alum [ˈəlʌm]　n. 明矾，白矾
aluminum [əˈluːmənəm]　n. 铝
alkaloid [ˈælkəlɔɪd]　n. 生物碱
tetrathiocyanodiaminochromate　四硫氰基二氨铬酸铵，雷氏铵盐
liquorice [ˈlɪkərɪs]　n. 甘草，甘草根
saponin [ˈsæpənɪn]　n. 皂苷，皂素
semipermeable [semɪˈpɜːmjəbl]　adj. 半透性的
cathode [ˈkæθˌəʊd]　n. 阴极，负极
parchment [ˈpɑːtʃmənt]　n. 羊皮纸
cellophane [ˈseləˌfeɪn]　n. 玻璃纸
volatilization [vɒˌlætɪlaɪˈzeɪʃən]　n. 挥发，发散
collodion [kəˈləʊdiən]　n. 火棉胶(药品名)；胶棉
anhydrous [ænˈhaɪdrəs]　adj. 无水的
anhydrous ethyl alcohol　无水乙醇

formaldehyde [fɔːˈmældəˌhaɪd] n. 甲醛；甲醛水溶液
rinse [rɪns] vt. 漂洗；冲洗
fractionation [ˌfrækʃəˈneɪʃən] n. 分馏法
boiling point 沸点
gush [gʌʃ] vi. 喷涌；迸出
azeotropic [əˌziːəˈtrɒpɪk] adj. 共沸的，恒沸点的
mixture [ˈmɪkstʃə] n. 混合，混杂
recrystallization [riːˌkrɪstəlaɪˈzeɪʃən] n. 再结晶(作用)，重结晶(作用)
recrystallize [riːˈkrɪstəlaɪz] vi. (使)再结晶
dropper [ˈdrɒpə] n. 滴管，点滴器
oscillate [ˈɒsəˌleɪt] vt. 使振荡，使振动
dissolution [ˌdɪsəˈluːʃən] n. 溶解，融化
Erlenmeyer flask 爱伦美氏(烧)瓶，锥形烧瓶
oven [ˈʌvən] n. 烤箱，烤炉
filtrate [ˈfɪltreɪt] v. 过滤，筛选
　　　　　　　　　n. 滤出液
glass rod 玻璃棒
multiple-low-dose 少量多次的
flammable [ˈflæməbəl] adj. 易燃的，可燃的
coinstantaneous [ˈkəʊɪnstænˈteɪnjəs] adj. 同时发生的，同时的
furfural [ˈfɜːfəræl] n. 糠醛
analyte [ˈænəlaɪt] n. (被)分析物，分解物
pivot [ˈpɪvət] n. 中枢；支点
drive pipe 套管
spring [sprɪŋ] n. 弹簧
reproducibility [rɪprəˌdjuːsəˈbɪlɪtɪ] n. 重复能力，可重现性
environment-friendly 环境友好的

Chapter 2
Technology of Chromatographic Separation

Chromatography is a technology based on different physical properties of different materials. All chromatographic systems are made up of two phases: one is stationary phase which is either solid material or components contained in solid material; the other is mobile phase which is flowing material, such as water and all kinds of solvents. When the mixture passes through stationary phase along with solvents (or mobile phase), the distribution of different components is different because of the variety of their physical and chemical properties which leads to different interaction of two-phase components (adsorption, interaction and dissolution). With the solvent moving forward, different components redistribute in two phases. Components which have weak force with stationary phase move forward fastly. Conversely, components which have strong force with stationary phase move forward slowly. Collecting liquid in steps, you can get each component of the sample (see tab. 2-1, tab. 2-2 and tab. 2-3).

Tab. 2-1   Classification by two-phase state

stationary phase	mobile phase	
	liquid	gas
liquid	liquid-liquid chromatography	gas-liquid chromatography
solid	liquid-solid chromatography	gas-solid chromatography

Tab. 2-2   Classification by chromatographic theory

name	isolation principle
adsorption chromatography	Ingredients are adsorbed on the surface of adsorbent in stationary phase with different adsorption ability.
partition chromatography	Ingredients' partition coefficients are different in stationary phase and mobile phase.
ion exchange chromatography	Stationary phase is ion exchange resin with different affinities to different components.
gel chromatography	Stationary phase is macroporous gel. Degree of obstruction is connected with molecular size of components.
affinity chromatography	Stationary phase only adsorbs one ingredient which has certain specialization.

Tab. 2-3 Classification by different operation forms

name	operation form
column chromatography	Pack stationary phase into column, and make the sample move straight ahead in one direction.
thin layer chromatography	Smear stationary phase evenly on thin layer plate, and spread out with mobile phase after spotting.
paper chromatography	Use filter paper as stationary phase, and spread out with mobile phase after spotting.
thin film chromatography	Produce thin film using polymeric organic absorbent. Its principle is similar to that of paper chromatography.

1. Adsorption Chromatography

Adsorption chromatography is a method that separate different materials according to different adsorption capacity. Commonly used adsorbents are alumina, silica gel, polyamide, etc. Liquid-solid adsorption chromatography is a common method which is especially suitable for the separation of samples with medium molecular weight (less than 1000Da, low volatility), especially for liposoluble constituents. Generally speaking, it isn't suitable for separating samples with high molecular weight such as proteins, polysaccharides or ionic hydrophilic compounds. Separation effect of adsorption chromatography is decided by adsorbent, solvent and characteristic of separated compounds.

1.1 Adsorbent

Commonly used adsorbents are silica gel, alumina, activated carbon, magnesium silicate, polyamide, diatomite, etc.

(1) Silica gel: Silica gel used for chromatography is a kind of porous substance with the structure of cross-linked siloxane. At the same time, there are many silanol groups on the surface of particles. The adsorption effect of silica gel is based on the amount of silanol groups. Silanol groups can adsorb moisture through the formation of hydrogen bonds. So the adsorption effect of silica gel decreases with the increasing of moisture content.

If moisture content is over 17%, its adsorption capacity will be very weak and it can't be used as adsorbent. But it can be used as supporter in distribution chromatography. The silica gel is activated at the temperature of 100~110℃, which can remove the water from silicon surface because of the adsorption of hydrogen bonds. However, When the temperature reaches 500℃, silanol groups will be dehydrated and form siloxane bond, and silica gel will lost the adsorption capacity and no longer has the nature of adsorbent for ever. So the activation temperature of silica gel should not be too high (water will be lost over 170℃).

Silica gel is a kind of acidic adsorbent which can apply to neutral or acid compositions. At the same time, silica gel is a kind of weak acidic cationic exchange agent whose silanol groups can release the weak acidic hydrogen ions. When encountering strong alkaline compounds, it will adsorb alkaline compounds because of ion exchange reaction.

(2) Alumina: Alumina may have alkalinity (may be mixed with sodium carbonate) which is beneficial to separating some basic natural ingredients such as alkaloids. But basic alumina should not be used for separating aldehyde, ketone, acid, and lactone because alkaline alumina can react with the compositions such as isomerization, oxidation, elimination, etc. Neutral alumica can be made by removing weak alkaline impurities in alumina and rinsing with water to neutral. Neutral alumina still belongs to the basic alumina which is applicable to the separation of acid composition. Treating alumina with dilute nitric acid or dilute hydrochloric acid not only can neutralize the alumina containing alkaline impurities, but also can make the surface of the alumina particles contain the anion of NO_3^- or Cl^-, which is suitable for separating acid compositions because of the property of exchange agent. Granularity of alumina used for column chromatography is 100~160 mesh. Separation effect is poor if granularity is smaller than 100 mesh; If granularity is more than 160 mesh, solvent velocity will be too slow, and then it is easy to cause diffusion of the spectrum band. Generally speaking, the ratio of dosage between samples and alumina is 1 : (20~50); the ratio between the inner diameter of the column and length of the column is 1 : (10~20). Eluting velocity of the solvent should not be too fast. When ml number of liquid flowing from the column every 0.5~1 hour is equal to the number of the adsorbent weight (g), the velocity is suitable.

(3) Activated carbon: It is a nonpolar adsorbent which is widely used in separation. Generally speaking, its pretreatment steps are as follows: rinse with hydrochloric acid, then rinse with ethanol and water, and dry at 80℃ at last. Activated carbon used for chromatography should be granular. Activated carbon powder should be packed in column with diatomite as filter aid lest flow velocity is too slow. Activated carbon is mainly used for separation of water-soluble ingredients, such as amino acids, carbohydrates and some glycosides. The adsorption effect of activated carbon is strongest in aqueous solution and poorest in organic solvent. So eluting power of water is poorest, but eluting power of organic solvent is strongest. For example, When eluting with alcohol-water, the eluting power will increase with progressive increase of ethanol concentration. Its adsorption rule is as follows: The adsorption capacity of aromatic compounds are larger than that of aliphatic compounds. The adsorption capacity of macromolecular compounds is larger than that of small molecules. Using the adsorption difference will separate water soluble aromatic material and aliphatic material, monosaccharide and polysaccharide, amino acid and polypeptide.

1.2 Solvent

Choice of solvent for chromatography impacts separation effect of components. The solvent (single agent or mixed solvents) used in the column chromatography is known as eluent; then the solvent used in thin layer chromatography or paper chromatography is often called developer. Select suitable eluent according to separated materials and adsorbent properties. When polar adsorbent is used for chromatography, select weak polar solvent if separated material is weak polar. On the contrary, select polar solvent if separated material is strong polar. The weak polar eluent should be selected if polar material is separated by weak adsorptivity adsorbent (using diatomite or talcum powder instead of silica gel).

The low polar solvent should be selected to dissolue the sample in order to adsorb separated components. Gradually increasing the polarity of solvent is a very slow process (called gradient elution) which makes the adsorbed compositions in column chromatography eluted one by one. Increasing the polarity too fast (namely the gradient is too big) will not obtain satisfactory separation effect. Eluting power of the solvent sometimes can be represented by dielectric constant (ε) of the solvent. The higher the dielectric constant is, the stronger the eluting power becomes. But the elution order only applies to polar adsorbent, such as silica gel, alumina. In the case of nonpolar adsorbent such as activated carbon, elution order is adverse to the above order. The adsorption force in hydrophilic solvent is greater than that in lipophilic solvent.

1.3 Properties of Separated Materials

Properties of separated materials, adsorbent and solvent are factors of affecting chromatography. When adsorbent and eluent are designated, separation effect is relative to the structure and properties of separated materials. Take polar sorbents as an example, the higher polarity of the compositions, the stronger adsorbility of the sorbents.

Certainly, the whole view of chemical compositions is important. More polar groups can improve the probability of adsorption; less carbon atoms of homologue will also have stronger adsorption. In short, the relationships among properties of separated materials, adsorption intensity of adsorbents and properties of solvents should be taken into account.

Operating method is as follows:

(1) Packing column: Clean and dry a chromatography column, add several glass beads wrapped with gauze in the bottom of the column, and then put a layer of adsorbent cotton. There are two kinds of packing column methods.

①Dry column method: Add adsorbent into the column with a funnel and do not stop during the whole operation; a trickle is formed which flows into column slowly. Also use a rubber mallet to tap the column and make the loading more even. After packing the column well, open the low piston, then add eluent to discharge the air in the column, and keep a certain space on the top of column.

②Wet column method: Add the eluent in the column, open the low piston, and make the eluent flow out slowly. Then add the adsorbent slowly and continuously into the column (or blend adsorbent with appropriate eluent to form liquid suspension and add it in the column). Depending on gravity and the movement of the eluent, the adsorbent generates free sediment in the column. Add the outflow in the column, and keep a certain liquid level. Then add a small piece of filter paper or a few cottons on the top of adsorbent. Keep a certain liquid level according to the sample dosage.

(2) Adding the sample: Dissolve the separated sample in a little eluent which will be packed

in the column and blend into a sample solution, and add it in chromatography column. The sample which is insoluble in the eluent should dissolve in volatile solvent and is added into appropriate adsorbent that is not more than 1/10 of all adsorbent. After mixing them evenly, remove the solvent, add the adsorbent containing the sample to the top of the column (always keep a certain liquid level), and then cover with a layer of adsorbent or glass beads at last.

(3) Elution.

①Atmospheric elution: The top of chromatography column is not sealed and is always connected with the atmosphere. Open the low piston of the column, keep eluent velocity within 1~2 drops per second. Each collected eluent has the same volume. Add the eluent constantly (or use separating funnel to control the speed which is similar with velocity of the column). If single solvent can not separate the sample, mixed solvents (no more than three kinds of solvents) usually can be used by gradient elution. As far as gradient elution is concerned, elution power increases from weak to strong gradually. Check each eluent with thin layer chromatography or paper chromatography; combine the eluents containing the same composition. Further concentration and recrystallization can often get monomer composition. If it is still the mixture of several components which is not easy to form monomer composition crystal, further chromatography separation methods should be sought.

② Vacuum elution: Fix a chromatography ball to the column, connect it with a nitrogen bottle, and elute in 0.5~5 kg/cm^2 pressure. The column used in chromatography is hard glass column. Particle diameter of adsorbent is 200~300 mesh. It can be used in thin layer chromatography of silica gel H, alumina, fine polyamide, activated carbon, etc. Its separation effect is higher than that of classic column chromatography.

2. Distribution Column Chromatography

It is a separation method that ingredients of the mixture have different distribution in two immiscible liquids. It is similar to continuous countercurrent extraction, but the difference is that the former fixes a solvent to a solid material which can only fix solvents and doesn't have adsorption capacity. So it is called support agent or supporter, and the solvent fixed by support agent is called stationary phase. Solvent used for elution is called mobile phase. In the process of elution, mobile phase flows through support agent and contacts with the stationary phase. Different distribution coefficient of sample ingredients in the two phase leads to different downward movement speed. Soluble compositions move rapidly in mobile phase and move slowly in stationary phase, which is the principle of distribution column chromatography.

2.1 Choice of Support Agent

Support agent for distribution column chromatography should have the following features: it is neutral porous powder, no adsorption effect, and insoluble in chromatographic solvent systems; it can adsorb stationary phase (more than 50% support agent), and mobile phase can flow through it freely and do not change its composition. Commonly used agents are as follows:

(1) Hydrated silica gel: Silica gel containing more than 17% water will lose adsorption capacity and can be used as support agent of distribution chromatography. Silica gel which adsorbs half of its own weight water is still in powder form.

(2) Diatomite: Diatomite can adsorb water of its own weight and is still in powder form. It almost has no adsorption, and is packed easily.

(3) Cellulose: It can adsorb water of its own weight and is still in powder form.

2.2　Choice of Stationary Phase

Hydrophilic compositions can be separated by normal-phase distribution chromatography whose stationary phase is composed of water and all kinds of water solution (such as acid, alkali, salt, buffer, methanol, formamide, etc.). Lipophilic compounds can be separated by reverse-phase distribution chromatography whose stationary phase is strong lipophilic solvents, such as silicone oil, liquid paraffin, etc.

2.3　Choice of Mobile Phase

In normal-phase distribution chromatography, insoluble solvents (or has a little solubility) is often used as mobile plase, such as petroleum ether, cyclohexane, benzene, chloroform, acetic acid, n-butanol and isoamyl alcohol, etc. During the elution course, the hydrophily of mobile phase increases from weak to strong. Then in reverse-phase distribution chromatography, water, methanol and ethanol are often used as mobile plase. The hydrophily of mobile phase reduces from strong to weak during the elution course.

2.4　Operation

(1) Packing column: Add the solvent of stationary-phase and support agent in a beaker, mix it evenly, filter with buchner funnel, remove excess stationary phase, then pour it in mobile phase, and stir vigorously to make two phases reach the saturated balance. Then add mobile phase which is saturated by stationary phase in chromatography column, and pack support agent carrying stationary phase in column by wet column method.

(2) Adding the sample: The dosage ratio of the sample to support agent is 1 to 100~1000. The weight of the sample will be less than that of adsorption chromatography. The steps are as follows. Dissolve the sample in a little mobile phase, and add it on the top of the column. If the sample is difficult to dissolve in mobile phase and easily dissolve in stationary phase, it should be dissolved in a little stationary phase and adsorbed by support agent before added in the column. At last, put the treated sample on the top of the column. If the sample is insoluble in two-phase solvents, other appropriate volatile solvents can dissolve it. Then mix it with support agent, remove the solvent, and pack the column after adding stationary phase by the ratio of 1 : (0.5~1) between support agent and stationary phase.

(3) Elution: Elution method is the same with adsorption column chromatography, but mobile phase must be saturated by stationary phase. Otherwise a lot of mobile phase flowing through the support agent can dissolve support agent, which breaks the

chromatographic balance. Then there is only support agent left and is hard to reach the purpose of separation.

3. Ion Exchange Chromatography

Ion exchange chromatography (IEC) is a column chromatography. Its principle is that the different affinities between exchangeable ion in ion exchange agent and the various separated ions in surrounding materials can promote ion exchange and reach the purpose of separation. The method can analyze many ion compounds; it has advantages such as high sensitivity, good repeatability and selectivity, high separating rate etc. It is usually used for the separation of many ionic biological molecules including protein, amino acid, peptide, nucleic acid, etc.

Compounds are usually separated by IEC in a glass tube packed by ion exchange agent which is a kind of synthetic polymer with many ionized groups. According to the different electric charges of these groups, it can be divided into ion exchange agent and cation exchange agent. When the separated ions in solution pass through the ion exchange column, different ions will bind with electric parts competitively on the ion exchange agent. The velocity of passing through the column is decided by the affinity and ionization degree of ion exchange agent, properties and concentration of different competitive ions in solution.

Ion exchange agent is composed of matrix, electric parts and countra-ion, which does not dissolve in water but releases countra-ion. At the same time, it can combine with other ions or ion compounds. Its physical and chemical properties don't change after combining with ions or ionic compounds.

Ion exchange reaction between ion exchange agent and ions or ion compounds in water solution is reversible. Assuming that RA represents cation exchange agent, dissociative cation A^+ in solution will generate reversible exchange reaction with cation B^+: $RA + B^+ \leftrightarrow RB + A^+$. This reaction reaches the balance at high speed and equilibrium shifting according to law of mass action.

Generally speaking, the exchange between ions in solution and ion exchange agent has the following regularities: the stronger electrical property, the more to exchange. For the cationic resin, exchange capacity of ions diluting solution at normal temperature and pressure increases with the enlargement of electrovalence, such as $Na^+ < Ca^{2+} < Al^{3+} < Si^{4+}$. If electrovalence is the same, exchange capacity increases with the enlargement of atomic number, such as $Li^+ < Na^+ < K^+ < Pb^+$. In diluting solution, binding force order of ions in strong alkali resin with negative group is as follows: $CH_3COO^- < F^- < OH^- < HCOO^- < Cl^- < SCN^- < Br^- < CrO_4^{2-} < NO^{2-} < I^- < C_2O_4^{2-} < SO_4^{3-} <$ citrate. Binding force order of ions in weak acid anion exchange resin with negative group is as follows: $F^- < Cl^- < Br^- < I^- < CH_3COO^- < MnO_4^{2-} < PO_4^{3-} < AsO_4^{3-} < NO_3^- <$ tartrate anion $<$ citrate $< CrO_4^{2-} < SO_4^{2-} < OH^-$.

Binding force of zwitterion such as protein, nucleotide and amino acid with ion exchange agent depends on its physical and chemical properties and ion state under special conditions: If pH<pI, it can be adsorbed by cation exchange agent; Conversely, if pH>pI, it can be adsorbed by anion exchange agent; If pI is the same, and pI>pH, the higher pI, the stronger alkaline, the easier the adsorption is by cation exchange agent.

General principles of choosing ion exchange agent are as follows:

(1) Choice of anion or cation exchange agent is decided to charge properties of separated materials. If separated material has positive charge, we should choose cation exchange agent; If separated material has negative charge, we should choose anion exchange agent; If separated material is zwitterion, we should choose exchange agent generally according to charge property in its stable pH range.

(2) Strong cation exchange agent has wide pH range, which is often used for preparation of deionized water or separation of some stable materials in solution with extreme pH.

(3) Ion exchange agent in the state of electroneutrality often has some counterions. Choice of ion exchange agent depends on binding force between ion exchange agent and counterion. In order to improve the exchange capacity, we generally should choose counterion with smaller binding force. Accordingly, strong acid and alkaline ion exchange agent should choose respectively the type H and OH; weak acid and alkaline ion exchange agent should choose respectively the type Na and Cl.

(4) Hydrophobic or hydrophilic matrix of exchange agent has different effects on separated materials. Therefore, It will affect the stability of separated materials and separation effect. Generally, separating macromolecular substances can use exchange agent with hydrophilic matrix whose adsorption and elution are mild to separated materials so that its activity is not easily damaged.

4. Gel Chromatography

Gel chromatography is also called molecular sieve chromatography; its separation principle is that different ingredients is separated according to molecular size when the mixture passes through a gel chromatography column with the mobile phase. It has the following advantages: simple equipment, convenient operation, good repeatability, high sample recovery rate. In addition to the separation or purification of protein, nucleic acid, polysaccharide and hormone, it still can be used to determine the protein's relative molecular mass and for sample desalination and concentration.

Gel is a kind of margarid granular material which has uncharged porous structure with three dimensional space. Each granular subtle structure and mesh diameter keep uniform (like a sieve), which makes small molecule enter the gel mesh and big molecule excluded from the granule. When the mixture of different size molecules is added in the column which is packed by the former gel granule, the separated compositions will flow along with the eluent. Macromolecular materials flow in the gap of gel granules along with the eluent mobile, which makes them have short process and high mobile speed, and makes them eluted from the chromatography column firstly; small molecules can pass through the gel mesh into the internal granules and then spread out, which makes them have long process and low mobile speed, and make them eluted out at last. If two or more molecules with different relative molecular mass can enter the gel mesh, they will still be separated because different exclusion and diffusion of components make them have different path and time in the column, which can reach the purpose of separation (see fig. 2-1).

○ indicates porous filler granule
● indicates macromolecule
• indicates small molecule

Fig. 2-1 Principle of gel chromatography

Commonly used gels are crosslinking sephadex, agarose gel, polyacrylamide gel, etc.

5. Thin Layer Chromatography

Thin layer chromatography (TLC) is a simple, fast and trace chromatography method. Commonly, add adsorbent of column chromatography on a flat surface such as glass to form a thin layer which is called TLC. Its principle is similar to that of column chromatography (see fig. 2-2).

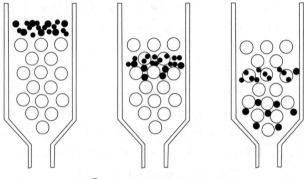

Fig. 2-2 Thin layer chromatography

5.1 Characteristics

TLC and column chromatography are similar.

5.2 Choice of Adsorbent

Adsorbent of TLC is the same with that of column chromatography, but it needs more finer granularity and homogeneous property, generally more than 250 mesh. Adsorbent used for TLC or prefabricated thin layer doesn't require very high activity, and usually Ⅱ or Ⅲ level is suitable. The development distance is decided by granularity. The finer granularity, the shorter development distance (usually less than 10 centimeter). Otherwise, it can cause chromato-diffusion and influence the separation effect.

5.3 Choice of Developer

If adsorbent activity of TLC is a fixed value (such as Ⅱ or Ⅲ level), the separating effect of TLC depends on the choice of developer. According to the different polarities, liposoluble constituents of natural medicine chemical composition can be roughly divided into non-polar, weak polar, moderate polar and strong polar ingredients.

5.4 Special Thin Layer

Separation or check of some special compounds sometimes needs a few special thin layers.

(1) Fluorescent thin layer: When some compounds are colorless, do not show fluorescence under UV lamp and have no proper chromogenic reagent, fluorescent thin layer which is made of adding fluorescent substances in adsorbent can be used for TLC. Place it under UV lamp, check the sample chromatography position according to the principle that thin layer plate shows fluorescence but sample point does not show fluorescence. Commonly used fluorescent substances are usually inorganic substances. One of fluorescent substances shows fluorescence under the 254 nm UV light, such as zinc silicate intensified by manganese. The other shows fluorescence under the 365 nm UV light, such as zinc sulphide and cadmium sulphide intensified by silver.

(2) Complex thin layer: TLC of silver nitrate is used to separate series of compounds with the same number of carbon atoms and unequal C—C double bonds, such as unsaturated alcohol and acid. The main mechanism is that C—C double bond can form complex with silver nitrate, but saturated C—C bond can't form complex. Chromatography of saturated components has highest Rf value because they have the weakest adsorption. Rf value of components containing a C—C bond is higher than that of components containing a C—C double bond, and Rf value of components containing a triple bond is also higher than that of components containing a C—C double bond. In addition, for a double-bond compounds, the *cis*-form is easier to complex with silver nitrate than *trans*-form. Therefore, it can also be used to separate *cis-trans* isomers.

(3) Acid-base thin layer and pH buffering thin layer: In order to change the original acid or alkaline of adsorbent, preparation of thin layer should use dilute acid or dilute alkali to replace water. Because silica gel is weak acid which sometimes has bad effect on the separation of alkaline substances (alkaloids), such as hardly developing or trailing, you can use a dilute alkali solution (0.1~0.5 mol/L NaOH) to prepare alkaline silicon thin layer. For example, when the separation of mucronatine takes silica gel as adsorbent and the developer ratio of chloroform-acetone-methanol is 8 : 2 : 1, Rf value is less than 0.1. When taking alkaline silica gel thin layer as the adsorbent with the same developer, Rf value is 0.4, which indicates mucronatine is an alkaline alkaloid.

5.5 Application

In the study of chemical ingredients of Chinese herbal medicine, TLC is mainly used in the pretreatment, identification and exploring the separation conditions of column chromatography. Choosing the separation conditions of TLC should be based on different kinds of properties and known conditions of compositions. Because it can separate some impurities with high selectivity, TLC makes the pretreatment results more reliable. In addition, standard substances in TLC are very important. If the standard substance and the sample in TLC have the same Rf value and color, it indicates the sample and standard substance are the same component, but it is essential to check the component with chemical reaction and infrared spectrum.

Exploring the conditions of column chromatography with TLC should firstly consider the choice of adsorbent and solvent, and then consider the elution subsequence. TLC still can be used to check the composition and relative content of components in the sample. Appropriate separation conditions in TLC can be used for dry column chromatography. During the course of the separation with TLC, better Rf range is less than 0.85 and more than 0.05. In addition, TLC is also applied to measuring the authenticity of Chinese herbal medicine, quality control and resource survey, controling the process of chemical reaction, checking the by-product of reaction, intermediate analysis, preparation of chemical medicine and examination of impurities, offering clinical examination and biochemical tests, poison analysis and so on.

6. Paper Chromatography

Paper chromatography (PC) is a kind of partition chromatography taken filter paper as support agent. Fiber of filter paper has strong affinity with water and adsorbs about 22% water. 6% to 7% water is combined with cellulose hydroxyl by hychrogen bond. Because the affinity between fiber of filter paper and organic solvents is very weak, stationary phase is fiber of filter paper and water, mobile phase is organic solvent in chromatography. Separation of mixture in PC produces two effects:one is that solute is distributed between the combined water and organic phase through the filter paper (namely liquid-liquid separation); The other is that solute is distributed between the fiber of filter paper and the mobile phase (namely solid-liquid distribution). Obviously the separation of mixture is the result of the effect of this two factors (see fig. 2-3).

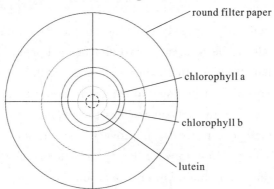

filter paper, Developer:petroleum ether-ether-methanol (30 : 10 : 0.5)

Fig. 2-3　Radialized PC of spinach extract

In practice, one end of filter paper after spotting is immersed in mobile phase which generates penetration and expansion from one end of the filter paper to another end because of capillary action. When mobile phase passes the place of spotting, the solute in the sample is distributed between mobile phase and the water attached to filter paper according to the respective distribution coefficient. A part of the solute leaves origin point along with mobile phase, moves into a non-solute area, and restarts the distribution; the other part of the solute enters the water phase. During the course of constant flow of mobile phase, the solute is distributed constantly and moves in the flow direction of mobile phase (see fig. 2-4). Usually use relative migration rate (Rf) to represent the moving ability:

Rf= (migration length of components from origin) /(migration length of solvents from origin)

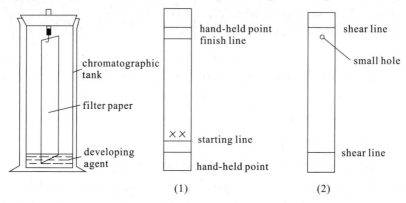

Fig. 2-4 Vertical developing of PC

If filter paper, solvent, temperature and other experimental conditions are constant, Rf value of the material is invariant, and it does not change with the change of moving distance of solvent. The relationship between Rf and distribution coefficient K is as follows: $Rf= 1/(1+\alpha K)$. α is a constant decided by the nature of filter paper. It shows the following laws: the larger K value, the smaller Rf value, which indicates the solute mainly dissolves in stationary phase; Conversely, the smaller Rf value, the larger Rf value, which indicates the solute mainly dissolves in mobile phase. Rf value is an important index of the qualitative analysis.

If the sample that contains more solutes or has similar Rf values in single-phase paper chromatography is not easy to be separated, two-dimensional paper chromatography can be used. The method is that dry the filter paper and rotate it 90° to spread out in another solvent system after it spreads out in a special solvent system in a direction, then take out the filter paper and dry it after the solvent reaches the required distance, and check color reaction at last. This method can greatly improve the separation effect when the solute can't spread out entirely in the first solvent. Paper chromatography is also combined with zone electrophoresis, which can obtain better separation effect and is called the fingerprint spectrum method.

7. Gas Chromatography

Gas chromatography (GC) is a separation method used widely in column chromatography which takes inert gas as mobile phase. The separation principle is based on distribution differences of the sample components in two phases (see fig. 2-5).

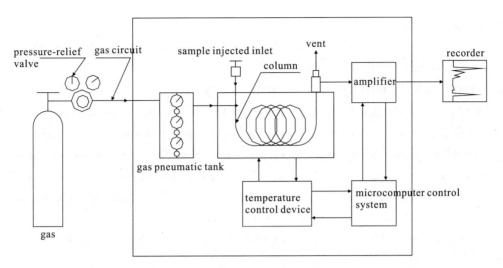

Fig. 2-5 Flow-process diagram of GC

Advantages of GC: High selectivity which can separate isomers and isotopes with similar structure; high sensitivity which can analyze the material with 10^{-11} content and identify the impurity with 1 ppm or even 1 ppb in trace analysis; high separation efficiency.

Although GC can separate complex mixture, its qualitative ability is bad. Usually the sample is qualitatively analyzed according to the retention features, so it is difficult to analyze completely unknown components or components without standard. With the qualitative analysis development of MS, IR and NMR, using the online spectrometry technology at present which is combined with other qualitative or structure analysis method will solve the problem of qualitative difficulty. Gas chromatography-mass spectrometry (GC-MS) is the first commercial hyphenated instrument.

A 50 m long capillary chromatographic column is used in modern gas chromatography (inner diameter of 0.1~0.5 mm). Its stationary phase is usually a kind of crosslinking silicon which adheres to the capillary wall and forms a layer of film. In normal operating temperature, its property is similar to that of liquid membrane and is much more solid. Mobile phase (carrier gas) is usually nitrogen or hydrogen. Different components have different distribution capabilities in carrier gas and silicon so as to achieve the purpose of selective separation. The separation effect of most biological macromolecules is influenced by column temperature, which can be kept constant (isothermal, usually 50~250℃). More often a temperature raising procedure is set (such as a rise from 50℃ to 250℃ at 10℃ per minute). Samples are injected into the top of column through an injection hole containing gas valve. The products of the column are detected by the following methods:

(1) Flame ionization detection (FID): Eluting gas flows through the flame that can make any organic compounds ionized, and it can be detected by a fixed electrode near the top of the flame.

(2) Electron capture detection: Use a kind of radioactive isotope that emits beta rays to detect the trace (pmol) electrophilic complex.

(3) Spectrophotometer detection: Including mass spectrometry (GC-MS) and far

infrared spectroscopy (GC-IR).

(4) Conductance detection: The change of ingredients in eluting gas will cause resistance change of platinum cable.

8. High Performance Liquid Chromatography

High performance liquid chromatography (HPLC) is a multipurpose chromatographic method which can use varieties of stationary phases and mobile phases, and can separate the components according to different molecular sizes, polarities, solubilities or adsorption characteristics in specific types of molecules. HPLC is generally composed of solvent tank, high-pressure pump (single pump, two pumps, four pumps etc.), chromatographic column, sampler (manual or automatic), detector (ultraviolet detector, refractive index detector, fluorescence detector etc.), data processor or chromatographic working station etc. (see fig. 2-6)

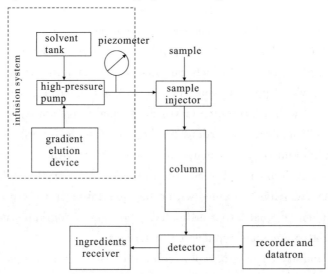

Fig. 2-6　Device composition of HPLC

Its core unit is high-pressure resisting chromatographic columns which are usually made of stainless steel, and all the units and the valves are made of high-pressure resisting materials. Choice of solvent system includes the following conditions. Isocratic elution: only use a solvent (or mixed solvents) in the whole process of analysis; Gradient elution: use the gradient procedure controlled by a microprocessor to change different ratios of the mobile phase.

Because of the advantages of high speed, sensitivity and multi-purpose etc, HPLC has became a method used for small molecular separation. The commonly used method is inverse distribution chromatography. Macromolecular separation (especially protein and nucleic acid) usually needs a "biological fit" system such as Pharmacia FPLC system. This kind of chromatography replaces stainless steel components with titanium, glass or plastic, and uses the lower pressure to avoid the loss of biological activity. It can also be separated by ion exchange chromatography, gel permeation chromatography (GPC) or hydrophobic chromatography.

Chapter 2　Technology of Chromatographic Separation

New Words and Phrases

chromatography [ˌkrəʊməˈtɒgrəfɪ]　*n.* 色谱分析法
adsorbent [ædˈsɔːbənt]　*n.* 吸附剂
silica gel　硅胶
alumina [əˈljuːmɪnə]　*n.* 氧化铝，铝土
magnesium silicate　硅酸镁
polyamide [ˌpɒlɪˈæmaɪd]　*n.* 聚酰胺
adsorption [ædˈsɔːpʃən]　*n.* 吸附(作用)
polysaccharide [ˌpɒlɪˈsækəraɪd]　*n.* 多聚糖
hydrochloric acid　盐酸；氢氯酸
granularity [ˌgrænjuˈlærɪtɪ]　*n.* 粒度
activated carbon　活性碳
aqueous [ˈeɪkwɪəs]　*adj.* 水的，水成的
polypeptide [ˌpɒlɪˈpeptaɪd]　*n.* 多肽
elute [ɪˈljuːt]　*vt.* 洗提
macromolecular [ˌmækrəʊməʊˈlekjʊlə]　*adj.* 大分子的
dielectric constant　介电常数，电容率
diatomaceous earth　硅藻土
talcum powder　滑石粉
pack column　装柱
elution [ɪˈljuːʃən]　*n.* 洗提；洗脱
porous [ˈpɔːrəs]　*adj.* 能穿透的；有毛孔或气孔的
hydrated [ˈhaɪdreɪtɪd]　*adj.* 含水的，与水结合的
diatomite [daɪˈætəmaɪt]　*n.* 硅藻土
cellulose [ˈseljʊˌləʊs]　*n.* 纤维素
anion [ˈænaɪən]　*n.* 阴离子
anionic [ˌænaɪˈɒnɪk]　*adj.* 阴离子的
cation [ˈkætaɪən]　*n.* 阳离子
cationic [ˌkætaɪˈɒnɪk]　*adj.* 阳离子的
tartrate [ˈtɑːtreɪt]　*n.* 酒石酸盐
citrate [ˈsɪtrɪt]　*n.* 柠檬酸盐
zwitterion [ˈtsvɪtəraɪən]　*n.* 两性离子
gel [dʒel]　*n.* 凝胶
sephadex [ˈsefədeks]　*n.* 交联葡聚糖
agarose [ˈɑːgərəʊs]　*n.* 琼脂糖
polyacrylamide [ˌpɒləˈkrɪləmaɪd]　*n.* 聚丙烯酰胺
prefabricated [ˌpriːˈfæbrɪkeɪtɪd]　*adj.* (建筑物、船等)预制构件的
developer [dɪˈveləpə(r)]　*n.* 显色剂，展开剂

fluorescent [fluə'resnt]　*adj.* 荧光的；发荧光的
　　　　　　　　　　　　　n. 荧光灯；日光灯
inorganic [,ınɔː'gænık]　*adj.* 无机的；无活力的
zinc silicate　硅酸锌
manganese ['mæŋgə,niːz]　*n.* 锰
cadmium sulphide　硫化镉
acid-base　酸碱的
alkaline ['ælkəlın]　*adj.* 碱性的，碱的；含碱的
　　　　　　　　　　　　n. 碱度，碱性
mucronatine ['muːkrəneıtaın]　*n.* 猪屎豆碱；短尖碱
migration length　迁移长度
piezometer [,paıə'zɒmıtə]　*n.* 压力计，压强计
hydrophobic [,haıdrəʊ'fəʊbık]　*adj.* 疏水的
permeation [,pəːmı'eıʃən]　*n.* 渗入，透过
sampler ['sæmplə]　*n.* 采样器；样板
spectrophotometer [,spektrəʊfə'tɒmıtə]　*n.* 分光光度计
platinum ['plætnəm]　*n.* 铂
electrophilic [ı,lektrəʊ'fılık]　*adj.* 亲电子的
radioactive isotope　放射性同位素
infrared ['ınfrə'red]　*adj.* 红外线的
　　　　　　　　　　　　n. 红外线
conductance [kən'dʌktəns]　*n.* 电导系数
isocratic elution　等度洗脱
gradient elution　梯度洗脱

Experiment 1　Extraction and Isolation of Phenolic Compounds from *Ilex purpurea* Hassk

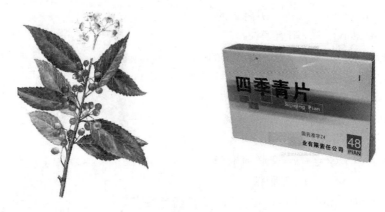

Fig. 2-7　Plant and preparation of *Ilex purpurea* Hassk

1. Experimental Purpose

(1) Master the method and principle of atmospheric pressure column chromatography.

(2) Understand the application of atmospheric pressure column chromatography in the separation of natural chemical compositions.

2. Experimental Principle

Protocatechuic aldehyde (3,4-dihydroxybenzaldehyde) is the main antianginal active component in purpleflower holly leaves (see fig. 2-7), which has the effect of expanding coronary artery and increasing coronary blood flow. Its melting point is 153~154℃, and it is very soluble in ethanol, acetone, ethyl acetate, ether and hot water, soluble in cold water, and insoluble in benzene and chloroform. It is hygroscopic and easily oxidized to change color in water.

Protocatechuic acid (3,4-dihydroxybenzoic acid) exists in purple flower holly leaves or other plants. It is a white to brown crystalline powder, its color varies in the air, and its melting point is 198~200℃. It is soluble in water, ethanol, ether, acetone and ethyl acetate, and hardly soluble in benzene and chloroform. It has antibacterial effect and has different degrees of inhibitory effect on *Pseudomonas aeruginosa*, *Escherichia coli*, *Salmonella Typhi*, *Dysentery bacilli*, Alcaligenes, *Bacillus subtilis* and *Staphylococcus aureus* in *vitro* tests. It also has expectorant and anti-asthmatic effect. It is used for the treatment of chronic bronchitis in clinic.

Protocatechuic acid   Protocatechuic aldehyde   2,4-Dinitrophenylhydrazine

2,4-dinitrophenylhydrazine is red crystalline powder that is slightly soluble in water, ethanol, and soluble in acid. Its melting point is 197~198℃. It is used in explosive manufacture, or used as a chemical reagent to identify aldehydes and ketones whose integrated substance is 2,4-dinitrophenylhydrazone that produces yellow or red crystals easily seen by human eyes. The experiment is done as the test method for aldehyde; its reaction process is as follows:

If the orange spots are detected in the eluent, use ammoniacal silver nitrate reagent to detect protocatechuic acid, which makes the silver ions in the solution of ammonia complex reduced into metallic silver by pyrocatechol hydroxyl group of protocatechuic acid ($Ag^+ \rightarrow Ag\downarrow$) and black spots appear. It can also be heated to promote reaction.

3. Experimental Procedure

(1) Take 20 g purple flower holly leaves, add 70% ethanol to reflux extraction for 1 h

and 0.5 h one after another, purify it by NKA-8 macroporous resin with the ratio of 1∶0.5 (resin∶crude drug), elute with 70% ethanol, and evaporate the eluent to dryness at low temperature.

(2) Take 6 g silica gel (pass 100 to 160 mesh, activity grade V) and pack column by dry column method.

(3) Take 5 mg sample to dissolve in 5 ml eluent by heating. After filtering, add the filtrate to the top of the column with a pipette.

(4) Eluent: petroleum ether-ethyl acetate (4∶6).

(5) Collecting eluent: 10 ml per fraction (about 10 fractions) with a small triangular flask.

(6) Detection: Take a small silicone CMC-Na plate, draw small lattices as the table 2-4, drop the eluent on the lattice with a capillary, and then drop the detection reagent of 2,4-dinitrophenylhydrazine and ammoniacal silver nitrate on corresponding sample points. Observe the results, and drop detection reagent only on another group of lattices as blank contrast.

Tab. 2-4 Thin-layer blocks of CMC-Na in the color reaction of purple flower holly leaves

blank reagent											
sample + reagents											
blank reagent											
sample + reagents											

From the reaction results we can determine which fraction contains protocatechuic aldehyde, which fraction contains protocatechuic acid, or blank fraction. The fractions are respectively concentrated and identified by TLC. Their conditions are as follows: Silica gel CMC-Na thin layer plate; Developer: chloroform-acetone-methanol-acetic acid (7∶2∶0.5∶0.5); Chromogenic reagent: 2% ferric chloride of ethanol solution.

Merge the same fractions, recover the eluent to small volume at normal pressure, recrystallize filter cake with ethanol, and get the crystal after filtering. Take a little crystal to dissolve in ethanol, identify it by TLC and observe whether it is the monomer. If it is the monomer, you can measure its melting point for preliminary identification and determine IR spectrum contrast to standard map if it is known compounds.

Record each stream bit of reaction and TLC results (draw map), write income monomer's melting point data. Preliminarily judge what kind of compound is the separated monomer.

4. Notice

4.1 Ammoniacal Silver Nitrate Reagent (Tollens Reagent)

Add 2 ml 5% silver nitrate solution to a clean test tube, drop one drop of 10% sodium hydroxide solution. Then add 20% aqueous ammonia and shake it for a while until the precipitate of silver oxide dissolves completely. In order to get the sensitive reagent, ammonia should not be excessive.

This reagent should be prepared before application because long preservation will decompose it and produce a precipitate with highly explosive property.

The test solution is dropped on the filter paper, then you can drop the fresh prepared reagent, and heat it at 100℃ for 5 to 10 min. If dark brown appears, we can infer that the solution contains aldehyde group of reducing sugar.

4.2　2,4-Dinitrophenylhydrazine Reagent

Preserve 0.2% of 2,4-dinitrophenylhydrazine in 2 mol/L hydrochloric acid solution or 0.1% of 2,4-dinitrophenylhydrazine in 2 mol/L hydrochloric acid ethanol solution.

5. Experimental Supplies and Arrangement of Class Hour

Experimental supplies: chromatography column, small conical flask, suction tube, pipette tube, small funnel, glass rod, NKA-8 macroporous resin, chloroform, acetone, methanol, acetic acid, ethanol, ammonia, dinitrophenylhydrazine, hydrochloric acid, sodium hydroxide, petroleum ether, ethylacetate, ferric chloride, silica gel etc.

Arrangement of class hour: to be completed within 6 class hours.

6. Questions

(1) Why do we choose the acid condition when checking the carbonyl group with 2,4-dinitrophenylhydrazine?

(2) What are the main factors of affecting Rf value of the sample during the course of TLC?

New Words and Phrases

phenolic [fɪˈnɒlɪk]　*adj.* 苯酚的
coronary [ˈkɒrəˌnerɪ]　*n.* 冠状动脉
artery [ˈɑːtərɪ]　*n.* 动脉, 要道
oxidize [ˈɒksɪˌdaɪz]　*vt.* 使氧化; 使生锈
inhibitory [ɪnˈhɪbɪtərɪ]　*adj.* 禁止的, 抑制的
Pseudomonas aeruginosa　铜绿假单胞杆菌
Escherichia coli　大肠杆菌
Salmonella Typhi　伤寒沙门氏杆菌
Dysentery bacilli　痢疾杆菌
alcaligenes [ælkəˈlɪdʒəniːz]　*n.* 产碱杆菌属
Bacillus subtilis　枯草芽孢杆菌
Staphylococcus aureus　金黄色酿脓葡萄球菌
vitro [ˈvɪtro]　（活）体外, 试管内
expectorant [eksˈpektərənt]　*n.* 祛痰剂
　　　　　　　　　　　　　　adj. 化痰的
asthmatic [æzˈmætɪk]　*adj.* 气喘的, 患气喘的
　　　　　　　　　　　　　n. 气喘患者, 哮喘患者
bronchitis [brɒnˈkaɪtɪs]　*n.* 支气管炎
protocatechuic aldehyde　乙醛

ferric chloride 三氯化铁
chromogenic reagent 显色试剂
filter cake 滤饼,滤后沉淀
lattice ['lætɪs] *n.* 格子框架
              vt. 把……制成格子状
aldehydes ['ældɪhaɪdz] *n.* 醛
dinitrophenyl [daɪnaɪtrəʊ'fenɪl] *n.* 二硝基苯基
hydrazone ['haɪdrəzəʊn] *n.* 腙
dinitrophenylhydrazine [daɪnaɪtrəʊfenɪlhaɪdreɪ'zɪ] *n.* 二硝基苯肼

Experiment 2 Isolation of Pigments from Red Pepper

1. Experimental Purpose

Master the theory and method of separation and extraction of natural products by TLC and column chromatography.

2. Experimental Principle

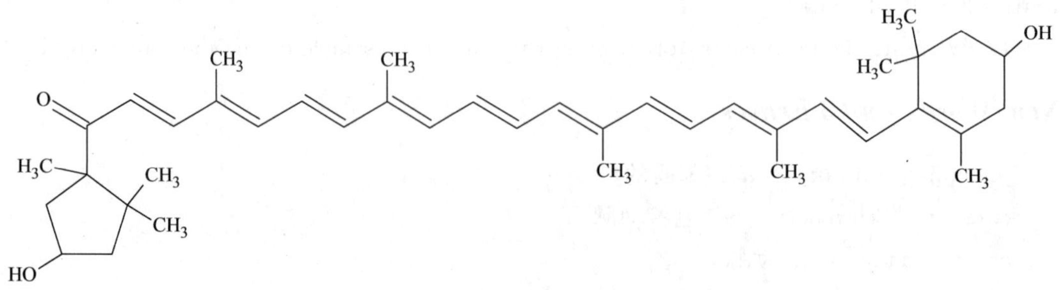

Capsanthin

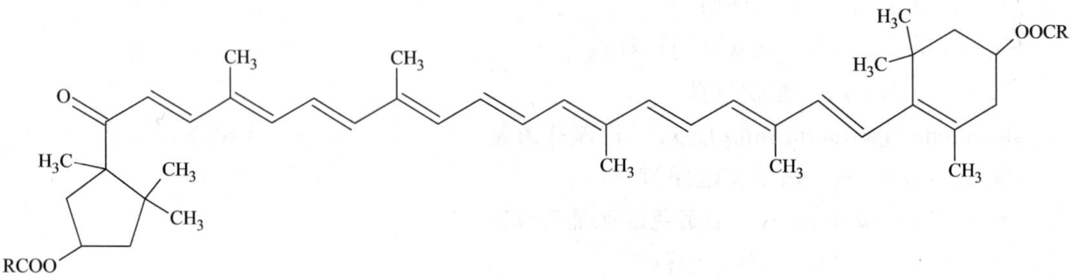

Capsanthin fatty acid ester

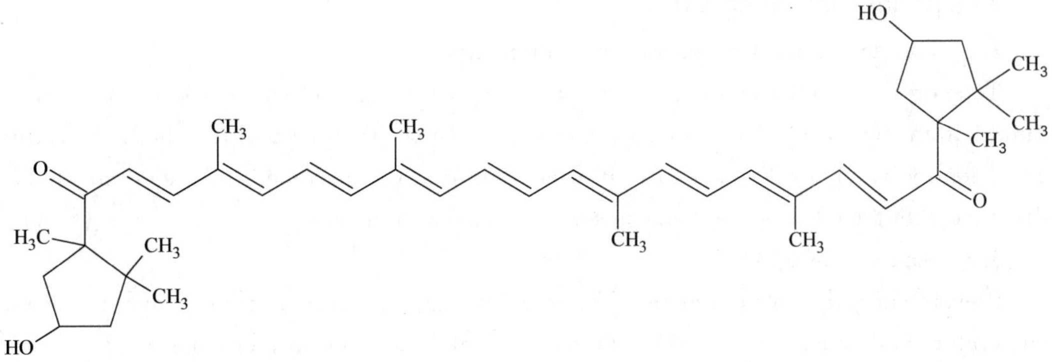

Capsorubin

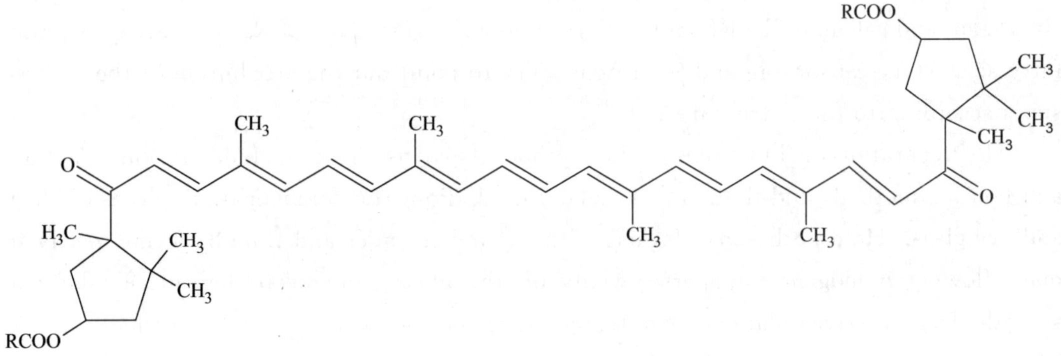

Capsorubin fatty acid ester

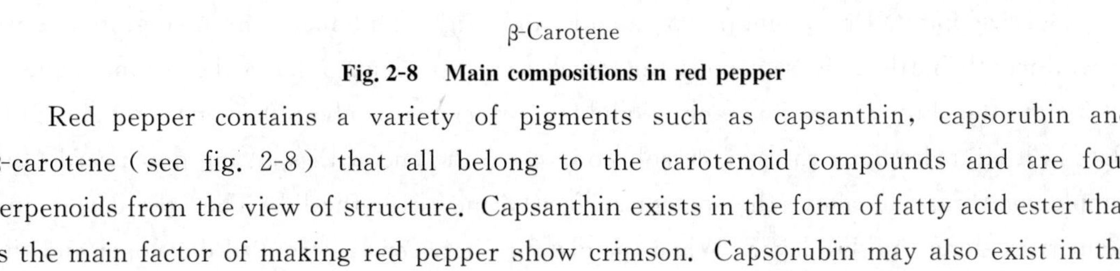

β-Carotene

Fig. 2-8　Main compositions in red pepper

Red pepper contains a variety of pigments such as capsanthin, capsorubin and β-carotene (see fig. 2-8) that all belong to the carotenoid compounds and are four terpenoids from the view of structure. Capsanthin exists in the form of fatty acid ester that is the main factor of making red pepper show crimson. Capsorubin may also exist in the form of fatty acid ester.

In the experiment, we extract the pigments from red pepper with dichloromethane as the solvent, concentrate and analyze it by TLC, then isolate the red pigments with column chromatography, and determinate their preliminary structures with infrared spectroscopy.

3. Experimental Procedure

3.1 Extraction and Concentration of Pigments

Take dry red pepper and cut into pieces, weigh 1 g cracked pepper and put in a 50 ml round bottom flask, add 10 ml dichloromethane and two or three zeolites, bath the reflux extraction by water for 20 min, filter it after cooling to room temperature, concentrate the filtrate to about 1 ml, and get the concentrated mixed pigments.

3.2 Analysis of TLC

Prepare six thin layer plates of silica gel-CMC-Na (2.5 cm×7.5 cm), dry it at room temperature and activate it at 105℃, take a plate and drop the former concentrated mixed pigments with a flat capillary, develop it with the mixture of one volume of petroleum ether (30~60℃) and three volumes of dichloromethane as developer, record each spot size, color and calculate the Rf value. Three known largest spots of Rf value are capsanthin fatty acid ester, capsorubin and β-carotene. Try to point out the attribution of these three spots according to their structures.

(1) Preparation of TLC plate: The method of paving plates includes rubbing method and pouring method, and the latter is usually used. Pour the homogenate to pieces of clean and dry glass. Hold both ends of glass with the index finger and thumb, shake gently to make flowing homogenate disperse evenly on the glass, and keep the surface flat and smooth. Dry the paved plate at room temperature and then bake it at 105℃ for half an hour in an oven, cool and preserve it in a dryer.

(2) Droping the sample: Take a TLC plate, and draw a line gently used for dropping the sample solution on the place of 1.0 cm from the edge with a soft pencil. Drop the obtained crude red pigment in a small conical flask, and then add 5 to 10 drops of methylene chloride to dissolve it (or the above filtrate). Select the capillary with flush mouth pipe to drop the sample solution, and touch gently the dropping place. If a drop is not enough, you can redo it several times after the sample solvent evaporates, but you should make sure that the spreading diameter of the sample is not more than 2 mm.

(3) Developing: Developing is operated in an airtight container (chromatographic tank or wild-mouth bottle). Firstly pour the developer (petroleum ether : dichloromethane = 1 : 3) into the chromatographic tank (liquid layer thickness is about 0.5 cm). Put the TLC plate in it after dropping the sample solution, place the end with spotting downward (the sample point must be above the solvent surface), and cover the lid. Then the developing agent rises along the thin layer. When the distance between the front of developer and the top of the TLC plate is about 1 cm, remove the plate, mark the leading edge of developer with a pencil fastly, and then dry it in a well-ventilated place or with a hair drier.

(4) Calculation of the Rf: The ratio the distance of compound moving in the TLC plate to the distance of developer moving forward is called Rf value.

3.3 Column Chromatography

As shown in fig. 2-9, choose the columns with internal diameter of 1 cm and long of 20 cm, and add silica gel 10 g (passing the sieve of 100 to 200 mesh) and dichloromethane to pack column. Drop the concentrated mixed pigments with a dropper to the top of the column, carefully rinse the inner wall and use the mixture of petroleum ether (30~60℃)-dichloromethane (3∶8) to elute it, and receive the first three ribbons that flow out of the column with different receiving bottles. Stop elution when the third ribbon flows completely from the colum.

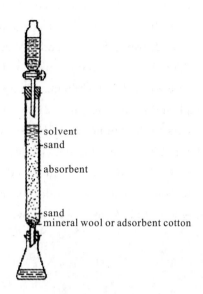

Fig. 2-9 Column chromatography device

(1) Packing column: Wet column method and dry column method can also be used in the experiment. If choosing dry column method, pack 8 g silica gel (100~200 mesh) to a dropper with a piston or column chromatography that contains 10 ml dichloromethane, expel air bubbles, and add a little clean sand (about 3 mg). Then unscrew the piston to make some dichloromethane flow out and its liquid level is slightly higher than the upper layer of the sand. If choosing wet column method, add 8 g silica gel in methylene chloride and stir into a paste, pour it slowly into a column, and beat the lower part of the column with a rubber stopper gently to make the packing tight. When the packing reaches 3/4 height of the column, add quartz sand with the thickness of 0.5 cm. The whole operation should keep the liquid level not lower than the upper layer of sand.

(2) Adding sample: When the solvent level reaches the upper surface of quartz sand, you can immediately add 1 ml of the sample solution along the column wall, and wash away the colored substances on the column wall.

(3) Elution: Elute the pigment (pigmented ring will appear in column chromatography) with dichloromethane. β-carotene moves down firstly due to its small polarity. Chlorophyll, lutein, and capsanthin that have high polarity will be kept in the upper end of the column and form different ribbons. When the first ribbon flows out of the column, change another flask and continue to elute until the eluent is colorless. Collect the eluate of 2 ml per fraction. After eluting the red pigment, you can stop elution or continue to elute the second component, namely yellow pigment, and then merge the same solution and evaporate for dryness.

3.4 Detection of Column Efficiency and Ribbon

Take three silica gel thin layer plates, mark the starting line, and drop the sample with different flat capillaries. Drop two kinds of spots in each plate: one is the mixed pigment concentrate, and the other is the first, second or third ribbon respectively. Still use the petroleum ether and dichloromethane (1 : 3) as developer. Compare the Rf value of each ribbon, and infer what compound each ribbon is.

3.5 Infrared Spectra and UV Adsorption of the Red Pigments

Concentrate the red pigment and evaporate until it's dry thoroughly and draw infrared spectra using pellet technigue. Compare with the spectrum of standard substance, and try to explain why the region of 3100~3600 cm^{-1} has no adsorption peak. In addition, use the pigments to determine the UV spectrum and assure that the λ_{max} has two distinct adsorption peaks in 470nm and 447nm. IR data indicates that the component contains the group of methyl (2925 cm^{-1}、2850 cm^{-1} and 1462 cm^{-1}), carbonyl (1747 cm^{-1}), carbon-carbon double bond (3020 cm^{-1} and 1700 cm^{-1}), *cis*-structure (710 cm^{-1}) and carbon-oxygen single bond (1162 cm^{-1}), as shown in fig. 2-10 and fig. 2-11.

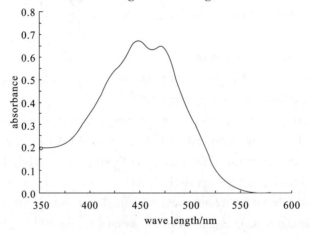

Fig. 2-10 UV-visible spectra map of capsanthin

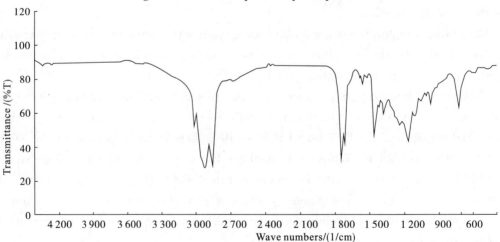

Fig. 2-11 IR spectra map of capsanthin

4. Notice

(1) The concentration of the sample solution should be appropriate because too high concentration could easily cause the tailing of spots, and too low concentration causes the

diffusion of spots owing to large volume. The distance between the two points should be about 1 cm, so the spot diameter of 2 mm is appropriate.

(2) The developer of TLC is relative to the polarity, solubility and adsorbent activity of the sample. The higher the polarity of developer, the greater its eluting ability and the larger its Rf value.

(3) The ratio of diameter to height of column is 1 : (5~10). Anhydrous anaerobic column commonly uses generally alumina as stationary phase because a large number of exposed hydroxyl groups in silica gel make the sample decomposed easily especially for metal organic compounds and phosphorus compounds.

(4) Smearing the lubricant on the piston below the column will pollute the product.

(5) There is no difference between dry packing column and wet packing column as long as we can pack it tightly. In most cases, some small air bubbles have little influence on the separation effect. But the cracking of stationary phase in column will affect seriously the separation, even make the experiment invalid.

5. Experimental Supplies and Arrangement of Class Hours

Experimental supplies: chromatography column, small conical flask, suction tube, pipette tube, small funnel, glass rod, red pepper, round bottom flask, dichloromethane, thin layer plate, petroleum ether, chromatographic tank, dropper, silica gel, infrared spectrophotometer, ultraviolet spectrophotometer etc.

Arrangement of class hours: to be completed within 6 class hours.

6. Questions

(1) Why do we control the temperature below 50℃ when extracting the crude red pigment in a water bath?

(2) Why do we stuff the adsorbent cotton at the bottom of column when packing column? What issues should we pay attention to?

New Words and Phrases

red pepper 红辣椒

capsanthin [kæpˈsænθɪn] *n.* 辣椒红

capsorubin [ˈkæpsəˌrubɪn] *n.* 辣椒玉红素

carotene [ˈkærətiːn] *n.* 胡萝卜素

carotenoid [kəˈrɒtənɔɪd] *n.* 类胡萝卜素

terpene [ˈtɜːpiːn] *n.* 萜烯,萜(烃)

ester [ˈestə] *n.* 酯

pepper [ˈpepə] *n.* 胡椒;辣椒

homogenate [həˈmɒdʒɪneɪt] *n.* 均匀混合物,(组织)匀浆

methylene chloride 二氯甲烷

hair drier 吹风机

dichloromethane [daɪkləː'rəmeθeɪn]   n. 二氯甲烷
unscrew [ʌn'skruː]   vt. 旋开，松开
stir [stɜː]   vt. & vi. （使）移动；搅拌
chlorophyll ['klɔːrəfɪl]   n. 叶绿素
lutein ['luːtɪən]   n. 叶黄素
carbonyl ['kɑːbənɪl]   n. 羰基
methyl ['meθɪl]   n. 甲基

Experiment 3   Extraction and Isolation of Chlorophyll in the Green Leaves

1. Experimental Purpose

Master the principle and method of extracting and separating chlorophyll by column chromatography.

2. Experimental Principle

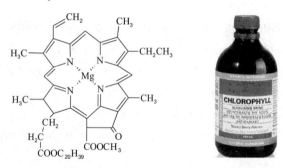

Fig. 2-12   Chlorophyll's structure and preparation

Chlorophyll (see fig. 2-12) exists in green plant cells. Chlorophyll usually integrates with protein and turns into a chloroplast in the plant cell, which is free when the plant cell dies. The pigments in green leaves include chlorophyll and carotenoid. The content of the former is four times of that of the latter, So the leaves are often green. According to modern studies, chlorophyll has active effects of sanguification, providing vitamins, detoxification and disease resistance, etc.

In this experiment, column chromatography is used to separate chlorophyll, carotene and lutein in the green leaves. Pigments in green leaves are fat-soluble, which are soluble in acetone, ethanol, ether, chloroform, petroleum ether and other solvents that can be used as extraction solvent. The free chlorophyll is very unstable and is sensitive to light and heat. It can be hydrolyzed into bright green chlorophyllin salts, phytol and methanol in dilute alkali solution. Under acidic conditions, Magnesium ions in the porphyrin ring can be replaced by hydrogen ions and generate dark green or green-brown pheophytin.

3. Experimental Procedure

3.1   Extraction of Pigments in Green Leaves

Weigh 1~2 g green leafy vegetables, place them in a mortar, add silica and calcium carbonate and grind into powder, then add 10 ml petroleum ether-acetone (1 : 1 in volume), continue to grind into paste, stand a while until forming precipitation, and suck the supernatant into a separatory funnel with a sucker. Add 10 ml petroleum ether (30～60℃), and then add 30 ml saturated sodium chloride solution, shake evenly until the solution is layered, and separate the brine layer. Use 30 ml saturated salt water to wash for one time, separate the brine layer again, and shift the pigment extract of green leaves to a conical flask. Add a little anhydrous sodium sulfate and dry 15 minutes, pour the filtrate into a evaporating dish, evaporate the solvent to dryness in a water bath, dissolve it with 2～3 ml petroleum ether (60～90℃), and then we can get the concentrated extract of pigments in green leaves.

3.2 Column Chromatography of Pigments in Green Leaves

Pave a layer of cotton wool at the bottom of a clean column with a funnel on its top, keep the alumina evenly flow into the column through the funnel, and don't stop operation during the course of adding the alumina. Tap on the glass tube gently to make the packing evenly, cover the surface of the alumina with a layer of anhydrous sodium sulfate after finishing the loading.

Suck the extract into the column, use petroleum ether and acetone (9 : 1 in volume) to elute the carotenoids when the yellow ribbon reaches the 1/4 height of the column, wash and then elute the chlorophyll with acetone and collect it in a beaker.

3.3 Properties of Chlorophyll

(1) Reacting with acid: Take 2～3 ml acetone extract and 5 drops of dilute hydrochloric acid, and observe the phenomenon after oscillating.

(2) Reacting with alkali: Take 2～3 ml acetone extract and 5 drops of dilute alkali solution, and observe the phenomenon after oscillating.

4. Notice

(1) The brine has an effect on extraction of substances which are soluble in water and acetone, but insoluble in petroleum ether. Adding salts can avoid the emulsification of petroleum ether.

(2) Ratio of diameter to height of the chromatographic column is usually 1 : (20～30).

(3) Separating 1 g sample needs 20～50 g aluminum oxide whose height is generally 3/4 height of a glass column.

5. Experimental Supplies and Arrangement of Class Hours

Experimental supplies: green leafy vegetables, glass powder (place broken glass in a iron mortar and grind into powder, pass through the sieve of 20 mesh, remove the irons with concentrated hydrochloric acid, then neutralize the acid with sodium hydroxide, and finally rinse to neutral with distilled water and dry it in an oven), petroleum ether (30～60℃), petroleum ether (60～90℃), alumina (neutral, 100～200 mesh), anhydrous sodium sulfate, acetone, saturated sodium chloride solution, 5 mol/L hydrochloric acid, 0.5 mol/L sodium hydroxide, mortar, separating funnel, evaporating dish, chromatography column, conical flask, and funnel.

Arrangement of class hours: to be completed within 6 class hours.

6. Questions

(1) Why choose the fresh green leaves?

(2) What's the purpose of adding the silica and calcium carbonate when grinding the leaves?

New Words and Phrases

chloroplast ['klɔːrəʊplæst] *n.* 叶绿体

carotenoid [kə'rɒtənɔɪd] *n.* 类胡萝卜素

hydrolyze ['haɪdrəlaɪz] *vi.* 水解

porphyrin ['pɔːfərɪn] *n.* 卟啉

pheophytin [ˌfiːə'faɪtɪn] *n.* 脱镁叶绿素

mortar ['mɔːtə] *n.* 研钵

sodium chloride 氯化钠

brine [braɪn] *n.* 盐水;海水

anhydrous [æn'haɪdrəs] *adj.* 无水的(尤指结晶水)

alkali ['ælkəˌlaɪ] *n.* 碱

tap [tæp] *vt.* 轻敲;轻打

phytol ['faɪtɒl] *n.* 叶绿醇

silica ['sɪlɪkə] *n.* 硅石,二氧化硅

calcium carbonate 碳酸钙

magnesium [mæg'niːziəm] *n.* 镁(金属元素)

leafy ['liːfiː] *adj.* 多叶的

sieve [sɪv] *n.* 筛子;滤网

concentrated hydrochloric acid 浓盐酸

neutralize ['njuːtrəlaɪz] *vi.* 中和

saturate ['sætʃəreɪt] *vt.* 浸透,使饱和

sodium hydroxide 氢氧化钠

evaporating dish 蒸发皿

Chapter 3
Technology of Structural Identification

1. Introduction

In the last half of the 20th century, spectroscopy has become a basic course of organic structural chemistry. Ultraviolet (UV) spectrum developed in the 1930s and infrared (IR) spectrum developed in the 1940s provide effective methods for chromophore and functional group of organic compounds. Researchers can use thimbleful sample and nondestructive experiments to get the structural information. In the 1950s, the development of mass spectrometry (MS) has a revolutionary impact on the organic structural chemistry. The MS testing can provide the molecular formula and structural information of the compound by cracking.

Nuclear magnetic resonance (NMR) has largest influence on the organic structural chemistry, and the influence is rapid and shocking. In recent 50 years, the development of organic spectrum especially NMR technology improves the method of structural identification of natural products. Spectrum technology becomes the most effective and reliable method of studying molecular internal secrets.

20 years ago, both 2D NMR technology such as HMBC (Heteronuclear Multiple-Bond Correlation), COSY (Correlation Spectroscopy), and pulse sequence newly developed by spectroscopist are rarely high and new technologies. But in recent years, these technologies applied on NMR spectrum on sale have become routine methods. As we know, morphine was separated by Serturner in 1806. But its structure was determined in 1952, and the process spends 150 years. Another example is brucine (or strychnine) whose structure identification spends more than half a century (1891~1946) and requires a number of painstaking effort of several generations of chemists. Because the main method of identifying the structure at that time is wet chemistry.

Strictly speaking, UV and IR belong to the spectrum, while MS is a kind of mass spectrum of the particle instead of spectrum, and NMR belongs to the spectrum. In the early years, they are called the four spectra.

1.1 Background Information of the Sample Structure

Most components in natural medicine are known so that structure identification is fast and easy relatively as long as there are enough literatures. A small number of new compounds are unknown compounds, and these compounds only have new substituent groups or different stereoscopic structures.

(1) Sample source and reference: Reference relates to sample source such as kingdom, division, class, order, family, genus and species of the plant. Spectrum data of known compounds is a necessary reference for studying the structure, but literature time, used instrument and the methodology of the structure must be taken into account.

(2) Properties of sample compounds: Properties of sample compounds include liquid, solid, crystalline morphology, melting point, boiling point, color, fluorescence, features of column chromatography, TLC features, paper chromatography features, HPLC features, color reaction, optical activity, solubility, purity, etc. Combine with reference background to infer the structure type of the sample is an important method for getting the skeleton information of the sample.

(3) Skeleton Information of the Sample: Skeleton information of the sample can be gotten from the above data and experimental results, which helps researchers to understand the process of structural identification quickly. If you don't get the skeleton information, more spectrum data should be used to obtain the information.

1.2 Chemical Method of the Structural Identification (Wet Chemistry)

In view of the fact that spectrum technology has improved the structural identification method of natural products, chemical method will play a secondary role in structural identification. But in many cases, chemical transformation and derivation are very beneficial and even necessary for the structural modification, synthesis and other fields.

1.3 Ultraviolet and Infrared Spectrometry

(1) UV/Vis spectrum: UV/Vis spectrum method is simple and it supplies less structure information such as the information of conjugated chromophore and auxochrome. Generally speaking, it is difficult to infer reliable molecular skeleton with UV/Vis spectrum. There is a big difference in UV absorption peaks even if carbon skeletons are the same when conjugated systen is interrupted. Even their molecular weights have great difference, they will have almost the same UV spectral lines so long as the two compounds have the same chromophore.

(2) Infrared spectroscopy (IR): In the 1950s－1970s, IR was the most important method of structural identification of organic compounds such as flavones, anthraquinones, triterpenoids and steroids, but now it is important to identify functional groups especially for carbonyl, carboxylic acid or acid anhydride, the size of the carbonyl group ring, group identification of CN, NCO, NCS and sulphone, sulfoxide, sulfo-group, nitro-group, hydroxyl, etc. A point worth emphasizing is that the fingerprint function of IR is convenient and reliable to identify compound on the premise of having standard spectra and reference substance.

Most important and most commonly used infrared spectroscopy in structural identification is FT-IR and grating IR. Especially the early standard spectra is basically grating IR.

The followings should be paid attention to for the IR spectrum analysis: peak position, peak profile, peak intensity and determination conditions. Peak position is the adsorption frequency, which can be expressed with cm^{-1}; peak profile is the shape of the peak, which is probably fat, thin, blunt or sharp; peak intensity is generally classified into strong (s), moderate (m) and weak (w); determination conditions mainly include liquid membrane and KBr pellet.

1.4 Mass Spectrometry (MS)

MS is an important method of structural identification, which has higher sensitivity than that of NMR and IR. MS can be used for the determination of molecular weight or molecular formula. The commonly used methods of structural determination are divided into the following ways according to different ionization mode.

(1) Electron impact mass spectra (EIMS) and high resolution electron impact mass spectra (HREIMS): EIMS and HREIMS are the most widely used MS methods used for structural identification, which can determine molecular weight, molecular formula, the elemental composition of debris ions and molecular fragmentation pattern. But it is difficult for EIMS to identify the components that have no or very weak molecular ion peak, such as thermal unstable compounds, large polarity compounds, and high molecular weight compounds.

(2) Fast atom bombardment (FAB) and high resolution fast atom bombardment (HRFAB): FAB and HRFAB are suitable for determination of extremely low volatile and strong polar organic compounds, thermal unstable compounds, and high molecular weight compounds.

(3) Field desorption (FD): M peak and MH peak usually exist in FD spectra, which generally applies in low molecular weight and strong polar compounds.

(4) Chemical ionization (CI): CI and EI have the same heat source which is only suitable for analysis of the samples that are volatile or difficult to decompose by heating. But it usually gets molecular weight information if molecular ion peak can not be observed in EIMS.

(5) Electrospray ionization (ESI): ESI is suitable for analysis of peptide, protein, nucleic acid, glycoprotein etc.

(6) Atmospheric pressure ionization (APCI): APCI is suitable for qualitative analysis of small molecular compounds and pharmacokinetic studies.

(7) Matrix assisted laser desorption ionization (MALDI): MALDI is used for analysis of peptide and protein, glycoprotein, DNA fragments, polysaccharide, etc.

EIMS can provide the most information in different ionization sources. If you want to use the least sample to get the most structural information, EIMS is taken into account firstly. In most cases, EIMS can not only determine molecular weight and molecular formula, but also get abundant information of fragmental debris whose elemental composition can be measured by HREIMS. If the sample has stable molecular skeleton and clear fragmentation regularity, using EIMS to infer the molecular structure is often very effective.

(8) Gas chromatography-mass spectrometry (GC-MS): GC-MS has become one of the

powerful means of structural identification for natural organic components. Almost all the components separated by GC can get satisfactory map by GC-MS, even if the sample content is only ng (10^{-9}).

(9) Liquid chromatography-mass spectrometry (LC-MS, HPLC-MS): LC-MS is very suitable for polar molecular separation and structural identification. It is indispensable analytical instrument that analyzes compounds with large molecular weight or strong polarity.

1.5 Nuclear Magnetic Resonance (NMR)

(1) NMR solvent: Determination of NMR spectra usually uses deuterium reagent. Chemical shift of these solvents and the water can be easily checked in common textbooks.

(2) One dimensional nuclear magnetic resonance (1D-NMR): The most common 1D-NMR is ^{1}H NMR, ^{13}C NMR, DEPT and NOE subtractive spectroscopy.

①Recognition method of active hydrogen: In ^{1}H NMR spectra, active hydrogen signal changes frequently, such as sharp peak, wide peak, some peak integral area decreased obviously, overlapping peak, some peak almost consistented with baseline etc. The reasons for the above phenomenon are as follows: Internal cause has to do with molecular structure, and external cause relates to sample concentration, temperature, solvent, and the water content in the sample. Several methods of identifying the hydrogen signal are as follows:

Ⅰ. Heavy water exchange: Heavy water exchange is the most classic and common method of discriminating the hydrogen signal.

Ⅱ. Identifying active hydrogen signal by H-C COSY spectra: Because active hydrogen does not usually connect with carbon directly, the proton signal should be the active hydrogen peak.

Ⅲ. Identifying active hydrogen by variable-temperature experiment: When active hydrogen signal overlaps other signals, heating experiment will make active hydrogen signal move toward high field. Comparing the map determined under normal temperature with the map determined at high temperature, we can identify active hydrogen signal.

②Water peak suppression: Using heavy water or dilute solution to determinate ^{1}H NMR will produce strong solvent signal, which disturbs chemical shift, water peak chemical shift and signal close to the sample. Water peak suppression technique can be used to suppress or eliminate water peak and solvent peak.

③Proton homonuclear spin decoupling spectra: It is a kind of common and important double resonance experiment. When line splitting is very complex, this technique can simplify the map, infer the relationship between the mutual coupling signals, and find hidden signal and get coupling constant, etc.

④1D NOE difference spectra: In the different spectra, all signals which are not affected will disappear, and then show the enhanced signal and a strong frequency signal.

⑤Notice in comparing measured data and literature data or maps: At first, observe whether deuterium reagents are the same. If solvent are different, chemical shift has certain difference because of the solvent effects. Secondly observe whether internal standard is consistent. Different internal standards cause different chemical shift directly.

⑥Conventional ^{13}C NMR spectra: Broadband decoupling experiment can determine regular ^{13}C NMR spectrum. Because fragmentation arising from the coupling of ^{1}H nuclear and ^{13}C nuclear is eliminated, ^{13}C nuclear signal turns into a narrow single peak, and makes ^{13}C signal-to-noise ratio connected with proton increase greatly.

⑦Off-resonance decoupling spectra (OFR): The early phase of OFR is used to measure the number of hydrogen connected with carbon.

⑧Distortionless enhancement by polarization transfer (DEPT) spectra: DEPT spectra is the most ideal technique to identify the number of hydrogen connected with carbon.

(3) Two-dimensional nuclear magnetic resonance (2D NMR).

①Homonuclear correlation spectroscopy (HOMCOR).

Ⅰ. H and H correlated spectroscopy (H-H COSY): H-H COSY is a powerful tool of determining the coupling relationship between associating protons, which is equivalent to many homonuclear spin decoupling experiment. Correlation peak(or cross peak) of H-H COSY mainly reflects the coupling relationship between 2J and 3J, occasionally has remote correlation peak.

Ⅱ. Phase sensitive H-H COSY (PH H-H COSY): Compared with H-H COSY, PH H-H COSY is pure adsorption line, which greatly improves resolution and signal-to-noise ratio.

Ⅲ. Total correlation spectroscopy (TOCSY): TOCSY can find the relevant information of all hydrogen nucleuses in the same coupling system, that is to say, hydrogen nuclear signal can find the correlation peak of all protons in the same spin system.

②2D heteronuclear correlated NMR spectroscopy.

Ⅰ. H and C correlated spectroscopy(H-C COSY): H-C COSY spectra is relevant to ^{1}H NMR and ^{13}C NMR signal and has the same function with HMQC and HSQC. Its map is more intuitive and easier to be analyzed.

Ⅱ. Heteronuclear multiple quantum correlation(HMQC) and heteronuclear single quantum correlation (HSQC): Their functions are the same with H-C COSY. They are reverse experiments with high sensitivity. HSQC has more advantages. But with much dosage of the sample, we should apply H-C COSY.

Ⅲ. Heteronuclear multiple bond correlation (HMBC): HMBC can not reflect correlation peak of an interval of one bond between C atom and H atom, but can distinguish correlation peak of an interval of two or three bonds between C atom and H atom.

Ⅳ. Correlation spectroscopy via long range coupling (COLOC): Intensity of long range coupling peak depends on the corresponding coupling constant value. If the coupling constant is often so small that related peak can not be determined, changing experimental parameters can help get an ideal map.

(4) Application of liquid chromatographic-nuclear magnetic resonance or high performance liquid chromatography-nuclear magnetic resonance (LC-NMR, HPLC-NMR). In recent years, LC-NMR hyphenated instrument has come into the chemist's laboratory. It has a strong function of HPLC separation and NMR spectrum. These maps provide much information which can be used for structural identification.

2. Method of Structural Identification

2.1 Search and Validation of Background Information

All kinds of background information about the structure of the sample from literature retrieval and chemical experimental results, and various spectrum experimental data are very important, but they must be repeatedly proven to be reliable.

Inferring the type of compounds from maps is basically how to solve the problem of the signal ownership if the molecular structure is known. You should start from the chemical shift or coupling type, and then gradually spread out to other identification. Preliminary analytic conclusion must be verified in the analytical process. Finally, all kinds of information must be coincided with each other, a series of arguments must be logical, thus you will get the correct conclusion. Characteristic structural information always has all kinds of independent experimental data and (or) evidence, which support with each other. With the increase of molecular structure complexity, there will be more characteristic information.

2.2 Structural Identification

(1) Background knowledge of structural skeleton: Researchers of natural products chemistry should form good habits of reading monograph in order to follow the tracks of the literature, learn new technology continuously, and accumulate the spectrum data and spectroscopic characteristics.

(2) About molecular formula: Molecular formula is not necessarily determined firstly because all sorts of spectra can directly get the interpretation of the structure. If molecular formula has been gotten, it means we have elemental composition and unsaturated degree which bring convenience to the next structure analysis. If the sample is too little and/or has poor purity, you had better use high resolution mass spectrometry with proper source of ionization to determine molecular formula instead of burning analysis.

(3) To determine the structure should start with what kind of spectrum: It is better to determine ^{1}H NMR, ^{13}C NMR, MS spectrum through carefully analysis and comparison with literature data. If the fast appraisal result is known compounds, too many tests are not needed. If components can't be judged, it requires some more spectrum determinations. In many cases, the gotten sample only has several milligrams, which requires great care. In the condition of several milligrams, molecular formula should be determined by HREIMS or HRFAB instead of burning analysis. After determining several routine NMR spectra, we should be careful to keep NMR sample tube for further

determination, such as IR spectrum and specific rotation. Of course, we should save the liquid membrane or KBr pellet of IR for recycling.

(4) Inferring molecular skeleton: Putting forward "job structure" (or assumed structure) is the key to structural determination.

①Judging the skeleton structure according to the sample source, color reaction, chromatography behavior, references and spectrum datum is the most commonly used method.

②Compared with the collected similar structure and characteristic spectral datum, you can find similarities and deal with the differences.

③How to obtain the information of skeleton structure from map: From all sorts of spectrum maps, especially ^{1}H NMR and ^{13}C NMR spectrum can reveal the skeleton information. Simultaneously, "spectrum distribution characteristic" is the important basis of identifying organic skeleton type.

(5) Using NMR for searching purpose skeleton: Using NMR for searching purpose skeleton is fast and practical, especially for compounds of exclusive color reaction.

(6) Enantiomer and diastereomer: NMR can't distinguish enantiomers, but it can tell the differences between the diastereomers.

(7) Excessive enantiomers: When a kind of enantiomer is excessive, using chiral NMR shift reagents can completely separate their two kinds of NMR signal enantiomers.

(8) Confirming the structure at last: Using reference substances can easily finish confirmation for known compounds. Original literature datum can confirm the structure in the condition of short reference substances.

For new compounds, besides the reliable method and data, it is essential to cite similar data in the literature in order to give evidence. All NMR signal should give accurate assignment or do it as much as possible, but data of IR, MS don't need to be explained fully.

New Words and Phrases

thimbleful [ˈθɪmblfʊl]　*n.* (酒等的)极少量

nondestructive [ˌnɒndɪsˈtrʌktɪv]　*adj.* 非破坏性的

heteronuclear [ˌhetərəˈnjuːklɪə]　*n.* 异质核糖核酸

multiple-bond　多键

spectroscopist [spektˈrɒskəpɪst]　*n.* 光谱学家

morphine [ˈmɔːfiːn]　*n.* 吗啡

skeleton [ˈskelɪtn]　*n.* 骨骼

auxochrome [ˈɔːksəkrəʊm]　*n.* 助色团

conjugate [ˈkɒndʒʊgeɪt]　*vt.* 结合；使成对
　　　　　　　　　　　　adj. 共轭的；结合的

flavone [ˈfleɪvəʊn]　*n.* 黄酮

anthraquinone [ˌænθrəkwɪˈnəʊn]　n. 蒽醌
triterpenoid [traɪˈtɜːpɪnɒɪd]　n. 三萜系化合物
steroid ['sterɒɪd]　n. 类固醇；甾族化合物
carboxylic [ˌkɑːbɒkˈsɪlɪk]　adj. 羧基的
sulphone ['sʌlfəʊn]　n. 砜
sulfoxide [sʌlfˈɒksaɪd]　n. 亚砜
nitro ['naɪtrəʊ]　n. 硝基
resolution [ˌrezəˈluːʃən]　n. 分辨率
peptide ['peptaɪd]　n. 肽；缩氨酸
nucleic acid　核酸
glycoprotein [ˌɡlaɪkəʊˈprəʊtiːn]　n. 糖蛋白
pharmacokinetic　adj. 药物代谢动力学的
matrix ['meɪtrɪks]　n. 基质；母体；子宫
polysaccharide [ˌpɒlɪˈsækəraɪd]　n. 多糖；多聚糖（等于 polysaccharid）
baseline ['beɪslaɪn]　n. 基线；底线
ultraviolet [ˌʌltrəˈvaɪələt]　adj. 紫外的；紫外线的；产生紫外线的
　　　　　　　　　　　　　　n. 紫外线辐射；紫外光
infrared spectroscopy　红外光谱学，红外线分光镜
nuclear magnetic resonance　核磁共振
mass spectrometry　质谱学，质谱测量，质谱分析
homonuclear [hɒməˈnjuːklɪə(r)]　adj. 同核的，共核的
bombardment [bɒmˈbɑːdmənt]　n. 炮击，轰炸
hydroxyl [haɪˈdrɒksɪl]　n. 羟基
milligram ['mɪlɪɡræm]　n. 毫克（千分之一克）
enantiomer [ɪˈnæntɪəʊmə]　n. 对映（结构）体；对映异构体
diastereomer [daɪəˈstɪərɪəʊmə]　n. 非对映异构体；非对映体

Chapter 4
Extraction and Separation of Various Compositions

Section 1 Saccharides

Experiment 1 Extraction of Lentinans

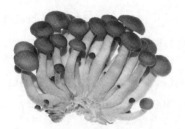 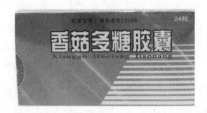

Fig. 4-1 Shiitake mushroom and its preparation

Shiitake mushroom originates from fruiting body of *Lentinus edodes* (Berk.) *sing* in tricholomagambosum (see fig. 4-1), which is the world second edible fungi and special local product in our country known as "*shanzhen*". It is a kind of fungus which grows in woods and has delicious taste, fragrant smell, and rich nutrition, therefore it has the fame of "plant queen". It contains much ergosterin which has the effect of prophylaxis and treatment for rickets; and lentinan which has molecular formula of $(C_{42}H_{70}O_{35})_n$ and can increase the immunization and inhibit the growth of cancer cell; and 40 species of enzymes from six groups of enzymes in the world which can make up the short of enzyme in human body; and aliphatic acid which can lower the blood fat.

1. Experimental Purpose

Master the method of separating polysaccharide compounds with hydrothermic boiling.

2. Experimental Principle

Polysaccharide is soluble in hot water and insoluble in ethanol above 60%, which can be extracted with hot water. Precipitate it with ethanol and remove the alcohol-soluble impurities because hot water can also extract proteins which can be removed by ethanol.

3. Experimental Procedure

3.1 Creation of Standard Curve

It is used in the method of phenol sulfuric acid, which takes glucose as the standard substance. Weigh 14.8 mg glucose that is dried at 105℃, place it into a 100 ml volumetric flask, add some water to dilute it to scale, take respectively 0 ml, 0.4 ml, 0.6 ml,

0.8 ml, 1.0 ml, 1.2 ml, 1.4 ml, 1.6 ml, 1.8 ml of it and add the water to 2.0 ml, then add 1 ml 5% phenol solution, add quickly 5 ml of concentrated sulfuric acid, shake evenly and stand for 20 minutes. Cool it to room temperature. Take the distilled water as blank, measuring the absorbance at 490 mm and drawing the standard curve can get the regression equation as follows: $y = 0.006x + 0.032$, $R = 0.9991$, linear range $0 \sim 266.4$ μg. Its experimental data can be seen in table 4-1.

Tab. 4-1 Drawing of standard curve

dosage of glucose solution/ml	0	0.4	0.6	0.8	1.0	1.2	1.4	1.6	1.8
A_{490}	0.005	0.016	0.020	0.019	0.029	0.031	0.041	0.044	0.049

3.2 Extraction

Take dried mushroom and grind it, weigh 20 g of it to place in a 250 ml beaker, add 100 ml distilled water, heat it to boiling on a asbestosed wire gauze and stir simultaneously for 30 min, filter it with a vacuum air pump, extract the residue with 100 ml distilled water for 30 min, merge the two filtrate, and concentrate it till 20 ml. Then dissolve it in 95% ethanol, stir and cool it to room temperature, put it aside for 1 h, centrifuge at 4000 r/min for 10 min, dry precipitate with a vacuum air pump, and get the crude lentinan.

3.3 Expulsion of Protein

Add 50 ml hot water (100℃) to the crude lentinan, stir it for solubility, add 10 ml Savag solution, shake violently for 10 min, stand for 10 min, centrifuge at 4000 r/min for 10 min, take supernatant fluid of the solution, add Sevag solution and do it repeatedly for 5 times.

3.4 Purification

Place the crude lentinan in a beaker, add 50 ml distilled water for solubility, add isometric CTAB (cetyl trimethyl ammonium bromide or hexadecyl trimethyl ammonium bromide, HTAB) with the concentration of 0.15 mol/L and boric acid buffer, stand for 10 min, centrifuge at 4000 r/min and get the precipitate. Add 2 mol/L ethanol for solubility, stand for 10 min, centrifuge at 4000 r/min, take supernatant and add 1% isometric methanol, stand for 24 h, filter it with a vacuum air pump, and get the purified letinan.

3.5 Experimental Results

(1) The weight of crude lentinan is about 3.46 g.

(2) Take 0.01 g dry lentinan, prepare 100 ml solution, take 1 ml solution to determine the absorbance according to the procedure of upper operation taking distilled water as the blank solution at the wavelength of 490 mm, and use the standard curve to calculate the content of lentinan.

4. Notice

(1) If the lentinan is a little gray, it may be caused by the impurities.

(2) Method of preparing Sevag solution: Add methenyl trichloride as the 1/5 volume of the lentinan solution, then add n-butyl alcohol as the 1/5 volume of methenyl

trichloride, shake violently, centrifuge for 20 min, remove the denatured protein of the interface between aqueous layer and Savag solution layer. The method is mild to the lentinan, but you need to repeat it for five times.

(3) Preparation of 0.15 mol/L of CTAB and boric acid buffer: Prepare the boric acid buffer firstly as follows: take 1 g boric acid and dissolve in 100 ml water whose pH is 5. Then weigh 5.5 g CTAB and add 100 ml of the former boric acid buffer, and stir it evenly.

5. Experimental Supplies and Arrangement of Class Hour

Experimental supplies: mushroom, glucose, ethanol, phenol, sulfuric acid, UV-Vis spectrophotometer, water bath, methenyl trichloride, n-butyl alcohol, CTAB, boric acid.

Arrangement of class hour: to be completed within 6 class hours.

6. Questions

(1) What is the principle of extracting lentinans?

(2) What are the main factors affecting the extraction efficiency of lentinans?

New Words and Phrases

shiitake mushroom   香菇
fungi ['fʌŋgaɪ]   n. (fungus 的复数)真菌(如蘑菇、霉菌)
prophylaxis [ˌprɒfɪ'læksɪs]   n. 预防
ricket ['rɪkɪt]   n. 大错;失风;佝偻病
lentinan ['lentɪnæn]   n. 香菇多糖
aliphatic [ˌælɪ'fætɪk]   adj. 脂肪族的
hydrothermic [haɪdrəʊ'θɜːmɪk]   adj. 热水的
precipitate [prɪ'sɪpɪteɪt]   vt. 使沉淀
　　　　　　　　　　　　 n. 沉淀物;结果,产物
standard curve   标准曲线
regression equation   回归方程式
centrifuge ['sentrɪfjuːdʒ]   n. 离心机
　　　　　　　　　　　　 vt. 使离心
supernatant [sjuːpə'neɪtənt]   adj. 浮在表面的
isometric [ˌaɪsəʊ'metrɪk]   adj. 等大的,等容积的
cetyl trimethyl ammonium bromide   十六烷基三甲基溴化铵
boric acid buffer   硼酸缓冲液

Experiment 2 Extraction of Saccharide in Ephedra

Ephedra is a traditional Chinese medicinal material (see fig. 4-2), which is from herbaceous stem of family Ephedraceae and has three different species as follows: *Ephedra sinica* Stapf, *Ephedra intermedia* Schrenk et C. A. Mey. and *Ephedra equisetina* Bge. According to the document of ancient books, it has the effect of inducing diaphoresis, dispersing the lung-qi and relieving asthma and diuresis, which can be used for the treatment of diseases such as cold, cough, asthma and edema as a traditional Chinese medicine. There are lots of chemical compositions in Ephedra such as alkaloids, flavonoids, volatile oil, organic acids and saccharide etc., in which saccharide has the effect of lowering the blood lipid and protecting the liver.

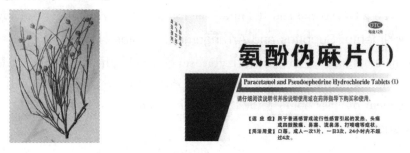

Fig. 4-2　Plant and preparation of Ephedra

1. Experimental Purpose

Master the principle and method of decoction and alcohol sedimentation technique in the process of extracting saccharides in Ephedra.

2. Experimental Principle

On the basis of the properties of saccharides which are easy to dissolve in the hot water, but don't dissolve in over 60% ethanol, saccharides can be extracted by hot water and impurities can be eliminated by alcohol sedimentation. Then the useless protein can be removed by the papain and Sevag method.

3. Experimental Procedure

3.1　Creation of Standard Curve

Phenol-sulfuric acid method: take glucose as the standard, weigh 4 mg glucose with exquisite precision, place it in a measuring flask, add some distilled water and dilute it to scale. Take the former glucose solvent of 0.4 ml, 0.6 ml, 0.8 ml, 1.0 ml, 1.2 ml, 1.4 ml, 1.6 ml, 1.8 ml, add the distilled water to 2.0 ml, then add 1 ml 6% phenol, shake it, add 5.0 ml concentrated sulfuric acid, shake it, and stand for 5 min. Then heat it for 15 min in water bath, take it out and cool it to the room temperature (25℃). Simultaneously, take 2.0 ml distilled water as the blank reagent, add the corresponding solvent in the former order. Measuring the absorbance at 490 nm and drawing the standard curve can get the regression equation. Its experimental data can be seen in fig. 4-3.

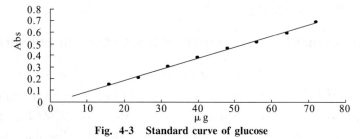

Fig. 4-3　Standard curve of glucose

3.2 Extraction

Take 20 g smashed ephedra material, place it in a 1000 ml round-bottom flask, then add 14 times distilled water of it and reflux for 4 h at 100℃ in a water bath, and cool it to room temperature. Filter it, add the distilled water as the former same volume to the residue, and extract it twice. Combine the filtrate, enrich it to 20 ml in a vacuum state at 50℃. Agitate the supernatant, add 95% ethanol three times to make the liquid concentration attain 75%, stand for 24 h at 4℃. Keep centrifuging for 20 min at 3000 r/min, collect the precipitation, rinse it with anhydrous alcohol, then keep centrifuging for 20 min at 3000 r/min, collect the supernatant, dry it at low temperature, and get the ephedra saccharides.

3.3 Expulsion of Protein

Add distilled water and dilute the ephedra saccharides to form 5% water solution, then add papain to keep the concentration at 1%(W/V), sustain enzymolysis for 2 h. Filter it, add the Sevag reagent as one third volume of the filtrate, keep oscillating for 30 min, stand a while, centrifuge at 2000 r/min and get off the infra-protein. Then add three-time ethanol, centrifuge and separate the precipitation, dissolve it with a little water, dry it at low temperature and get the purified ephedra saccharides.

3.4 Experimental Results

Weigh 8 mg ephedra saccharides which are dried to constant weight at 60℃ with exquisite precision, dissolve it in double distilled water, dilute it to 100 ml. Take 2 ml ephedra saccharides solution, operate according to the content in item 3.1, repeat the determination three times, calculate the content of glucose in the sample with the regression equation, and the saccharides content as the following formula:

Content of saccharides(%) = $C \times D \times f \times 100 / W$, C is the glucose concentration of the sample solution (mg/ml); D is the dilution ratio of saccharides (ml); f is calculation factor; W is the weight of the sample (mg).

4. Notice

(1) Methods of trichloroacetic acid and enzyme also can be used for expulsion of protein.

(2) Determination of calculation factor: Weigh 25 mg ephedra saccharides which are dried to constant weight at 60℃ with exquisite precision, place it in a 100 ml volumetric flask, and add distilled water to the flask scale. Then take 2 ml solution and place it respectively in five volumetric flasks of 25 ml, add the water and dilute it to the scale. On the basis of absorbance of the solution and the regression equation, the glucose content of five samples of the saccharides can be calculated, and then get the calculation factor according to the following formula: $f = W/(C \times D)$. W is the saccharides weight; C is the glucose concentration of the saccharides solution; D is the dilution ratio of the saccharides.

5. Experimental Supplies and Arrangement of Class Hour

Experimental supplies: ephedra, glucose, ethanol, phenol, sulfuric acid, UV-Vis spectrophotometer, water bath, methenyl trichloride, n-butyl alcohol, papain.

Arrangement of class hour: to be completed within 6~9 class hours.

6. Questions

(1) Why do we stir the solution constantly when adding the ethanal to precipitate the saccharide in ephedra?

(2) What are the other methods for extracting saccharide in ephedra?

New Words and Phrases

papain [pə'peɪn] n. 木瓜蛋白酶
ephedra ['efədrə] n. 麻黄属植物
saccharide ['sækəraɪd] n. 糖,糖类
diaphoresis [ˌdaɪəfə'riːsɪs] n. 发汗
asthma ['æsmə] n. 气喘,哮喘
diuresis [ˌdaɪjʊə'riːsɪs] n. 多尿,利尿
edema [ɪ'diːmə] n. 水肿,瘤腺体
phenol ['fiːnɒl] n. 苯酚
supernatant [ˌsjuːpə'neɪtənt] n. 上清液
enzymolysis [enzaɪ'mɒlɪsɪs] n. 酶解(作用)
oscillate ['ɒsɪleɪt] vt. 使振荡,使振动

Section 2　Phenylpropanoids

Experiment 1　Extraction, Isolation and Identification of Esculin and Esculetin in Ash Bark

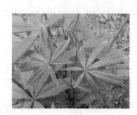 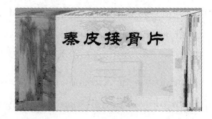

Fig. 4-4　Plant and preparation of Ash Bark

Ash bark is the dry bark or trunk bark from plants of Oleaceae such as *Fraxinus rhynchophylla* Hance., *F. chinensis* Roxb., *F. szaboana* Lingelsh. and *F. stylosa* Lingelsh(see fig. 4-4). Ash bark is bitter and slightly cold. It has the effect of eliminating heat, dampness and astringing, which is mainly effective for warm and heating dysentery, swelling and pain of eyes.

Ash bark contains a variety of lactones, saponins, tannins, etc., which mainly include esculin, esculetin, fraxin and fraxetin (see fig. 4-5) that have many physiological activity of antibacterial and anti-inflammatory. For example, esculetin has a better therapeutic effect for bacillary dysentery, acute enteritis and reducing fever. It is suitable for children because it is low toxic with little side effect and not bitter.

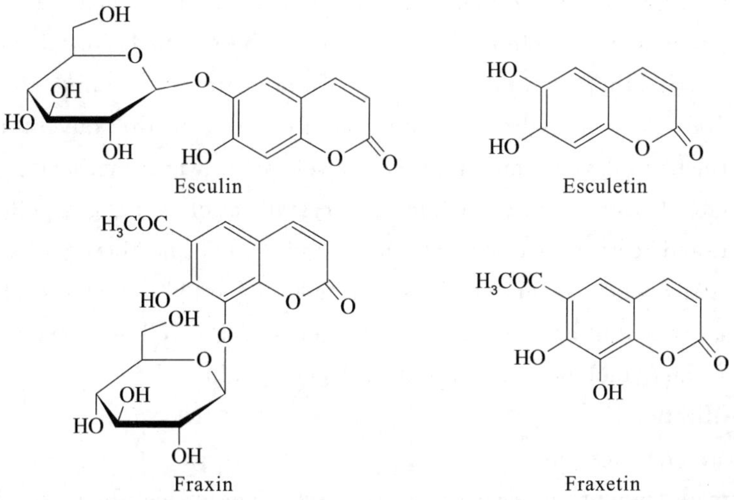

Fig. 4-5 Main chemical components in Ash Bark

(1) Esculin that is also known as Ma-su bark glycosides has white powdered crystal and a m. p. of 205~206℃. It is easily soluble in hot water (1 : 15), soluble in ethanol (1 : 24), slightly soluble in cold water (1 : 6 or 1 : 10), difficultly soluble in ethyl acetate, and insoluble in ether and chloroform. It is hydrolyzed by dilute acid, and blue fluorescence appears in aqueous solution.

(2) Esculetin is yellow needle like crystal and has a m. p. of 276℃. It is soluble in boiling ethanol, sodium hydroxide solution and ethyl acetate, slightly soluble in boiling water, and almost insoluble in ether and chloroform.

(3) Fraxin has a m. p. of 205℃.

(4) Fraxetin has a m. p. of 227~228℃.

1. Experimental Purpose

(1) Master the effect of liquid-liquid extraction in the separation of coumarin glycosides and aglycones.

(2) Be familiar with the basic operation of the recrystallization well.

2. Experimental Principle

Esculin and esculetin can dissolve in boiling ethanol so that they can be extracted by boiling ethanol, and then use the different solubility in ethyl acetate for separation.

3. Experimental Procedure

3.1 Extraction

Take 150 g crude powder of ash bark and place it in a Soxhlet extractor, add 400 ml 95% ethanol and reflux for 2 hours, get the ethanol extract, recover the solvent under reduced pressure to ointment, and get the total extract.

3.2 Separation

Add 40 ml water to the ointment and dissolve it, shift it to a separatory funnel, extract it twice with isometric chloroform, evaporate the residual chloroform of the water layer. Add isometric ethyl acetate and extract it three times, combine the ethyl acetate solution, dehydrate with anhydrous sodium sulfate, recover the solvent under reduced pressure to ointment to dryness and dissolve the residue in warm methanol. Concentrate it to the appropriate dosage, stand a while for crystallization, and get yellow needle-like crystal. Filter it and recrystallize with methanol and water, and then get esculetin.

Concentrate the water layer which is extracted by ethyl acetate to the appropriate dosage, stand a while for crystallization, and get slightly yellow crystal. Filter it and recrystallize with methanol and water, and then get esculin.

3.3 Identification

(1) Chemical identification.

① Take small amount of esculetin and esculin and place them in two test tubes respectively, and add 1 ml ethanol to dissolve them. Then drop 2~3 drops of 1% iron trichloride solution so that it turns dark green, and then drop 3 drops of concentrated ammonia and add 6 ml water, so that the color becomes dark red under sunlight.

② Take a little esculetin and esculin, place them in two test tubes respectively, add 2~3 drops of the methanol solution of hydroxylamine hydrochloride, then add 2~3 drops of 1% sodium hydroxide solution, heat it for a few minutes in a water bath, cool it, then adjust its pH to 3~4 by hydrochloric acid, add 1~2 drops of 1% iron trichloride solution, so that it turns red to purple.

③ Reaction of Gibb's or Emerson: Do it as the content of Chapter 5.

(2) Observe the fluorescence: Take a drop of methanol solution of esculin and esculetin and drop on the filter paper respectively, observe the fluorescence under ultraviolet light at 254 nm. Then drop one drop of sodium hydroxide solution on the original spot, and observe the change of the fluorescence.

(3) Identification of TLC.

Adsorbent: silica gel G.

Samples: standard substances of esculin and esculetin and their homemade alcohol solution.

Developer: acetic ether-methanol-1% ethylic acid solution (7:3:0.1).

Color:

① Observe the results under $UV_{254\,nm}$ lamp. Gray fluorescence appears for esculin, and taupe appears for esculetin.

② Spray the diazotized p-nitroaniline solution, and the color becomes onyx.

Results: Rf of esculin is 0.04, while Rf of esculetin is 0.28.

4. Notice

(1) There are so many varieties of ash bark, some of which don't contain coumarin.

You should distinguish their original plant varieties.

(2) Pay attention to avoid emulsification when shaking the separating funnel during the course of extraction, and rotate it gently.

(3) The fluorescence of coumarin under UV lamp in TLC can be identified.

5. Experimental Supplies and Arrangement of Class Hour

Experimental supplies: reflux device, solvent recovery device, filtration device, 250 ml separating funnel, Erlenmeyer flask (500 ml, 250 ml, 50 ml), separation chamber, filter paper, zeolite, ash bark, 95% ethanol, chloroform, ethyl acetate, methanol, hydroxamic acid iron reagent, Gibb's reagent, Emerson reagent.

Arrangement of class hour: to be completed within 6 class hours.

6. Questions

(1) How to tell esculin from esculetin when they appear in TLC as two major fluorescent spots?

(2) How to make sure that natural medicines contain coumarins using the easiest method?

New Words and Phrases

ash bark　秦皮

oleaceae ['əʊlɪəsɪˌiː]　*n.* 木樨科

astringe [ə'strɪndʒ]　*vt.* 使……收缩

dysentery ['dɪsənˌteriː]　*n.* 痢疾;脏毒

tannin ['tænɪn]　*n.* 鞣酸,丹宁酸

esculin ['eskjʊlɪn]　*n.* 七叶灵,马栗树皮苷

esculetin [ˌeskjʊ'liːtən]　*n.* 七叶亭,七叶苷原

fraxin ['fræksɪn]　*n.* 白蜡树苷

fraxetin ['fræksɪtɪn]　*n.* 皮亭

anti-inflammatory [ˌæntɪ ɪnflə'meɪtəri]　*adj. & n.* 抗炎的(药)

coumarin glycoside　香豆素糖苷

aglycone [ə'glaɪˌkəʊn]　*n.* 糖苷配基

ointment ['ɔɪntmənt]　*n.* 软膏,药膏

dehydrate [ˌdiː'haɪdreɪt]　*vt.* 使……脱水

hydroxylamine hydrochloride　盐酸羟胺

sodium hydroxide　氢氧化钠

taupe [təʊp]　*n.* 灰褐色

Erlenmeyer flask　锥形烧瓶;爱伦美氏烧瓶

hydroxamic acid iron　异羟肟酸铁

Experiment 2 Extraction, Isolation and Identification of Paeonol

Cortex moutan is the dry root bark of *Paeonia suffruticosa* Andr. in Ranunculaceae (see fig. 4-6). In addition, it is also from the root bark of *Paeonia suffruticosa* Andr. var spontanea Rehd, *Paeonia papaveracea* Andr., *Cynanchum pariculatum* (Bge) Kitag, *Paeonia szechuanica* Fang, and *Paeonia potanini* Kom.

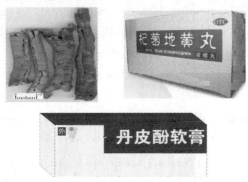

Fig. 4-6 Plant and preparation of Cortex Moutan

It has the effect of removing pathogenic heat from blood, activating blood circulation and removing blood stasis. It is used for hyperthermic plaque, hematemesis, night fever abating at dawn, non-sweat hectic fever due to *yin* deficiency, amenorrhea or dysmenorrhea, pyogenic carbuncle and traumatic injury. Its main ingredients are paeonol (1.9% ~ 2%), paeonoside, paeonolide, apiopaeonoside etc. Then, it contains a little volatile oil (0.15% ~ 0.4%) and phytosterols.

$$\begin{array}{ll} \text{Paeonol} & R=H \\ \text{Paeonol glycosides} & R=\text{glucose} \\ \text{Paeonol original glycosides} & R=\text{glucose-arabinose} \end{array}$$

(1) Paeonol: Its molecular formula is $C_9H_{10}O_3$. It is a kind of white needle-like crystal and has a m.p. of 49.5~50.5℃. It is soluble in ethanol, ether, acetone, chloroform, benzene, and slightly soluble in water and volatile, which can be used for steam distillation.

(2) Paeonoside: Its molecular formula is $C_{15}H_{20}O_8$. It is colorless columnar crystal (in ethanol) and has a m.p. of 81~82℃. It is soluble in water, alcohol, acetone, ethyl acetate, and soluble slightly in chloroform and benzene.

(3) Paeonolide: Its molecular formula is $C_{20}H_{28}O_{12}$. It is colorless columnar crystal (in ethanol-ethyl acetate) and has a m.p. of 157~158℃. It is soluble in water, alcohol, acetone, ethyl acetate, and slightly soluble in benzene and petroleum ether.

1. Experimental Purpose

(1) Master the method of extracting paeonol by steam distillation.

(2) Be familiar with the method of chromatographic detection and qualitative identification.

(3) Understand the method of identifying paeonol in Qiju Dihuang Pills.

2. Experimental Principle

(1) Paeonol is volatile and can be distilled with water vapor. Meanwhile, it is difficult to dissolve in cold water so that it will crystallize when it is cold.

(2) Paeonol that dissolves in ether is a kind of active ingredient of eight herbs in Qiju Dihuang Pills, which can be extracted by ether and inspected by phenolic color reaction contrasted to Cortex Moutan extract and standard substance of paeonol.

3. Experimental Procedure

3.1 Extraction and Isolation of Paeonol

Take 150 g commercial cortex moutan, grind it, add 700 ml distilled water, 10 ml ethanol and 40 g sodium chloride, distill it after soaking. Collect about 300 ml distillate, cool it, put it aside overnight, get white needle-like crystal, filter it, dry and weigh it. If the crystal is not pure, add 95% ethanol to dissolve it (about 15 times of coarse crystal), filter it and add four times amount of water to make the solution milky white, stand a while and a large number of white needle-like crystals. If white crystal can't be gotten and only the precipitate of oil and bead-like materials appears in the extraction process, you can add a small amount of crystals and rub the flask sidewall, which can get a large number of paeonol crystals. Ether can be used to extract it several times, merge all the extract, add anhydrous sodium sulfate for dehydration, recycle the ether to small volume, stand a while for crystallization, rinse the crystal 2~3 times with a little water after filtration, dry it in a dryer and weigh it.

3.2 Identification of Paeonol

(1) Color reaction.

①Reaction of ferric chloride: Dissolve a little paeonol crystal in 1 ml ethanol, drop alcohol solution of 5% ferric chloride, and observe the phenomena.

②Reaction of concentrated nitric: Dissolve a little paeonol crystal in 1 ml ethanol, drop a few drops of concentrated nitric acid, and observe the phenomena.

(2) TLC identification.

Thin chromatography plate: plate of silica gel G-CMC-Na.

Spotting: 10 μl ethanol solution of the sample and standard substance of paeonol.

Developer: cyclohexane-ethyl acetate (3 : 1).

Color: Spray it with alcohol solution of 5% ferric chloride acidized by hydrochloric acid solution, and blow it with hot winds till the spot color is clear.

3.3 TLC Identification of Paeonol in Qiju Dihuang Pills

Qiju Dihuang Pill that consists of wolfberry fruit, chrysanthemum, *Rehmannia glutinosa* and *cornus* is a kind of honeyed bolus or water-honeyed pill, which has the effectiveness of nourishing liver and kidney.

(1) Preparation.

①Preparation of the sample: Take 9 g honeyed bolus of Qiju Dihuang Pills (or 6 g water-honeyed pills), add 4 g diatomite and grind it evenly, add 40 ml ether and reflux 1 h, filter it, remove the ether of the filtrate, add the residue into 1 ml ethanol, and get the sample solution.

②Preparation of standard substance: Add homemade paeonol and standard paeonol into ethanol and get the solution containing 1 mg paeonol per 1 ml solution.

(2) TLC identification: Its conditions are the same with 2.2.

4. Notice

(1) The content of paeonol has more to do with Cortex Moutan's producing area and collecting seasons. Generally speaking, it has higher content when it is harvested in spring in Sichuan province. You can increase or reduce the dosage of Cortex Moutan according to its content.

(2) Paeonol is easily soluble in water and slightly soluble in cold water, which is easy to trigger crystal precipitation in cold conditions and adhere to the sidewall of condenser pipe because initial fraction of paeonol has high concentration. Adding ethanol can make it soluble and flow into receiving flask.

(3) Adding sodium chloride can significantly improve the speed of distillation, and reduce the extraction time.

5. Experimental Supplies and Arrangement of Class Hour

Experimental supplies: cortex moutan, Qiju Dihuang Pills, 95% ethanol, sodium chloride, ferric chloride, standard paeonol, cyclohexane, ethyl acetate, diatomaceous earth, ether; steam distillation unit, reflux extraction device, developing tank, thin layer plate.

Arrangement of class hour: to be completed within 6 class hours.

6. Questions

(1) What chemical components can we extract with steam distillation?

(2) How to identify the main components of Chinese patent medicine?

New Words and Phrases

paeonol [piːˈəʊnəʊl]   *n.* 芍药醇

cortex moutan   丹皮

pathogenic [ˌpæθəˈdʒenɪk]   *adj.* 引起疾病的

stasis [ˈsteɪsɪs]   *n.* 停滞,静止

hyperthermic plaque   热斑

hematemesis [ˌhiːməˈtemɪsɪs]   *n.* 吐血,咯血

abating [əˈbeɪtɪŋ]   *v.* 减少,减去

hectic [ˈhektɪk]   *n.* 肺病热患者;潮红

yin deficiency 阴虚
amenorrhea [eɪˌmenəˈriːə] *n.* 无月经(因生病或怀孕),停经
dysmenorrhea [ˌdɪsmenəˈriːə] *n.* 月经困难,痛经
pyogenic [ˌpaɪəʊˈdʒenɪk] *adj.* 生脓的,化脓的
carbuncle [ˈkɑːbʌŋkl] *n.* 红榴石,红宝石;痈
traumatic [trɔːˈmætɪk] *adj.* 外伤的,损伤的
paeonoside [piːˈəʊnəˌsaɪd] *n.* 芍药糖苷
paeonolide [piːˈəʊnəˌlaɪd] *n.* 芍药交酯
apiopaeonoside [æpiːəʊpiːˈnəʊsaɪd] *n.* 丹皮酚新苷
phytosterol [faɪˈtɒstərɒl] *n.* 植物甾醇类
Qiju Dihuang Pills 杞菊地黄丸
needle-like *adj.* 针状的
recycle [ˌriːˈsaɪkl] *vt.* 回收利用;使再循环
concentrated nitric acid 浓硝酸
wolfberry [ˈwʊlfbəri] *n.* 薄叶西方雪果
Chinese wolfberry 枸杞
chrysanthemum [krɪˈsænθəməm] *n.* 菊花;菊属
rehmannia 地黄
honeyed bolus 蜜丸
sidewall [ˈsaɪdwɔːl] *n.* 边墙,侧壁

Section 3 Quinones

Experiment 1 Extraction and Isolation of Anthraquinones from Chinese Rhubarb

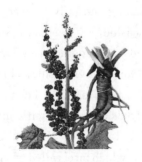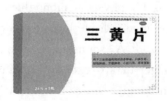

Fig. 4-7 Plant and preparation of Chinese Rhubarb

As a kind of conventional Chinese medicine, Chinese rhubarb is the rhizome of *Rheum Palmatum* L., *Rheum tanguticum* Maxim. ex Balf, or *Rheum officinale* Baill. in Polygonaceae plant (see fig. 4-7). It mainly contains anthraquinones, which have the effect of purgation and antibiosis.

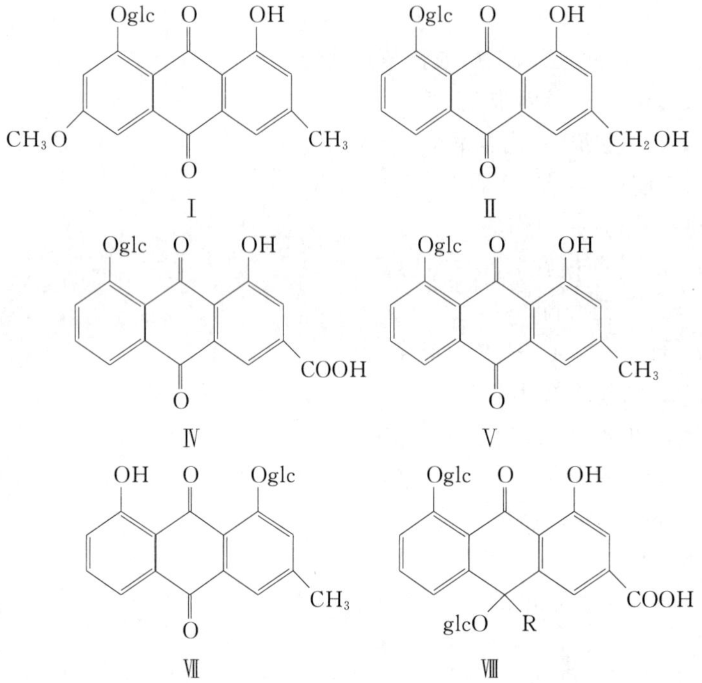

R=H: rhein glycoside C   R=OH: rhein glycoside B
R=OH: rhein glycoside A   R=H: rhein glycoside D

I: Physcion monoglucoside   II: Aloe-emodin monoglucoside   III: Emodin monoglucoside
IV: Rhein monoglucoside   V: Chrysophanol monoglucoside   VI: Emodin-1-O-β-D-glucopyranosyl emodin
VII: Chrysophanol-1-O-β-D-glucopyranosyl emodin

Fig. 4-8 Compositions of hydroxyl anthraquinone glycoside from Chinese Rhubarb

Hydroxyl anthraquinone glycosides can be seen in figure 4-8. Chinese rhubarb has several anthraquinone derivatives which have purgative effect, in which glycosides are major components. Purgative effect of Chinese rhubarb is proportional to its content of combined rhein. Anthraquinone glycosides with strong purgative effect are as follows: chrysophanol-1-monoglucoside, emodin-6-monoglucoside, aloe-emodin-8-monoglucoside, rhein-8-monoglucoside, physcion monoglucoside and anthraquinone derivatives of double glycosides such as emodin-di-O-glucoside, aloe-emodin-di-O-glucoside, chrysophanol-di-O-glucoside and sennoside A, sennoside B, sennoside C, sennoside D. The purgative effect of sennosides is stronger than that of anthraquinone glycosides, but their content is less than that of anthraquinone glycosides. In recent years, a Japanese, Nishioka, separates four new purgative compositions from Chinese rhubarb, which are called rhein glycoside A, rhein glycoside B, rhein glycoside C, and rhein glycoside D. In addition, it contains Chinese rhubarb tannic acid such as gallic acid (it is composed of free group and galloyl glucoside) and catechin, which have antidiarrheal effect that is quite opposite to purgative effect of anthraquinone derivatives.

Rhubarb aglycone mainly includes five kinds of free anthraquinones such as chrysophanol, emodin, rhein, aloe-emodin and physcion, which have almost no purgative effect. Their structures are as follows:

Chrysophanol	$R_1=CH_3$	$R_2=H$
Emodin	$R_1=CH_3$	$R_2=OH$
Rhein	$R_1=COOH$	$R_2=H$
Physcion	$R_1=CH_3$	$R_2=OCH_3$
Aloe-emodin	$R_1=CH_2OH$	$R_2=H$

1. Experimental Purpose

(1) Master the method of pH gradient extraction and the principle of extracting and isolating various anthraquinone aglycones in Chinese rhubarb.

(2) Learn the method of color reaction of anthraquinones and chromatography identification.

2. Experimental Principle

Chinese rhubarb's anthraquinone glycosides can be hydrolyzed into free hydroxy-anthraquinones and sugars on the condition of heating in acidic, which don't dissolve in water, but dissolve in ether, chloroform and other lipophilic organic solvents that used for extraction. Then separate them with pH gradient extraction method on the basis of different acidity of free hydroxyanthraquinones. They can also be separated by silica gel column chromatography according to different polarity of free hydroxyanthraquinones.

3. Experimental Procedure

3.1 Extraction of Free Anthraquinones

Weigh 10 g coarse powder of Chinese rhubarb, add 150 ml 20% H_2SO_4 aqueous solution, heat it in a electric furnace for one hour, cool it for a while, filter it with an air pump, dry at 70℃, grind and place it in a Soxhlet extractor, add 150 ml ether for reflux extraction for 2 hours, and then get the ether extract.

Rhein, aloe-emodin emodin, physcion and chrysophanol can be determined in the ether extract by TLC. You should choose silica gel-CMC cohesive plate as thin layer plate and petroleum ether(60~90℃)-ethyl acetate (7 : 3) as the developer to spread out in nearly level or vertical direction. We can see four spots under visible light and the yellow spot (Rf=0.9) is the mixture of chrysophanol and physcion which can't be separated in this condition. The other three spots (Rf order from high to low) are emodin (orange spot), aloe-emodin (yellow spot) and rhein (yellow spot).

3.2 pH Gradient Extraction

(1) Separation of emodin: Add ether extract to a 250 ml separatory funnel, use 40 ml 5% $NaHCO_3$ aqueous solution to extract it, and the aqueous layer becomes purplish red. Then separate the aqueous layer, repeat the extraction till the color fades away. Combine the aqueous layer, acidize it to pH 3 with concentrated hydrochloric acid, and get rhein precipitate. (Notice: add the acid solution slowly to prevent it from overflowing) After filtering, rinse it several times with water at first, and then rinse it with ice-cold acetone. Then dry it and crystallize for 2~3 times with glacial acetic acid or pyridine, and get

yellow needle-like crystal which can be inspected by melting point test, PC or TLC contrast to standard substance.

(2) Separation of rhein: Extract the remaining ether layer for several times by 40 ml 5% Na_2CO_3 aqueous solution per time, and the aqueous layer turns red. Then separate the aqueous layer, and repeat the extraction till the color fades away. Combine the aqueous layer, acidize it with concentrated hydrochloric acid, and get yellow precipitate. After filtering, rinse it several times with water at first, and then rinse it with ice-cold acetone to remove the colored impurities. Then dry it and crystallize for 2~3 times with glacial acetic acid or pyridine, and get orange needle-like crystal which can be inspected by melting point test, PC or TLC contrast to standard substance.

(3) Separation of aloe-emodin: Extract the remaining ether layer for several times by 40 ml 2.5% NaOH aqueous solution per time, and the aqueous layer turns red. Then separate the aqueous layer, and repeat the extraction till the color fades away. Combine the aqueous layer, acidize it with concentrated hydrochloric acid, and get yellow precipitate. After filtering, rinse it several times with water at first. Then dry it and crystallize for 2~3 times with glacial acetic acid or acetic ether, and get orange needle crystal which can be inspected by melting point test, PC or TLC contrast to standard substance.

(4) Separation of chrysophanol and physcion: Extract the remaining ether layer for several times by 50 ml 5% NaOH aqueous solution per time until no color is in alkaline water. Combine the extract, acidize it with concentrated hydrochloric acid and get precipitate. After filtering, rinse it to the neutral, dry it at low temperature. Then dissolve it in acetic ether, separate it with a silica gel column with petroleum ether (b.p. 60~90℃)-acetic ether(15 : 1) as the eluent. The substance eluted first is chrysophanol, and next is physcion. They are purified by acetic ether and crystallization, determinate the melting point and identify them by TLC. Another method is as follows: Dissolve the sample in a little petroleum ether, and use paper chromatography to separate it.

PC conditions: filter paper (7 cm×20 cm).

Developer: saturated petroleum ether (b.p. 60~90℃).

Developing pattern: ascending method.

Chromogenic reagent: 4% NaOH alcohol solution.

3.3 Separation of Chrysophanol and Physcion with Cellulose Powder Column Chromatography

(1) Preparation of the cellulose powder: Weigh 15 g filter paper (or the scraps of paper) which is cut into small pieces, add 300 ml dilute nitric acid (add 5 ml 65%~68% nitric acid every 100 ml water), heat it for hydrolysis (about 2 hours), filter it with an air pump (type G3 acidproof funnel), rinse the filter cake with distilled water to neutral, and then add some ethanol and ethyl ether to rinse it respectively. After removing the remaining ethyl ether, dry it at low temperature, smash it and sieve it by a 120 mesh sieve for preservation.

(2) Packing column: Weigh 8 g cellulose powder, use wet column method to pack column with saturated petroleum ether (b. p. 60~90℃).

(3) Adding the sample: Shift the sample carefully to the top of the column with a pipette.

(4) Elution: Elute with saturated petroleum ether (b. p. 60~90℃), divide into 10 ml samples, concentrate them respectively, check them by PC (PC conditions is ditto), combine the same fraction, and collect respectively chrysophanol and physcion. Use ethyl acetate to recrystallize the chrysophanol and determine its melting point.

3.4 Purification of Emodin with Silica Gel Column Chromatography

(1) Packing column: Take 10 g silica gel passed through 100~200 mesh, and pack the column with dry column method (size of column: 1.5 cm×8.5 cm).

(2) Adding the sample: Dissolve the coarse emodin extract in 5 ml petroleum ether (b. p. 60~90℃)-acetic ether (7 : 3), shift the sample solution to the top of the column with a pipette.

(3) Elution: Elute with petroleum ether (b. p. 60~90℃)-acetic ether (7 : 3), divide into 10 ml samples, and check it by TLC.

3.5 Identification of Chrysophanol

(1) Use guttate reaction to check reaction of chrysophanol with NaOH solution and $MgAc_2$ solution in the thin plate.

(2) Determination of chrysophanol ultraviolet spectrum.

(3) Use potassium bromide compressor method to determinate its infrared spectrum.

4. Notice

(1) Integrated anthraquinones is the major form of Chinese rhubarb, only a small part of them are free anthraquinones. In order to improve the yield of free anthraquinones, use the method combining acid hydrolysis with extraction.

(2) Two-phase extraction requires slow shake instead of violent shake, which costs a long time. But it can avoid serious emulsification phenomenon of affecting the separating effect. For example, rinsing chloroform with water is especially easy to trigger emulsification, which can be added into the sodium to separate two layers.

5. Experimental Supplies and Arrangement of Class Hour

Experimental supplies: 500 ml round bottom flask, beaker, dropper, rubber tubes, condensing tubes (30 cm), chromatography cylinder, wild-mouth bottle, Soxhlet extractor, 250 ml separating liquid funnel, Brinell funnel, suction filter bottle, ordinary filter paper, thin layer board, column, sprayer, widely pH test paper, 10~20 g Chinese rhubarb, $NaHCO_3$, Na_2CO_3, NaOH, sulfuric acid, ammonia, hydrochloric acid, ether and petroleum ether, ethyl acetate.

Arrangement of class hour: to be completed within 6 class hours.

6. Questions

(1) Briefly describe the relationship between the acidity and structure of the five free hydroxyanthraquinone compounds in Chinese rhubarb.

(2) What is the principle of pH gradient extraction? How to separate the five kinds of free hydroxyanthraquinone compounds in Chinese rhubarb?

New Words and Phrases

Chinese rhubarb　大黄

purgation [pɜːˈgeɪʃən]　*n.* 清除；净化

antibiosis [ˌæntɪbaɪˈəʊsɪs]　*n.* 抗菌（作用）

derivative [dɪˈrɪvətɪv]　*n.* 衍生物

chrysophanol [ˈkrɪsəfənəl]　*n.* 大黄酚

monoglucoside　葡萄糖苷

emodin [ˈemədɪn]　*n.* 大黄素，泻素

rhein [raɪn]　*n.* 大黄酸

aloe [ˈæləʊ]　*n.* 芦荟，芦荟油

sennoside [seˈnəʊsaɪd]　*n.* 番泻叶苷

gallic acid　五倍子酸，没食子酸

catechin [ˈkætɪtʃɪn]　*n.* 儿茶酚；儿茶酸

aglycone [əˈglaɪˌkəʊn]　*n.* 糖苷配基

hydrolyze [ˈhaɪdrəlaɪz]　*vi.* 水解

hydroxyanthraquinone [haɪˌdrɒksɪænθrəˈkwɪnəʊn]　*n.* 羟基蒽醌

purplish [ˈpɜːplɪʃ]　*adj.* 略带紫色的

glacial acetic acid　冰乙酸

pyridine [ˈpɪrɪdiːn]　*n.* 吡啶；氮（杂）苯

physcion [ˈfɪsʃn]　*n.* 大黄素甲醚

acetic ether　乙酸乙酯

dissolve [dɪˈzɒlv]　*vt.* 使溶解

cellulose [ˈseljəˌləʊs]　*n.* 细胞膜质，纤维素

melting point　熔点

boiling point　沸点

eluent [ˈeljʊənt]　*n.* 洗脱剂

Experiment 2　Extraction, Isolation and Identification of Emodin from Polygonum Cuspidate

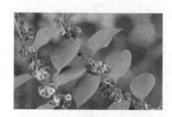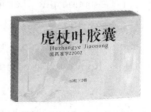

Fig. 4-9　Plant and preparation of Polygonum Cuspidate

Polygonum cuspidate is the rhizome or root of *polygonum cuspidatum* Siebet Zucc (see fig. 4-9), which has the effect of activating blood circulation and removing blood stasis, eliminating heat and detoxification, removing the phlegm and relieving cough. In recent years, it is used in the treatment of acute jaundice, reducing the blood fat, increasing white blood cells and platelets, and curing chronic bronchitis or other kinds of inflammations and burn injuries. It contains a lot of ingredients of anthraquinones and stilbenes.

Physical and chemical properties of known ingredients (see fig. 4-10) in the rhizome of polygonum cuspidate are as follows:

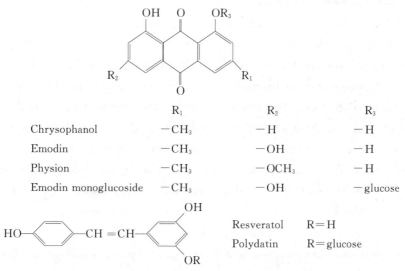

Fig. 4-10 Main components in Polygonum Cuspidate

(1) Chrysophanol: auratus flaky crystal (acetone) or needle crystal (alcohol), m. p. 196~197℃, it can be sublimated and is soluble in benzene, chloroform, acetic acid, ethanol, NaOH aqueous solution and Na_2CO_3 hot solution, and slightly soluble in petroleum ether and ethyl ether, insoluble in water, aqueous solution of $NaHCO_3$ or Na_2CO_3.

(2) Emodin: orange yellow needle crystal, m. p. 256~257℃, it can be sublimated and easily soluble in ethanol, soluble in aqueous solution of NH_4OH, Na_2CO_3 and NaOH, and hardly soluble in water.

(3) Physion: brick red needle crystal, m. p. 206℃, it can be sublimated and easily soluble in NaOH solution, soluble in benzene, chloroform, pyridine, toluene, slightly soluble in acetic acid, ethyl acetate, and ethyl ether, and insoluble in water.

(4) Emodin monoglucoside: light yellow needle crystal (precipitating in dilute ethanol, containing crystal water), m. p. 190~191℃.

(5) Resveratrol: colorless needle crystal, m. p. 256~257℃, 216℃, 264℃, it can be sublimated and is easily soluble in ethyl ether, chloroform, methanol, ethanol, acetone, etc.

(6) Polydatin (or piceid): colorless needle crystal, m. p. 223~226℃ (decomposition). It is easily soluble in methanol, ethanol, acetone, hot water, and soluble in acid ethyl

ester, Na_2CO_3 and NaOH aqueous solution, slightly soluble in cold water, and hardly soluble in ether.

1. Experimental Purpose

(1) Master the method of extracting hydroxyanthraquinones from polygonum cuspidate.

(2) Be familiar with the general operation technology of separating mixed hydroxyanthraquinones with silica gel column chromatography.

(3) Be familiar with main distinguishing reactions of hydroxyanthraquinone compounds.

2. Experimental Principle

This experiment is based on the property that free anthraquinones ingredients can dissolve in aqueous chloroform. Firstly, keep the material wet with strong acid solution, add aqueous chloroform for reflux extraction which can make combined anthraquinone (glycosides) ingredients hydrolyzed to free anthraquinone. In this way, the hydrolyzed anthraquinone along with the original existing free anthraquinone will be extracted by aqueous chloroform. Also according to the property that anthraquinone ingredients in polygonum cuspidate can dissolve in ethanol, use ethanol to extract it, and reflux with aqueous chloroform on the basis of the principle that free anthraquinones are soluble in hot aqueous chloroform, so that free anthraquinone, anthraquinone glycoside and other alcohol-soluble impurities with high polarity are separated respectively.

Hydroxyanthraquinone compounds have different acid-base properties. They can be separated, because those containing carboxyl group or many β-phenol hydroxyl groups can dissolve in sodium bicarbonate solution, and those containing one β-phenol hydroxyl group can dissolve in sodium carbonate solution, so the pH gradient method can be used to achieve separation. In addition, we can use silica gel column chromatography to achieve separation according to different polarities of different compounds. For example, because the polarity of emodin is higher than that of physcion, which leads to the tighter adsorption, emodin is eluted after physcion.

3. Experimental Procedure

3.1 Extraction of Free Anthraquinone

Method 1: Take 50 g coarse powder of polygonum cuspidate, add 50 ml 10% sulfuric acid solution, stir it and mix fully, and add 200 ml chloroform for reflux extraction in hot water bath for one hour, then filter it and get chloroform filtrate. The residue continues to be extracted as before with 200 ml chloroform for one hour, and then filter it. Combine two chloroform extracts in a round bottom flask, put several zeolites in it, recover the chloroform and dry in water bath (also under reduced pressure), and get red brown residue. Then put 30 ml benzene solution into a round bottom flask for reflux extraction in water bath for half an hour, filter it, shift benzene filtrate to an evaporating dish, add 3~5 g silica powder which is used in column chromatography, stir evenly and dry it in a ventilated place, and get even sample powder for column chromatography separation.

Method 2: Take 50 g coarse powder of polygonum cuspidate, add 500 ml 95% ethanol in it for reflux extraction for one hour, pour out the liquid, add 400 ml ethanol to extract for half an hour, combine two extracts, filter it, recover the filtrate until it has no alcohol, add 100 ml aqueous chloroform for the one-hour reflux extraction, and pour out the chloroform (if chloroform extract has deep color, then extract once more). Combine the extract, add 50 ml water in a separating funnel and rinse it for 2～3 times, then concentrate the chloroform to about 10 ml, pour it into a small conical flask while still hot, place it for crystallization and air pump filtration, and get the orange free anthraquinone.

3.2 Separation of Emodin with Column Chromatography

(1) Packing column: Take 10～15 g 100～160 mesh silica powder used for column chromatography, add it in a 20 mm×300 mm chromatography column whose bottom is covered with refined cotton, tap chromatography column lightly to make the silica gel powder in the column even, and then get a chromatography column filled with dry silica gel.

(2) Separation: Take the mixing powder of free anthraquinone and silica gel, add it into the top of the silica gel chromatography column carefully, tap it lightly to make the sample powder flat, and open the lower piston of the column. Add suitable benzene slowly to make the benzene slowly permeate the column, and then elute using benzene as eluent and collect the eluent with a conical flask under the column. After eluting for a white, we can see gradually a red ribbon and a brown ribbon in the upper of the silica gel column. When two ribbons are separated larger distance (more than 2 cm), continue to elute with ethyl acetate-benzene (2:8). Change the collection vessel and wait for the outflow of the first ribbon, control the rate of flow and collect the effluent liquid (15 ml each portion), and number each portion consecutively until two ribbons are all eluted. Check each portion by thin layer chromatography, combine them with the same spots, and respectively recover the solvent and concentrate it. Stand a while for crystallization, filter it and respectively collect the crystal. Physcion is eluted firstly, and emodin is eluted at last.

3.3 pH Gradient Separation of Emodin

Add about 100 ml ether in the anthraquinone, dissolve it completely (or use directly the chloroform extract), and then add 5% sodium carbonate solution to extract it for several times (20～30 ml every time) until the color is light red. Combine the extract, add hydrochloric acid to pH 2～3, precipitate out all emodin. Filter and rinse it, then drop dilute ethanol and rinse it by pumping. Crude emodin is recrystallized by pyridine or glacial acetic acid. Acidizing the extracted ether liquid by sodium carbonate (the method is the same with the above treatment of sodium carbonate solution) may get physion and other faintly acid anthraquinone ingredients.

3.4 Identification of Emodin

(1) Melting point: 256～257℃.

(2) Alkaline reaction: Take a little emodin, add 2 ml ethanol to dissolve it, and then add 2～3 drops of sodium hydroxide solution. The emodin solution turns red immediately,

but adding dilute hydrochloric acid to acid makes red disappear.

(3) Magnesium acetate reaction: Take a little emodin, add 2 ml ethanol to dissolve it, add several drops of magnesium acetate solution, and it turns orange red (or purple).

(4) Identification of TLC.

Adsorbent: silica gel-CMC thin layer plate.

Developer: benzene-ethyl acetate (8:2).

Reference substance: 1% emodin alcohol solution or 1% physcion solution.

Sample: 1% emodin alcohol solution and 1% physcion solution.

Chromogenic reagent: Observe under natural light firstly, and then observe after fumigating with ammonia.

4. Notice

(1) In the method of free anthraquinones extraction, combined hydroxyanthraquinone ingredients insoluble in chloroform are not extracted. Using 10% sulfuric acid and chloroform for reflux extraction in method one has the purpose of making combined anthraquinones change into free anthraquinones which are easy to be extracted by chloroform. In this way the anthraquinone ingredients are extracted completely.

(2) The dosage of silica gel in column chromatography depends on the content of the sample. The ratio of sample to adsorbent is 1:100 in general. But low dosage triggers poor separation effect. Excessive dosage certainly needs longer column which cause slower elution velocity.

(3) Wet column method needs to add benzene liquid in a chromatography column, then add silica gel through a funnel, and always keep benzene on the surface of silica gel. Dry column method is that add anthraquinones in a little acetone, add silica gel with lower activity, mix it evenly and stand a while. After removing the solvent under the condition of natural evaporation or at low temperature, add it to the top of column, and then elute with benzene.

(4) Using silica gel column chromatography to separate them is difficult because of the similar polarity of chrysophanol and physcion. If taking calcium hydrogen phosphate as adsorbent and petroleum ether as eluent, we can elute the chrysophanol and physcion in turn.

(5) According to general conventional column operation, this experiment should first use benzene to elute physcion, and then use the mixed solvent of benzene and ethyl acetate to elute emodin. But it was not necessary to change solvent after eluting all physcion in order to accelerate the progress of the experiment. In fact, we can change solvent so long as two ribbons are separated apparently.

(6) Ethyl ether is used many times in the experiment. Therefore, we must pay particular attention to prevent fire and absolutely forbid using ethyl ether near an open fire.

5. Experimental Supplies and Arrangement of Class Hour

Experimental supplies: crude powder of polygonum cuspidate, chloroform saturated by water, benzene, ethanol, silica gel for column chromatography (100~160 mesh), silica gel-CMC hard plate, benzene-ethyl acetate (8 : 2), ethyl ether, sodium carbonate, sodium hydroxide, hydrochloric acid, spot plate, 1000 ml round bottom flask, evaporating dish, chromatography column, test tubes, pear-shaped separatory funnel, refined cotton, circulating water pump, rotary evaporator, electric heating-jacket, water bath.

Arrangement of class hour: to be completed within 6 class hours.

6. Questions

(1) What properties do hydroxyanthraquinone ingredients have? According to its property, please explain the principle of extraction and separation.

(2) What is the principle of emodin's lye reaction and magnesium acetate reaction?

New Words and Phrases

detoxification [diːtɒksɪfɪ'keɪʃən] *n.* 消毒
staphylococcus [ˌstæfələʊ'kɒkəs] *n.* 葡萄球菌
flaky ['fleɪkɪ] *adj.* 薄片的;成片的
sublimate ['sʌblɪmət] *n.* 升华物
spot plate 滴试板
polygonum cuspidate 虎杖
sodium bicarbonate 碳酸氢钠,小苏打
heating-jacket 加热套
phlegm [flem] *n.* 冷静;镇定

Section 4 Flavonoids

Experiment Extraction, Isolation and Identification of Rutin

Rutin is also called rutinoside which widely exists in plant kingdom and is highly contained in the sophora flower bud and buckwheat leaves (see fig. 4-11) which can be used as the raw material of rutin extraction. Quercetin is called rutin aglycone, which can be made by the hydrolysis of rutin.

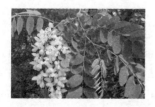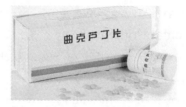

Fig. 4-11 **Sophora flower and its preparatim**

Flos sophora is the flower bud of *Sophora japonica* L. from legume plant, which was taken as hemostatic in ancient time. Rutin has the effect of reducing capillary permeability and is taken as effective adjunctive drug for prevention and control of hypertension in clinic. In addition, it has a certain therapeutic effect on some hemorrhage diseases caused by the radioactive hazard.

The content of rutin in flos sophora reaches 20%. It contains some saponins which can be hydrolyzed into betulin ($C_{30}H_{50}O_2$) and sophoradiol ($C_{30}H_{50}O_2$).

(1) Rutin: It is light yellow fine needle crystal, whose molecular formula is $C_{27}H_{36}O_{16} \cdot 3H_2O$. It has the following physical properties: melting point of 177~178℃, anhydride's melting point of 190℃ (incomplete), foaming and decomposition at 214~215℃. Rutin is soluble in hot water (1:200), hardly soluble in cold water (1:8000), and soluble in hot methanol (1:7), cold methanol (1:100), hot ethanol (1:30), cold ethanol (1:300). But it is hardly soluble in ethyl acetate, acetone and insoluble in benzene, chloroform, ether and petroleum ether etc. Rutin is soluble in the lye, which shows yellow and separates out after acidification.

Rutin

(2) Quercetin: Quercetin is a rutin aglycone, which is yellow crystal and has the molecular fomula of $C_{15}H_{10}O_7 \cdot 2H_2O$. It has the following physical properties: melting point of 313~314℃, anhydride's melting point of 316℃. It is soluble in hot ethanol (1:23), cold ethanol (1:300), glacial acetic acid, ethyl acetate, acetone and other solvents. It is insoluble in petroleum ether, benzene, ethyl ether, chloroform and water.

1. Experimental Purpose

(1) Master the principle and method of extracting flavonoid glycosides by alkali-solution and acid-isolation.

(2) Learn methods of extraction and separation of flavonoids ingredients, taking rutin as an example.

(3) Master the main properties of flavone ingredients and the identification methods of flavonoid glycoside, aglycone and sugar.

2. Experimental Principle

According to the properties of rutin such as containing many phenolic hydroxyls, showing acidity, soluble in basic aqueous solution, and hardly soluble in acid water, we can extract it from plants. In addition, we can also extract it with the water or alcohol according to its good solubility in water or alcohol.

3. Experimental Procedure

3.1 Extraction

Weigh 1~1.5 g lime powder, place it in a dry mortar, add 10 ml water and grind into emulsion for storage. Then take 20 g flos sophora, place it in a dry mortar and grind into coarse powder, shift it to a 500 ml beaker, add boiling 400 ml 0.4% borax aqueous solution, stir it and add the former lime milk to adjust the pH to 8~9, heat it for 30 min under slight boiling state, replenish the evaporated water, stand for 5~10 min, pour out the supernatant, and filter it with a gauze. Extract the residue once again, combine the filtrate, cool it to 60~70℃, adjust pH to 4~5 with hydrochloric acid, add 8 drops chloroform, stand for all the night, filter it with an air pump, wash 3~4 times with water, dry it in the air, and get the crude rutin.

3.2 Recrystallization

Take 2 g crude rutin, add 400 ml deionized water or distilled water, heat the water and keep boiling for 15 min, filter it immediately, stand overnight for crystallization (or cool it to crystallization), filter it with an air pump, and get refined rutin.

3.3 Hydrolysis of Rutin

Take 1 g rutin, add 80 ml 2% H_2SO_4, reflux them for 0.5~1 h with boiling water. Clear solution will be seen after heating for 10 minutes, gradually quercetin which is a yellow small needle crystal will precipitate, crystallize with an air pump (preserving 20 ml filtrate for checking monosaccharide), and wash out the acid with some water, then recrystallize with 10 ml 95% ethanol, and identify it by TLC.

3.4 Identification of Rutin, Quercetin and Sugar

(1) Physical and chemical reaction: Rutin belongs to flavonoid glycosides and has general reaction of flavonoid glycosides.

①Molisch reaction: Take a little rutin in a tube, add 0.5 ml ethanol to dissolve it, put it in equivalent 1% α-naphthol ethanol solution, shake it for a while, then add 0.5 ml sulfuric acid along with tube wall (don't shake after adding it), and observe whether a purple ring appears in the liquid interface.

②Fehling's reaction: Take a little rutin in a tube, add 0.5 ml ethanol to dissolve it, then add 1 ml Fehling reagent, heat it in a boiling water bath, and observe whether brick red precipitate appears. If not, add 1 ml concentrated hydrochloric acid, heat it for half an hour in water bath, and observe whether the precipitation appears or not. If it appears, remove it by filtering, add sodium hydroxide solution to alkaline, then add 1 ml Fehling reagent, heat it in a boiling water bath, and observe whether brick red precipitate appears.

③Hydrochloric acid-magnesium powder reaction: Take a little rutin in a tube, add 5 ml ethanol to dissolve it, take it in hot water, add a little magnesium powder, and then drop several drops of concentrated hydrochloric acid, heat it slightly, and observe the change of color.

④Iron trichloride reaction: Take a little rutin, dissolve it in water or ethanol, add one drop of 1% iron trichloride ethanol solution, and observe the change of color. It can also be done on the filter paper.

⑤Aluminium trichloride reaction: Drop some rutin ethanol solution on the filter paper, observe fluorescent under the UV lamp, then spray 1% aluminium chloride methanol solution, and observe fluorescent under the UV lamp (365nm) once again.

(2) TLC.

Sample: homemade rutin, quercetin.

Reference substance: rutin, quercetin.

Developer and color: take n-butyl alcohol-acetic acid-water (4 : 1 : 5 upper layer or 4 : 1 : 1), observe the color under visible light, and then observe the color under UV light; take 25% acetic acid solution, and observe the color after fumigating it with ammonia; take 85% acetic acid solution, and observe the color after spraying aluminium chloride reagent.

(3) Identification of sugar.

① TLC method: Take 20 ml the former hydrolysis filtrate, add fine powder (2.6 g) of $Ba(OH)_2$ and neutralize to pH 7, filter the generated precipitate of $BaSO_4$, and concentrate the filtrate to about 1 ml for dropping the sample.

Developer: n-butanol-acetic acid-water (4 : 1 : 5 upper layer or 4 : 1 : 1).

Reference substance: glucose and rhamnose solution.

Chromogenic agent: aniline-phthalic acid (bake for ten minutes at 105℃ after spraying the chromogenic reagent, and the brown or brown-red spots arise).

② Method of circular filter paper: Take 10 ml the former filtrate, add fine powder of $Ba(OH)_2$ (mix about 1～1.5 g barium hydroxide with 10 ml water, stir them evenly to emulsion) and neutralize to pH 7, filter the generated precipitate of $BaSO_4$, and concentrate the filtrate to about 1 ml for dropping the sample. Then take a circular filter paper, draw three straight lines through the center with a pencil and get six equal parts. Respectively drop the filtrate and reference substance of glucose and rhamnose solution in the spots at a distance (>0.5 mm) from the center. Tube a small filter paper, insert it into the former center to form capillary action, and then make a radial development with the developer of n-butanol-acetic acid-water (4 : 1 : 5, upper layer).

4. Experimental Supplies and Arrangement of Class Hour

Experimental supplies: beaker (100 ml, 500 ml); round bottom flask (100 ml, 150 ml); condenser pipe; suction flask; circulating water pump; UV lamp; 0.4% borax aqueous solution; lime milk; ethanol, methanol; 2% sulphuric acid, hydrochloric acid; barium hydrate; aluminium muriate; n-butanol : acetic acid : water (4 : 1 : 5 upper layer or 4 : 1 : 1); 25% acetic acid; 85% acetic acid; ethanol-water (7 : 3); reference substance of rutin, quercetin, glucose and rhamnose.

Arrangement of class hour: to be completed within 9～12 class hours.

5. Questions

(1) What structural unit of the rutin does Molisch reaction identify?

(2) If a compound shows positive in the above examination reaction, can we prove it is rutin? why?

(3) What is the result when rutin isn't hydrolyzed completely? What is the hydrolysis product?

（4）What is the factors of impacting output and quality in the process of rutin extraction? Why do we add borax solution?

New Words and Phrases

  rutin ['ru:tɪn] *n.* 芦丁
  sophora 槐属
  hemostatic [ˌhi:mə'stætɪk] *adj.* 止血的
           n. 止血剂
  flos [flɒs] *n.* 花
  hypertension [ˌhaɪpə'tenʃən] *n.* 高血压；过度紧张
  hemorrhage ['hemərɪdʒ] *n.* （尤指大量的）出血，失血
         vi. 大出血
  betulin ['betjʊlɪn] *n.* 桦木脑，桦木醇，白桦脂醇
  sophoradiol [səʊfə'reɪdɪəʊl] *n.* 槐花二醇
  anhydride [æn'haɪdraɪd] *n.* 酐
  lye [laɪ] *n.* 碱液
     vt. 用碱液洗涤
  flavonoid ['fleɪvənɒɪd] *n.* 类黄酮
  lime powder 石灰粉末
  borax ['bɔ:ræks] *n.* 硼砂
  crude [kru:d] *adj.* 粗糙的，粗杂的；天然的，未加工的
      n. 原材料，天然物质
  refined [rɪ'faɪnd] *adj.* 精炼的；精制的
       v. 精炼（refine 的过去式和过去分词）；精制
  naphthol ['næfθɒl] *n.* 萘酚
  iron trichloride 三氯化铁
  fumigate ['fju:mɪˌgeɪt] *vt.* 用化学品熏（某物）消毒
  rhamnose ['ræmnəʊs] *n.* 鼠李糖
  glucose ['glu:kəʊs] *n.* 葡萄糖，右旋糖
  sulfate copper 硫酸铜
  potassium sodium tartrate 酒石酸钾钠

Section 5 Terpenoids and Volatile Oil

Experiment 1 Extraction of Limonene from Orange Peel

  Orange peel which is also called yellow peel is the dry peel of fragrant citrus (see fig. 4-12). It is a kind of Chinese medicine that has acrid flavor and slightly bitter taste and the effect of relieving cough and reducing sputum acting on spleen and lung. The content of volatile oil in the peel is $1.5\% \sim 2\%$. Its volatile oil has many chemical components such as decanal, citral, limonene, octyl alcohol, poncirin, hesperidin, and naringin.

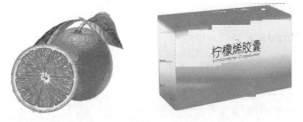

Fig. 4-12 Orange and its preparation

Limonene is also known as carvene whose structure is seen in the following picture. Pure limonene is a colorless liquid whose boiling point is 176～178℃. It has a pleasant smell of lemony aroma which can be used for soft drinks, ice cream, candy, baked goods, etc. It has effects of antitussive, expectorant, and bacteriostasis. In clinical practice, compound limonene is used in choleresis, stone dissolution, promoting the secretion of digest liquid and eliminating gas in the intestines.

Limonene

1. Experimental Purpose

(1) Master the method of extracting the limonene from orange peel.

(2) Be familiar with the general method of studying and identifying the monoterpene.

2. Experimental Principle

Limonene has good volatility, which is used for extraction by steam distillation.

3. Experimental Procedure

Take the peel of two oranges and cut into small pieces, put in a 500 ml three-necked flask, add 200～250 ml hot water in it, extract the limonene by steam distillation until the distillate volume reachs 60 ml. A thin layer of oil substance can be seen on the distillate. Shift the distillate to a separating funnel, extract three times with 10 ml dichloromethane, and combine the extract liquid in 50 ml dry conical flask. Add 2～3 g anhydrous sodium sulfate for dryness, filter and shift the solution to a 50 ml flask, continue to distill, and remove dichloromethane in a water bath. When the dichloromethane is distilled from the solution completely, use water pump to distill the residual dichloromethane in the solution under reduced pressure. At last, residual orange yellow liquid in the flask is orange oil that can be determined by gas chromatography, in which the content of limonene is about 95%. At the same time, you can determine the refractive index and the optical rotation.

4. Notice

(1) It is better to use fresh orange peel, because dried peel will have poor yield.

(2) The measurement of optical rotation should use 5% orange oil solution (diluted

with 95% ethanol). If the orange oil is insufficient, you can collect the extract from several portions. You can take the standard sample for comparison if necessary.

5. Experimental Supplies and Arrangement of Class Hour

Experimental supplies: dichloromethane, anhydrous sodium sulfate, two or three oranges, standard substance of limonene 500 ml three-necked flask, 50 ml conical flask, water bath, steam distillation device, gas chromatograph refractometer, polarimeter, vacuum pump, suction flask, 50 ml flask, buchner funnel, separatory funnel.

Arrangement of class hour: to be completed within 6 class hours.

6. Questions

What is the product of catalytic hydrogenation (two molecules) of d-limestone? Does the product have optical activity? Why?

New Words and Phrases

limonene ['lɪməˌniːn]   *n.* 柠檬烯
citrus ['sɪtrəs]   *n.* 柑橘属果树；柠檬，柑橘
spleen [spliːn]   *n.* 脾脏；坏脾气
meridian [məˈrɪdɪən]   *adj.* 子午线的；最高点的
decanal [dɪˈkeɪn(ə)l]   *n.* 癸醛
citral ['sɪtrəl]   *n.* 柠檬醛
octyl ['ɒktəl]   *n.* 辛基
poncirin [pɒnˈsaɪrɪn]   *n.* 枳属苷
hesperidin [heˈspɛrɪdɪn]   *n.* 橙皮苷
naringin ['nærɪngɪn]   *n.* 柚苷，柚皮苷
antitussive [ˌæntɪˈtʌsɪv]   *n.* 止咳药，镇咳药
　　　　　　　　　　adj. 能止咳的
expectorant [ɪksˈpɛktərənt]   *adj.* 化痰的
　　　　　　　　　　　n. 除痰剂
bacteriostasis [bækˌtɪərɪəˈsteɪsɪs]   *n.* 细菌抑制
choleresis ['kəʊlərəsɪs]   *n.* 胆汁分泌
intestine [ɪnˈtɛstɪn]   *adj.* 内部的；国内的
　　　　　　　　n. 肠
three-necked flask   三颈烧瓶
yield [jiːld]   *n.* 产量，产额
refractometer [ˌriːfrækˈtɒmɪtə]   *n.* 折射计；屈光仪
polarimeter [ˌpəʊləˈrɪmɪtə]   *n.* 偏振器，旋光计
suction flask   吸滤瓶
Buchner funnel   布氏漏斗
catalytic hydrogenation   催化氢化作用

optical rotation 旋光度,旋光性
refractive index 折射率
distillate ['dıstıleıt] n. 馏出物,馏出液

Experiment 2 Extraction, Separation and Identification of Andrographolide from *Andrographis paniculata*

Andrographis comes from the aboveground parts of *Andrographis paniculata* (Burm. f.) Nees in Acanthaceae (see fig. 4-13), which has the effect of clearing away heat, detoxification, diminishing inflammation and relieving pain. It mainly cures bacterial dysentery, urinary tract infection, acute tonsillitis, enteritis, faucitis, pneumonia and influenza. It can also cure the toxicity of sore, furuncle and trauma infection for external use. It contains a variety of diterpenoids compounds such as andrographolide, deoxyandrographolide, neoandrographolide and deoxyandrographolide, etc. Their structures and properties are as follows.

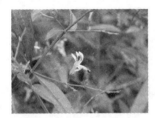

Fig. 4-13 Plant and preparation of andrographis

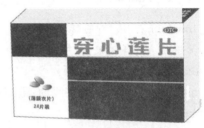

Andrographolide   Deoxyandrographolide   Neoandrographolide   Dehydroandrographolide

(1) Andrographolide: It has the molecular formula of $C_{20}H_{30}O_5$ and molecular weight of 350.44. It is colorless square or rectangle crystal whose flavour is extremely bitter and its melting point is 230~231℃. It is easily soluble in methanol, ethanol, acetone, and pyridine, slightly soluble in chloroform and ether, and hardly soluble in water, petroleum ether and benzene.

(2) Neoandrographolide: It has the molecular formula of $C_{26}H_{40}O_8$ and molecular weight of 480.58. It is colorless columnar crystal which is not bitter and has the melting point of 167~168℃. It is easily soluble in methanol, ethanol, acetone, pyridine, slightly soluble in water, and hardly soluble in benzene, ether, chloroform and petroleum ether.

(3) Deoxyandrographolide: It has the molecular formula of $C_{20}H_{30}O_4$ and molecular weight of 334.44. It is colorless flake crystal (acetone, ethanol or chloroform) or colorless

needle crystal (ethyl acetate) which is slightly bitter and has the melting point of 174~175℃. It is easily soluble in methanol, ethanol, acetone, pyridine, chloroform, soluble in ether, benzene, and slightly soluble in water.

(4) Dehydroandrographolide: It has the molecular formula of $C_{20}H_{28}O_4$ and molecular weight of 332.42. It is colorless needle crystal (30% or 50% ethanol) whose melting point is 204℃. It is easily soluble in ethanol, acetone, soluble in chloroform, slightly soluble in benzene, and almost insoluble in water.

1. Experimental Purpose

(1) Master the principle and method of extracting lipotropy compositions from *Andrographis paniculata* (Burm. f.) Nees.

(2) Be familiar with the principle and method of removing chlorophyll.

(3) Understand the main physical and chemical properties and identification method of lactones.

2. Experimental Principle

This experiment chooses ethanol as the extracting solvent on the basis of its property that lactones from andrographis are easily soluble in methanol, ethanol, and acetone. Andrographis contains a lot of chlorophyll which can be eliminated by activated carbon adsorption. Andrographolide and deoxyandrographolide are separated according to their different solubilities in chloroform. In addition, we can use different polarities of andrographolide, deoxyandrographolide and neoandrographolide to separate them by alumina column chromatography because their structures are difference.

3. Experimental Procedure

3.1 Extraction

Method 1:

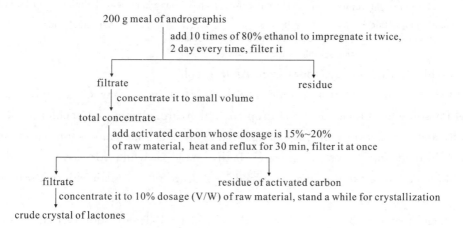

Method 2：

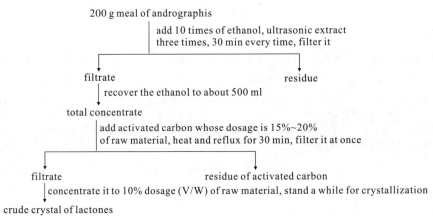

3.2 Purification

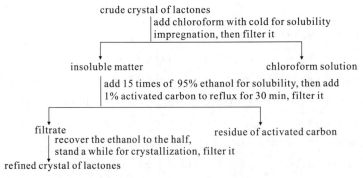

3.3 Separation

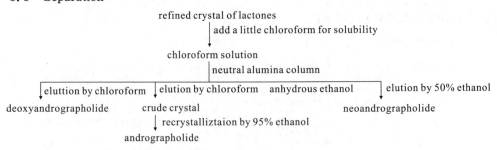

3.4 Identification of Lactones from Andrographis

(1) Hydroxamic acid iron reaction: Take several milligrams of crystal, add 1 ml alcohol for solubility, then add 2~3 drops of 7% hydroxylamine hydrochloride methanol solution, add 1~2 drops of 10% potassium hydroxide methanol solution to make it alkaline, heat it for 2 min in a water bath, stand a while for cooling, add dilute hydrochloric acid to make it acidic, then add 1~2 drops of 1% ferric chloride solution and mix well, so it turns mauve.

(2) Legal reaction: Take a little crystal and add 1 ml alcohol solution, add 2~4 drops of 0.3% nitrosyl iron sodium cyanide solution, then add 1~2 drops of 10% sodium hydroxide solution, so it turns purple.

(3) Kedde reaction: Take a little crystal and add 1 ml alcohol solution for solubility, then add 2 drops of basic 3,5-dinitrobenzoic acid, so it turns purple.

(4) Identification of lactones from andrographis.

　　Thin layer plate: silica gel H-CMC-Na.

　　Sample: ethanol solution of homemade lactones from andrographis.

　　Standard substance: ethanol solution of standard lactones from andrographis.

　　Developer:

　　①chloroform-methanol (9 : 1).

　　②chloroform-normal butanol-methanol (2 : 1 : 2).

　　Chromogenic agent: Spray the Kedde reagent and heat it for color.

4. Notice

(1) Lactone from andrographis is a kind of diterpenoid that has extremely unstable properties which trigger easily oxidation and polymerization to form resinous substances. Therefore, andrographis used for extraction should be new medicinal material produced in current years and the stem or leaf used shouldn't be wet or metamorphic, otherwise the content of lactones will reduce obviously to extremely low which is difficult to be extracted.

(2) During the course of using hot ethanol to extract total lactones from andrographis, many impurities such as chlorophyll, resin and inorganic salt will be extracted, which leads to difficulty of crystallization and purification. Therefore, this experiment uses cold impregnation and ultrasonic oscillation to deal with it.

(3) Crystallization of lactones from andrographis should be done under the condition of high concentration of ethanol, which gets better crystal form and crystal purification. When water content or viscosity of the solution is higher, it is often difficult to get the crystal.

5. Experimental Supplies and Arrangement of Class Hour

Experimental supplies: vacuum concentration device; beaker of 1000 ml, 500 ml, 100 ml, 10 ml; 10 ml tube; test-tube rack; counter balance; cylinder; triangular funnel; washing bottle; buchner funnel; water bath; 10 cm×20 cm thin layer plate; 10 cm×20 cm developing tank; capillary of spotting; UV lamp; glass rod; bone spoon; gauze; adsorbent cotton; spray bottle of chromogenic agent; small-sized air compressor; ultrasonic oscillator; chromatography column (ϕ1.5 cm); coarse powder of andrographis; filter paper; pH test paper; activated carbon; chloroform; neutral alumina used for column chromatography; 7% hydroxylamine hydrochloride methanol solution; potassium hydroxide methanol solution; dilute hydrochloric acid; 1% ferric chloride solution; 0.3% nitrosyl iron sodium cyanide solution; 10% sodium hydroxide solution; alkaline 3,5-dinitrobenzoic acid; silica gel H used for TLC; 0.2% CMC-Na, methanol; standard lactones from andrographis; developer of chloroform-methanol (9 : 1) and chloroform-n-butanol-methanol (2∶1∶2).

Arrangement of class hour: to be completed within 6 class hours.

6. Questions

(1) What other methods can be used for removing chlorophyll besides the method of activated carbon adsorption?

(2) What method can we use to separate total lactones? Try to compare the advantages and disadvantages of each method.

(3) What is the principle of Legal and Kedde reactions? What kind of structure does a compound have to cause positive reaction?

New Words and Phrases

acanthaceae [ˌækænˈθeɪsiː] *n.* 爵床科
andrographolide [ændrəʊgˈræphɒlɪd] *n.* 穿心莲内酯
deoxyandrographolide [diːɒksɪæændrəʊgˈræphɒlɪd] *n.* 去氧穿心莲内酯
neoandrographolide [niːəʊændrəʊgˈræphɒlɪd] *n.* 新穿心莲内酯
deoxyandrographolide [diːɒksɪə ændrəʊ ˈgræphɒlɪd] *n.* 去氧穿心莲内酯
lipotropy [ləˈpɒtrəpɪ] *n.* 抗脂(肪),亲脂
lactone [ˈlæktəʊn] *n.* 内酯
detoxification [diːˌtɒksɪfɪˈkeɪʃən] *n.* 去毒,消毒
dysentery [ˈdɪsənˌteriː] *n.* 痢疾
urinary tract infection 尿路感染
tonsillitis [ˌtɒnsəˈlaɪtɪs] *n.* 扁桃体炎
enteritis [entəˈraɪtɪs] *n.* 小肠炎
aucitis [fɒˈsaɪtɪs] *n.* 咽喉炎
pneumonia [njuːˈməʊnjə] *n.* 肺炎
influenza [ˌɪnflʊˈenzə] *n.* 流行性感冒
sore [sɔː] *adj.* 疼痛的;剧烈的
furuncle [ˈfjuːrʌŋkl] *n.* 疖
trauma [ˈtraʊmə] *n.* 创伤,损伤
diterpenoid [ˈdaɪtəpiːnɔɪd] *n.* 双萜类
impregnation [ˌɪmpregˈneɪʃən] *n.* 怀孕,受精
recover [rɪˈkʌvə] *vt.* 恢复;找回
hydroxylamine hydrochloride 盐酸羟胺
potassium hydroxide 氢氧化钾
nitrosyl [ˈnaɪtrəsɪl] *adj.* 亚硝酰基的
cyanide [ˈsaɪəˌnaɪd] *n.* 氰化物
sodium hydroxide 氢氧化钠
andro [ˈændrəʊ] *n.* 穿心莲内酯;雄烯二酮

dinitrobenzoic 二硝基苯的
resinous [ˈrezɪnəs] *adj.* 树脂的
oscillation [ˌɒsɪˈleɪʃən] *n.* 振荡；振动
viscosity [vɪˈskɒsətɪ] *n.* 黏性，黏度
bone spoon [bəʊn spuːn] *n.* 牛骨匙

Experiment 3 Extraction and Identification of Volatile Oil from Star Anise

Star anise which mainly distributes in Guangxi Province, Guizhou Province and Yunnan Province comes from dry ripe fruit of *Illicium verum* Hook. F. in magnoliaceae (see fig. 4-14). It contains 4%~9% of volatile oil, about 22% of fat oil (mainly exists in seeds) and protein, gum, resin, etc. The main chemical component in volatile oil is anisole, which is about 80%~90% of the total volatile oil. It is also called anethole because of precipitation after cooling. In addition, it still contains shikimic acid and a small amount of methyl chavicol and anisaldehyde, anisic acid, etc. Their structures and properties are as follows:

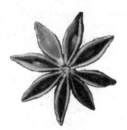
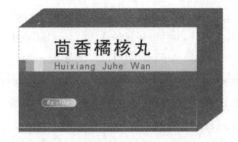

Fig. 4-14 Star anise and its preparation

(1) Anethole: It has the molecular formula of $C_{10}H_{12}O$ and molecular weight of 148.21. It is white crystal whose melting point and boiling point are respectively 21.4℃ and 235℃. It is miscible with ether and chloroform, soluble in benzene, ethylacetate, acetone, carbon disulfide and petroleum ether and almost insoluble in water.

(2) Shikimic acid: It has the molecular formula of $C_7H_{10}O_5$ and molecular weight of 174.15. It is colorless needle crystal (methanol-acetic ester) and has the melting point of 190~191℃. It is easily soluble in water, soluble in ethanol and hardly soluble in chloroform, benzene, petroleum ether.

Anisaldehyde

(3) Methyl chavicol: Molecular formula $C_{10}H_{12}O$, colorless liquid, b. p. 215~216℃.

(4) Anisaldehyde: It has the molecular formula of $C_8H_8O_2$ and two kinds of states: One is edge crystal with the melting point of 36.3℃, the boiling point of 236℃; another is liquid with the melting point of 0℃, the boiling point of 248℃.

(5) Anisic acid: It is a needle crystal and has the molecular formula of $C_8H_8O_3$, whose melting point is 184℃ and boiling point is 275～280℃.

1. Experimental purpose

(1) Master the method of steam distillation extraction of volatile oil.

(2) Be familiar with the qualitative identification of chemical components in volatile oil by TLC.

(3) Understand general identification method of volatile oil and the identification of volatile oil with unidirectional secondary thin layer chromatography.

2. Experimental Principle

Steam distillation is a general method of extracting volatile oil. Because the compositions of volatile oil are complex, which often contain functional groups such as alkane, olefins, alcohol, phenol, aldehyde, ketone, acid, ether etc., we can use some detection reagents in thin layer plate and do dropping tests to learn component types of volatile oil. Different components in volatile oil have different polarities. Generally speaking, hydrocarbons and terpenoids that do not contain oxygen have low polarity so that they are developed by petroleum ether in TLC; then oxygenic hydrocarbons and terpenoids whose polarities are so high that they can't be developed easily by petroleum ether, but they can be developed by the mixed solvent of petroleum ether and ethyl acetate. In order to separated each component of volatile oil in a piece of thin layer chromatography plate, it often can be developed with unidirectional secondary chromatography.

3. Experimental Procedure

3.1 Extraction and Separation of Anethole

Take 50 g coarse powder of star anise and place it in a round bottom flask, add appropriate water for moisture, and extract with general steam distillation. Another method is to shift the pounded star anise to a flask in a determination apparatus of volatile oil, add 500 ml distilled water and several glass beads, connect volatile oil determination apparatus and reflux condenser pipe, add some water from the top of condenser pipe to the graduation, and make the water overflow into the flask. Slowly heat it to boiling, stop heating when oil no longer increases, stand a while for cooling, and separate the oil layer. Put the oil in a refrigerator for 1 h and get white crystal, filter it at once, and squeeze it for dryness with a filter paper. The crystal is anethole, and the filtrate is the star anise oil.

3.2 General Identification

(1) Oil spots test: Take appropriate star anise oil and drop on a filter paper, stand a while at room temperature (or bake it by heating), and observe whether oil spots disappear.

(2) Dropping reaction of TLC plate: Take a silica gel G plate, draw the line as table 4-2, dilute the volatile oil with 5～10 times of ethanol, drop in each row of small grids with a capillary, then drop all kinds of inspection reagent respectively in the sample spots with a

dropper, and observe the color. Infer the type of chemical components of each volatile oil preliminarily.

Tab. 4-2 Dropping reaction of volatile oil in TLC

reagent / sample	1	2	3	4	5	6
star anise oil						
lemon oil						
clove oil						
peppermint oil						
camphor oil						
eucalyptus oil						
turpentine						
blank control						

Reagent
1. ferric trichloride reagent
2. 2,4-dinitrobenzene hydrazine reagent
3. alkalinepotassium permanganate reagent
4. vanillin-concentrated sulfuric acid reagent
5. 0.05% bromophenol blue reagent

(3) Unidirectional secondary developing of TLC: Take a piece of thin layer plate (6 cm×15 cm) of silica gel H-CMC-Na, draw the starting line which is 1.5 cm to the bottom of the plate and the finish line which is 8 cm to the bottom of the plate with a pencil. Dissolve star anise oil in acetone, use a capillary to drop in the starting line and form a long strip, develop to the finish line first with the developer of petroleum ether (30~60℃)-acetic acid ethyl ester (85∶15). Take the plate out, evaporate the developer, and then add the developer of petroleum ether (30~60℃) and develop close to the top of thin layer plate. Take the plate out, evaporate the developer, and spray the following chromogenic agents for color respectively:

①1% Vanillin-sulfuric acid reagent: It can produce purple and red with volatile oil.

②Fluorescein-bromide reagent: It indicates the existence of unsaturated compounds if yellow spots appear.

③2,4-Dinitrobenzene hydrazine reagent: It indicates the existence of aldehydes or ketones if yellow spots appear.

④0.05% Bromocresol green ethanol reagent: It indicates the existence of acid compounds if yellow spots appear.

4. Notice

(1) We can judge whether the volatile oil has been extracted completely by observing the degree of distillate turbidity. The original distillate has more oil which makes it obviously cloudy. With the reduction of oil dosage in distillate medium, turbidity also reduces until the distillate turns clear and even has no smell of volatile oil. We can stop distillation at this time.

(2) We should place the extract for cooling after extracting until oil and water are separated completely. Remove the oil layer and do not take out the water if possible.

(3) During the course of unidirectional secondary developing, we should use firstly the developer of high polarity, and then the developers of low polarity to develop. You should evaporate all the developer of the first developing to dryness, otherwise it will affect the polarity of second developer and the separation effect.

(4) Because volatile oil is easy to evaporate, the operation should be quick and timely during the course of TLC inspection.

(5) Spraying the chromogenic agent of vanillin-concentrated sulfuric acid should be done in the draught cupboard; don't operate in acidic conditions when using bromocresol green reagent.

5. Experimental Supplies and Arrangement of Class Hour

Experimental supplies: 100 ml and 10 ml beaker; 250 ml triangle flask; 10 ml test tube; test tube rack; counter balance; cylinder; washing bottle; distillation device; electric jacket; thin layer plate of 10 cm×20 cm; developing tank; capillary of dropping samples; UV lamp; glass rod; bone spoon; spray bottle of chromogenic agent; small-sized air compressor; coarse powder of star anise; filter paper; ferric trichloride reagent; 2,4-dinitrobenzene hydrazine reagent; alkaline potassium permanganate reagent; vanillin-concentrated sulfuric acid reagent (preparation before use); 0.05% bromophenol blue reagent; lemon oil; clove oil; peppermint oil; camphor oil; eucalyptus oil; turpentine; acetone; petroleum ether (30~60℃); ethyl acetate.

Arrangement of class hour: to be completed within 6 class hours.

6. Questions

(1) What is the principle of extracting and separating anethole from the star anise?

(2) What are the advantages of using dropping reaction to indentify general volatile oil?

(3) Why is the polarity of developer used at first time higher than that used at second time during the course of unidirectional secondary developing used for TLC detection of volatile components? What are the advantages of unidirectional secondary developing in TLC?

New Words and Phrases

star anise [stɑː ænɪs] 八角；大茴香

magnoliaceae [mæɡˈnəʊljəsiː] *n.* 木兰科

anethole [ˈænəθəʊl] *n.* 茴香脑

shikimic acid 莽草酸

methylchavicol 甲基胡椒酚

anisaldehyde [ˌænɪˈsældəhaɪd] *n.* 茴香醛

anisic acid 茴香酸

carbon disulfide 二硫化碳

unidirectional [ˌjuːnɪdɪˈrekʃənəl] *adj.* 单向的，单向性的

alkane [ˈælkeɪn] *n.* 链烷，烷烃

olefin [ˈəʊləfɪn] *n.* 烯烃，链烯

aldehyde [ˈældɪhaɪd] *n.* 醛，乙醛

oxygenic [ˌɒksɪˈdʒenɪk] *adj.* 氧的；含氧的

hydrocarbon [ˌhaɪdrəˈkɑːbən] *n.* 碳氢化合物

acetic acid ethyl ester 乙酸乙酯
vanillin ['vænɪlɪn] *n.* 香草醛
bromide ['brəʊˌmaɪd] *n.* 溴化物
dinitrobenzene [daɪˌnaɪtrəʊ'benziːn] *n.* 二硝基苯
hydrazine ['haɪdrəziːn] *n.* 肼,联氨
bromocresol [brɒmɒkrɪspl] *n.* 溴甲酚
turbidity 混浊度;浊度
finish line 终点线
vanillin [və'nɪlɪn] *n.* 香草醛,香兰素
draught cupboard 通风橱
counter balance 托盘天平
peppermint oil 薄荷油

Experiment 4 Extraction, Isolation and Purification of Geniposide from Gardenia

Gardenia comes from the dry ripe fruit of *Gardenia jasminoides* Ellis in rubiaceae (see fig. 4-15). It is bitter and cold in nature and innocuity. It has the effect of clearing heat, purging fire and cooling blood, which mainly cure the diseases of heating vacuity vexation and insomnia, jaundice, conjunctival congestion, pharynx pain, hematuria, sprain swelling and pain, etc. Its main chemical compositions have three types as follows: iridoid glycosides, organic acids and pigments. Gardenia contains a large number of iridoid glycosides which are mainly geniposides, also called gardenosides, which have the effect of anti-inflammatory, antipyretic, cholagogue and laxation effect, etc.

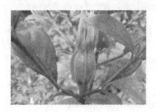
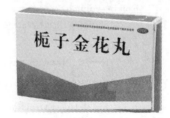

Fig. 4-15 Plant and preparation of Gardenia

Geniposide which has molecular formula of $C_{17}H_{24}O_{10}$ and melting point of 161~162℃ is colorless needle crystal and bitter. It is soluble in ethanol, water; slightly soluble in ethyl acetate, acetone, ether and carbon tetrachloride, and insoluble in chloroform, petroleum ether.

Geniposide

1. Experimental Purpose

(1) Master the principle and method of separating compounds by column chromatography of macroporous adsorption resin.

(2) Understand the method of using magnesia to adsorb and separate compounds.

2. Experimental Principle

Macroporous adsorption resin which is a kind of polymer adsorbent that does not contain exchange group and has macroporous structure is also a kind of lipophilic material. We can use macroporous adsorption resin to adsorb lower polarity compounds and remove hydrosoluble impurities such as sugar, and achieve the purpose of separation and purification through the gradient alcohol elution.

There are two types of methods of using the adsorption to separate and purify traditional Chinese medicine composition: one is to adsorb the separated and requisite materials, but does not adsorb impurities; the other is to adsorb impurities. Magnesium oxide is one of the commonly used adsorbent, which is used to adsorb requisite materials in this experiment.

3. Experimental Procedure

3.1 The Process of Extraction and Separation (see fig. 4-16)

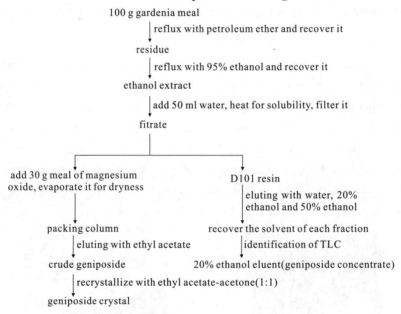

Fig. 4-16 Extraction and purification of geniposide

(1) Extraction: Take 100 g gardenia and put in a 1000 ml round bottom flask, add 200 ml petroleum ether to reflux 0.5 h, filter it with a vacuum pump. Add 200 ml 95% ethanol and reflux three times, 30 min each time, combine the extract, recover the ethanol at reduced pressure, and get the ethanol extract. Heat the ethanol extract for solubility, filter it, and get the filtrate which can be used in the following two experiments.

(2) Column chromatography of macroporous adsorption resin.

Pretreatment: Take a glass chromatography column of 1.8 cm × 28 cm, take 25 g D101 macroporous adsorption resin, add some water impregnate it for 30 min, pour it into the column, elute with 95% ethanol until the solution is not muddy after adding two times of water, and then rinse the column with water to remove the redundant alcohol for reservation.

Adding sample: Add prepared sample to the top of the column.

Elution: Elute by water firstly, detect the carbohydrate of effluent with Molisch reaction until the reaction has no carbohydrate or color is very weak, and then stop elution. Elute with 20% ethanol and 50% ethanol in turn, change the eluent when Molisch reaction shows negative. Concentrate three fractions at reduced pressure, and identify by TLC compared with standard substance. Geniposide mainly exists in 20% alcohol eluent, and get geniposide concentrate. In addition, there is also a small amount of geniposide in the water, but not in 50% ethanol elution solution.

(3) Magnesia adsorption: Take the filtrate into an evaporation pan, add 30 g magnesium oxide, evaporate to dryness at 60℃ in a water bath, and get magnesium oxide powder which is absorbed by the sample. Then load magnesia in a chromatography column, elute by 500 ml ethyl acetate, recover the solvent at reduced pressure, concentrate and recrystallize it in ethyl acetate-acetone (1 : 1), and get purified geniposide.

3.2　Identification by Silica Gel TLC

Sample: homemade and standard geniposide.

Developer: ethyl acetate-acetone-formic acid-water (5 : 3 : 1 : 1 or 5 : 5 : 1 : 1).

Chromogenic reagent:

①50% sulfuric acid ethanol solution.

②Ehrlich's reagent: Take 0.25 g paradimethylaminobenzaldehyde and dissolve in 50 g glacial acetic acid, 5 g 85% phosphoric acid and 20 ml water, and preserve it in a brown bottle.

4. Experimental Supplies and Arrangement of Class Hour

Experimental supplies: gardenia meal; round bottom flask; petroleum ether; vacuum pump; 95% ethanol; glass chromatography column; D_{101} macroporous resin; ethyl acetate; acetone; formic acid; sulfuric acid; glacial acetic acid; phosphoric acid.

Arrangement of class hour: to be completed within 6 class hours.

5. Questions

(1) What is the principle of separating compounds by macroporous adsorption?

(2) Why is there geniposide in water eluent?

(3) What is the principle of separation and purification with magnesia?

New Words and Phrases

gardenia [gɑːˈdiːnɪə]　*n.*　栀子

rubiaceae　茜草科

innocuity [ˌɪnəˈkjuːɪtɪ]　*n.*　无害；无毒

vacuity [væˈkjuːɪtɪ]　*n.*　空白；真空

vexation [vekˈseɪʃən]　*n.*　烦恼；恼火

insomnia [ɪnˈsɒmnɪə]　*n.*　失眠症

jaundice ['dʒɔːndɪs] n. 黄疸病
conjunctival [,kɒndʒʌŋk'taɪvə] adj. 结膜的
congestion [kən'dʒestʃən] n. 拥塞；充血
pharynx ['færɪŋks] n. 咽
hematuria [,hiːmə'tjʊrɪə] n. 血尿症
sprain [spreɪn] vt. 扭伤（关节）
iridoid [ɪərɪ'dɒɪd] n. 环烯醚萜苷；环烯醚萜
antipyretic [,æntɪpaɪ'retɪk] adj. 退热的，退烧的
cholagogue ['kɒləgɒg] n. 利胆剂
laxation [læk'seɪʃən] n. 松弛；松懈
magnesia [mæg'niːʃə] n. 氧化镁
polymer ['pɒləmə] n. 多聚物；聚合物
lipophilic [,lɪpə'fɪlɪk] adj. 亲脂性的
hydrosoluble [,haɪdrə'sɒljuːbl] n. 水溶（性）的
muddy ['mʌdɪ] adj. 泥泞的；模糊的
geniposide [dʒenɪ'pəʊsaɪd] n. 京尼平苷
paradimethylaminobenzaldehyde 对二甲氨基苯甲醛

Section 6　Triterpenoids

Experiment 1　Extraction and Identification of Glycyrrhizic Acid

Glycyrrhizic acid is a main effective ingredient in root or rhizome from *G. uralensis* Fisch., *G. inflata* Bat. or *G. glabra* L. (see fig. 4-17) Its content is about 7%～10%, which tastes very sweet and is also known as glycyrrhizin. In addition, liquorice also contains a variety of flavonoid constituents, such as liquiritigenin, isoliquiritigenin, liquritin, neoliquiritin, and neoisoliquiritin. Modern pharmacological studies show that liquorice preparations and glycyrrhizic acid have adrenal cortical hormone-like effect; Glycyrrhizic acid also has the effect of detoxification whose mechanism is that glycyrrhizin's hydrolysate can produce glucuronic acid which can integrate with toxicant. Accordingly, it has a good effect on peptic ulcer in clinic.

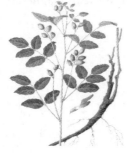
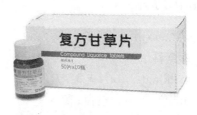

Fig. 4-17　Plant and preparation of Liquorice

1. Experimental Purpose

(1) Master the principle and method of extracting glycyrrhizic acid.

(2) Be familiar with the nature and identification of saponins.

2. Experimental Principle

Glycyrrhizic acid is a white columnar crystal (glacial acetic acid) whose melting point is 170℃. It is soluble in hot water, hot dilute ethanol, acetone and insoluble in ethanol and ether. It can be hydrolyzed into glycyrrhetinic acid and two molecules of glucuronic acid under the action of heat, pressure, and dilute acid.

Structural formula of glycyrrhizic acid

The principle of its extraction and purification is as follows: Glycyrrhizic acid exists in the form of potassium or calcium salt in raw materials. Because its salt is soluble in water, we can extract it with warm water and get glycyrrhetate, and then add sulfuric acid to precipitate glycyrrhizic acid which is difficult to dissolve in cold acid. Glycyrrhizic acid can dissolve in acetone, and then add potassium hydroxide to produce the crystal of tripotassium glycyrrhetate which is hard to be preserved because of moisture adsorption. We can add glacial acetic acid to make it turn into glycyrrhizic acid salt containing one potassium which has a fine crystalline and is easy to be preserved.

3. Experimental Procedure

3.1 Extraction of Glycyrrhizic Acid

Take 20 g licorice, add 150 ml water, percolate it in a water bath for 30 minutes. Filter it with cotton, and extract the residue once again with 100 ml water. Combine the filtrate and concentrate it to 40 ml, filter and remove the sediment, stand a while for cooling and add concentrated sulfuric acid, and stir it constantly until the precipitate of glycyrrhizic acid doesn't emerge. Stand a while and pour out the supernatant, rinse the lower brown viscous precipitate for four times, dry at room temperature, grind it into fine powder, and get crude glycyrrhizic acid.

Put the crude glycyrrhizic acid in a round bottom flask, reflux for 1 h with 50 ml ethanol, filter it, add 30 ml ethanol to the residue and reflux for 30 min, filter it and combine the filtrate, concentrate it to 20 ml, and cool it off. Add 20% KOH ethanol solution until it no longer has precipitate, and stir it simultaneously. Adjust pH value of the solution to 8, stand for a while and filter it, get precipitation of tripotassium glycyrrhetate dry in a desiccator and weigh it.

Put tripotassium glycyrrhetate in a small beaker, add 15 ml glacial acetic acid, heat it on a water bath for solubility, filter it at once, and add a little hot glacial acetic acid to rinse glycyrrhizic acid of the adsorption on the filter paper, cool it off and produce white crystal, filter it with a vacuum pump, rinse it with absolute alcohol, and get milky glycyrrhizic acid salt with monopotassium.

3.2 Experiments of Property and Chromatographic Examination

(1) Foam experiment: Take 2 ml of the aqueous solution of glycyrrhizic acid salt with monopotassium to a test tube, shake vigorously, stand a while for 10 min, and observe the foam.

(2) Reaction of acetic anhydride-concentrated sulfuric acid (Liebermann-Burchard reaction): Take a little glycyrrhizic acid salt with monopotassium to a white board, add 2~3 drops of ethylic acid for solubility, and then add half drop of concentrated sulfuric acid and observe the color change.

(3) Reaction of chloroform-concentrated sulfuric acid: Take a little glycyrrhizic acid salt and add 1 ml chloroform, and then add 1 ml concentrated sulfuric acid along the test wall; observe the color change and fluorescence in two layers of solution.

(4) Thin layer chromatography.

Adsorbent: silica gel G plate (activated at 100℃ for half an hour).

Developing solvent: n-butanol-acetic acid-water (6∶1∶3 upper layer).

Sample: standard glycyrrhizic acid salt with monopotassium, 70% ethanol solution of glycyrrhizic acid salt with monopotassium.

Chromogenic reagent: phospho-molybdic acid.

4. Notice

(1) Tripotassium glycyrrhetate must be preserved in a dryer because of its easily moisture adsorption.

(2) The developer must be evaporated to dryness before the color reaction in TLC.

5. Experimental Supplies and Arrangement of Class Hour

Experimental supplies: licorice, cotton, concentrated sulfuric acid, round bottom flask, reflux device, KOH, ethanol, pH test paper, beaker, glacial acetic acid, water bath, vacuum pump, chloroform.

Arrangement of class hour: to be completed within 6 class hours.

6. Questions

(1) What are color reactions of glycyrrhizic acid?

(2) During the course of extracting glycyrrhizic acid, what's the purpose of adding concentrated sulfuric acid?

New Words and Phrases

rhizome ['raɪzəʊm]   n. 根茎,根状茎
liquorice ['lɪkərɪs]   n. 甘草,甘草根
peptic ulcer   胃溃疡
desiccator   ['desɪkeɪtə]   n. 干燥器
viscous ['vɪskəs]   adj. 黏性的;半流体的

Experiment 2 Extraction, Isolation and Identification of Oleanolic Acid

Ligustrum lucidum as a Chinese medicine of strengthening and consolidating body resistance comes from the dry mature fruit of *Ligustrum lucidum* Ait. (see fig. 4-19) Its components of enhancing immune function are oleanolic acid, ursolic acid and acetyloleanolic acid. Then it still contains oleuropein, D-mannitol, stearic acid and vegetable wax. Oleanolic acid is pentacyclic triterpenoid compound which is widely distributed in the plant kingdom and exists in more than 150 kinds of plants in the form of free state, ester and glycoside. For example, it exists in the form of free state and combined with glycosides in *Ligustrum lucidum*. Its content of oleanolic acid is highest in august and reach 8.04%, but its content declines to about 2.5% with the mature of fruit.

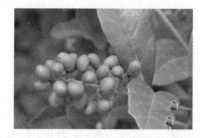
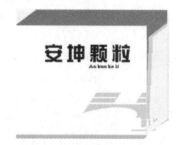

Fig. 4-18 Plant and preparation of *Ligustrum Lucidum*

In addition, oleanolic acid is a broad-spectrum anti-allergy drug which can inhibit the I and II type of hypersensitivity. It is also a good immunomodulator which has the effect of tumor inhibition, transaminase decrease, prevention and treatment of hepatitis and cirrhosis, hypoglycemic action, enhancing white blood cells and immunity enhancement.

Main ingredients of ligustrum lucidum are as follows:

(1) Oleanolic acid: $C_{30}H_{48}O_3$ (A), white needle-like crystals (95% ethanol), m. p. 305~306℃. It is soluble in hot methanol, ethanol, ether, chloroform, acetone and insoluble in water.

(2) Acetyl oleanolic acid: $C_{32}H_{50}O_5$ (B), white druse, m. p. 258~260℃. It is soluble in chloroform, ether, ethanol and insoluble in water.

(3) Ursolic acid: $C_{30}H_{48}O_3$ (C), white needle-like crystals (95% ethanol), m. p. 286~287℃. It is easily soluble in dioxane, pyridine, soluble in hot ethanol, slightly soluble in benzene, chloroform, ether, and insoluble in water.

1. Experimental Purpose

(1) Master the technology of extraction, separation and identification of triterpenoid saponins.

(2) Be familiar with the nature of triterpenoid saponins.

(3) Understand the method of two-phase solvent hydrolysis.

2. Experimental Principle

Using acid hydrolysis and extraction by chloroform to extract oleanolic acid on the basis of the principle that oleanolic acid exists in the form of free type or glycoside in the fruit.

3. Experimental Procedure

3.1 Extraction

Take 50 g meal from fruit peel and put in a round bottom flask, add 350 ml 15% hydrochloric acid solution and 250 ml chloroform, reflux and hydrolyze it for 2 h at 70℃ in a water bath, filter it and take chloroform to extract for preservation (rinse it with water to neutral and dehydrate it with anhydrous sodium sulfate, then filter it). Rinse the residue with water to neutral, filter it with a vacuum pump, and dry the residue to the moisture content of less than 10%. Place the dry residue in a round bottom flask, add 250 ml chloroform and reflux for 1 h. Combine two chloroform extracts which is kept 2 ml for identification of TLC, recover the remaining chloroform till it turns syrupy, shift it to a beaker while hot, and semisolid state appears after cooling.

3.2 Separation and Purification

Method 1: Take former substance of semisolid state to be rinsed by a little benzene in order to remove the fat-soluble ingredients and produce solid precipitation, filter it with a vacuum pump and get buff precipitate. Then reflux for 10 min with 100 times dosage (W/V) of 95% ethanol, filter it and concentrate the filtrate to small volume, stand a while and the coarse crystal appears which can be filtered with a vacuum pump for crude oleanolic acid. Recrystallizing it with 90% ethanol can get purer oleanolic acid.

Method 2: Rinse it with benzene as the method 1, get buff precipitate, add 10 times dosage of 5% sodium hydroxide solution and boil for 10 min, filter it after cooling, then rinse it 1~2 times with appropriate amount of hot water, filter it with a vacuum pump and get white precipitation, reflux with 95% ethanol, filter it at once, adjust the pH value to 1~2 with hydrochloric acid, and stand a while for crystallization. Filter it and get crude

Chapter 4　Extraction and Separation of Various Compositions

oleanolic acid. Recrystallizing it with n-hexane-ethanol (1 : 1) can get purer oleanolic acid.

3.3　Identification

(1)Color reaction: Take a little oleanolic acid and put in a test tube, add 1 ml acetic anhydride for solubility, drop several drops of sulfuric acid along the test wall, and a purple ring appears at the junction of the two liquid layers.

(2)Identification of TLC.

TLC plate: silica gel G-CMC-Na plate.

Dropping sample: chloroform extract of ligustrum lucidum, homemade oleanolic acid ethanol solution, standard oleanolic acid ethanol solution(1 mg/ml).

Developer: Choose either chloroform-acetone (95 : 5) or cyclohexane-ethyl acetate (8 : 2).

Color: Spray methanol solution of 10% sulfuric acid, bake to show color at 105℃, inspect it under sunlight and UV light (365nm).

4. Notice

(1)The content of oleanolic acid in *Ligustrum lucidum* is great difference because of different harvest seasons and different producing areas. You should increase or reduce the dosage of raw medicinal material according to the content.

(2)Controlling the dosage of benzene for rinsing the solution can avoid the loss of ingredients. You can replace benzene with petroleum ether.

5. Experimental Supplies and Arrangement of Class Hour

Experimental supplies: fruit peel, round bottom flask, hydrochloric acid, chloroform, reflux device, water bath, vacuum pump, beaker, benzene, pH test paper, acetic anhydride, oleanolic acid, acetone, cyclohexane, methanol, UV light.

Arrangement of class hour: to be completed within 6 class hours.

6. Questions

(1)What are the benefits of the peel as raw material?

(2)What is the principle of two-phase solvent hydrolysis?

(3)What is the significance of saponification reaction used in this experiment?

(4)What is the difference between oleanolic acid and ursolic acid? How to discriminate them in TLC? Try to tell their separation methods.

New Words and Phrases

　　oleanolic acid　石竹素,齐墩果酸
　　ursolic acid　乌索酸
　　acetyloleanolic acid　乙酰齐墩果酸
　　oleuropein [ˌəʊlɪˈjʊərəpiːn] *n.* 橄榄苦苷
　　stearic [stɪˈærɪk] *adj.* 硬脂的;硬脂酸的
　　mannitol [ˈmænɪtɒl] *n.* 甘露醇
　　pentacyclic [ˌpentəˈsaɪklɪk] *adj.* 五环的

broad-spectrum 广谱的；用途广泛的
allergy ['ælədʒɪ] n. 过敏性反应；厌恶
hypersensitivity [,haɪpəsensə'tɪvɪtɪ] n. 过敏症；高灵敏度
immunomodulator ['ɪmjʊnəʊmɒdjʊleɪtə] adj. 免疫调节剂
transaminase [træn'zæmɪneɪz] n. 转氨酶，氨基转移酶（等于 aminotransferase）
hepatitis [,hepə'taɪtɪs] n. 肝炎
cirrhosis [sɪ'rəʊsɪs] n. 硬化；肝硬化
hypoglycemic [,haɪpəʊglaɪ'siːmɪk] adj. 血糖过低的，低血糖症的
ligustrum lucidum 女贞
dioxane [daɪ'ɒkseɪn] n. 二氧六环；二氧己环
semisolid [,semɪ'sɒlɪd] adj. 半固体的 n. 半固体
buff [bʌf] n. 浅黄色；软皮

Section 7　Steroids

Experiment　Extraction and Identification of Diosgenin

Diosgenin is commonly known as Chinese yam saponin, which exists in plants of Dioscoreaceae. Its content is about 1%～3%. There are many species and resources of Diocoreaceae in China. Raw materials of diosgenin production mainly exist in *Dioscorea zingiberensis* C. H. Wright that is commonly known as turmeric (see fig. 4-19), and *D. nipponica* Makino that is commonly known as yam, whose rhizomes are raw materials for extracting diosgenin.

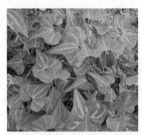
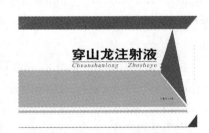

Fig. 4-19　Plant and preparation of *Dioscorea zingiberensis*

Dioscin belongs to steroidal saponins which can be hydrolyzed into diosgenin that is an important raw material of synthesizing steroid hormone and steroid contraceptive in modern pharmaceutical industry. Dioscin is amorphous powder or needle crystal whose melting point is 288℃. It is soluble in methanol, ethanol, and formic acid, hardly dissolve in acetone and weak polar organic solvents, and insoluble in water. Diosgenin is white powder whose melting point is 204～207℃. It is soluble in organic solvent, formic acid and insoluble in water.

1. Experimental Purpose

(1) Master the physical and chemical properties of steroidal sapogenins.

(2) Be familiar with the method of extracting and separating steroidal sapogenins (lipotropic and neutral compositions).

(3) Understand the inspection method of steroidal sapogenins.

2. Experimental Principle

This experiment is to extract diosgenin from the raw materials of *Dioscorea nipponica* Makino that contain a variety of steroid saponins which can be divided into water soluble saponins and water insoluble saponins. Total saponins can be hydrolyzed into diosgenin whose content is 1.5%~2.6%. Because diosgenin is insoluble in water and soluble in organic solvent, we can extract it from the original plant with continuous reflux extraction by petroleum ether.

3. Experimental Procedure

3.1 Preliminary Experiment

In the research of natural medicines or Chinese medicine chemical compositions, first of all you should know their chemical composition type in order to choose a proper extraction and separation method, which needs to be based on preliminary experiment of chemical compositions. Preliminary experiment is divided into systematic experiment and single experiment. Systematic preliminary experiment can check all kinds of compositions, while single preliminary experiment is a method of determination of components, which is used in this experiment. In order to find natural drugs or Chinese traditional medicines containing saponins, foam test and hemolysis test can be used for determination of saponins.

(1) Foam test: Take 1 g coarse powder of *D. nipponica*, add some water (1 : 10) and immerse it for 1 h or 30 min at 80 ℃ in a water bath, filter it and get the filtrate for the following test.

Take 2 ml test solution in a test tube, plug the tube mouth and shake it violently so that it produces a large number of persistent foam like honeycomb (it comfirms the existence of saponins).

(2) Hemolysis test: Take 1 ml 2% blood cell suspension, add 8 ml normal saline, and add 1 ml filtrate for foam test. Mix evenly and stand a while. The solution turns from muddy to transparent in a few minutes, and shows hemolytic phenomena (it comfirms the existence of saponins).

3.2 Extraction and Separation of Diosgenin

coarse powder of Rhizoma Dioscoreae Nipponicae (50 g)
↓ put it in a round bottom flask, add 250 ml water, 20 ml H_2SO_4, immerse it for 24 hours at room temperature, heat with mild fire and reflux for 4~6 hours, stand a while it for cooling, pour out the acid water solution

acid dregs of a decoction
↓ rinse 3 times with water, pour it into a mortar, add Na_2CO_3 powder, grind it repeatedly and adjust pH to neutral, rinse it with water, dry it

neutral residue
↓ dry for 12 h at low temperature(80 ℃)

dry residue
↓ put it into a mortar and grind into fine powder, then add it into soxhlet extractor and reflux 4~5 h with petroleum ether(60~90 ℃)

petroleum ether extract
↓ recover petroleum ether to 10~15 ml, put it quickly in a small triangle flask, stand a while for cooling, fiter it.

↓ filtrate   ↓ precipitate
                  ↓ rinse twice with a little cold petroleum ether, dry by fitering with a vacuum pump

crude diosgenin
↓ recrystallize it with anhydrous EtOH or $CHCl_3$-MeOH(9 : 1)

purified diosgenin
↓ make structural transformation

different kinds of steroids

3.3 Identification of Diosgenin

(1)Measurement of physical constants: Measure melting point and optical rotation.

(2)Chemical detection.

①Liebermann-Burchard reaction: Take appropriate sample and add 0.5 ml glacial acetic acid to dissolve it, and then add 0.5 ml acetic anhydride, stir it evenly, drop a drop of concentrated sulfuric acid along the wall of the test tube, observe and record the phenomenon.

②Salkowski reaction: Take appropriate sample and add 1 ml chloroform to dissolve it, then add concentrated sulfuric acid along the tube wall, put it respectively under visible and ultraviolet lamp, observe and record the phenomenon.

③Identification of UV.

UV $\lambda_{max}^{H_2SO_4}$ nm (logε): 334(3.68), 412(4.1), 512(3.52)

④Thin Layer Chromatography.

Adsorbent: silica gel-CMC-Na thin layer plate.

Sample: 5% homemade diosgenin ethanol solution.

Reference substance: 5% standard diosgenin ethanol solution.

Developer: benzene-ethyl acetate (8 : 2).

Chromogenic reagent: 5% phospho-molybdic acid ethanol solution, heating at 105 ℃ to get clear spots.

4. Notice

(1)Raw materials should be fully rinsed to neutral after acid hydrolysis in order to avoid carbonization during the course of drying.

(2) In the process of drying, you should crush caking and turn it over from time to time.

(3) In the process of continuous extraction, check whether the effective ingredients have been extracted completely. Drop a little extract in a white porcelain dish, evaporate the solvent, observe whether it has the residue, and then do the experiment of acetic anhydride-concentrated sulfuric acid. If the reaction is negative, it suggests that the extraction is finished.

(4) The solution containing protein and mucoid substance can also produce foam, but the foam disappears quickly.

(5) The melting point of crude diosgenin can be measured. It should be further recrystallized if the measurement is not qualified.

(6) Blank control should be set to make the phenomenon more clearly in hemolysis test. Its operation method is same as the former's; the only difference is to replace the sample solution with 1 ml physiological saline.

5. Experimental Supplies and Arrangement of Class Hour

Experimental supplies: Rhizoma Dioscoreae Nipponicae, round bottom flask, H_2SO_4, reflux device, mortar, Na_2CO_3, soxhlet extractor, petroleum ether, triangle flask, $CHCl_3$, MeOH, acetic anhydride, ultraviolet spectro photometer, silica gel-CMC-Na thin layer plate, standard diosgenin, benzene, ethyl acetate, phospho-molybdic acid.

Arrangement of class hour: to be completed within 6 class hours.

6. Questions

(1) What reactions can be used to identify steroid saponin?

(2) Try to design a kind of technological process of extracting Rhizoma Dioscoreae Nipponicae and explain the principle of extraction and separation.

(3) What issues should we pay attention to when using petroleum ether as extraction solvent?

New Words and Phrases

diosgenin [daɪˈɒdʒənɪn]　*n.* 薯蓣皂苷元
yam [jæm]　*n.* 薯蓣；甘薯
dioscoreaceae　*n.* 薯蓣科
turmeric [ˈtɜːmərɪk]　*n.* 姜黄,姜黄根
contraceptive [ˌkɒntrəˈseptɪv]　*adj.* 避孕的,避孕用的
dioscin [ˈdaɪəʊsɪn]　*n.* 薯蓣皂苷
honeycomb [ˈhʌnɪkəʊm]　*n.* 蜂窝,蜂巢
hemolytic [ˌhiːmɒˈlɪtɪk]　*adj.* 溶血的
porcelain dish　瓷盘,瓷蒸发皿
acetic anhydride　乙酸酐

Section 8 Alkaloids

Experiment 1 Extraction, Isolation and Identification of Oxymatrine

Sophora flavescen is the dried root of legume *Sophora flavescens* Ait. (see fig. 4-20), which has many effects such as heat-clearing and dampness-drying, disinsection and diuresis. In clinic, it is used for the treatment of disinsection, dysentery, hepatitis, urticaria, eczema, tracheitis, etc. Pharmacology experiment proves that total alkaloids of *Sophora flavescens* have activity of antiarrhythmic and anticancer, and oxymatrine has effect of anti-cancer and anti-aging. Its main chemical components are alkaloids and flavonoids. The main alkaloids are as follows: matrine, oxymatrine, sophoridine, sophocarpine. Their physicochemical properties are listed in tab. 4-3.

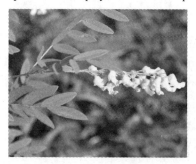
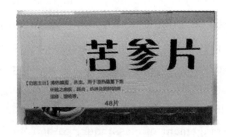

Fig. 4-20 Plant and Preparation of *Sophora flavescen*

^{13}C-NMR data of oxymatrine: 68.7(C-2), 17.0 (C-3), 25.9 (C-4), 34.3 (C-5), 66.6 (C-6), 42.4(C-7), 24.4(C-8), 17.0(C-9), 69.1(C-10), 52.8 (C-11), 28.3 (C-12), 18.5 (C-13), 32.7(C-14), 169.8(C-15), 41.6(C-17).

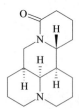 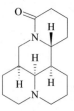 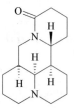

   Matrine   Oxymatrine   Sophoridine   Sophocarpine

Tab. 4-3 Physicochemical properties of alkaloids in *Sophora flavescens*

substance	formula	characters	m.p. (℃)	optical rotation	solubility
matrine	$C_{15}H_{24}N_2O$	white needle crystal	76	+39.11°	dissolve easily in alcohol and chloroform, dissolve in ether, benzene, water.
oxymatrine	$C_{15}H_{24}N_2O_2$	white square crystal	207~208	+47.7°	dissolve easily in water, ethanol, methanol, chloroform, don't dissolve in ether, benzene

Continued

substance	formula	characters	m. p. (℃)	optical rotation	solubility
sophoridine	$C_{15}H_{24}N_2O$	white prismatic crystal	106~108	−63.45°	dissolve easily in water, methanol, ethanol, carbon tetrachloride, etc.
sophocarpine	$C_{15}H_{22}N_2O$	white prismatic crystal	80~81	−29.44°	dissolve easily in water, methanol, ethanol, carbon tetrachloride, etc.

Extracting alkaloids from *Sophora flavescens* generally requires water, acidic water or ethanol. The crude extract can be purified by resin or acid-base method, and column chromatography is often used with alumina or silica gel.

1. Experimental Purpose

(1) Master the principle, operation and impact factors of the percolation method.

(2) Master the principle, characteristic and operation of the continuous reflux extraction.

(3) Learn the method of purification of the crude extract, and learn to analyze the principle of purification process.

2. Experimental Principle

Alkaloids in *Sophora flavescens* include matrine and oxymatrine. Their molecular structures all include two nitrogen atoms. One is the tertiary amine, the other is acid amide. Total alkaloids can react with acids to form salts. After extracting with acid water, alkaloids are in cationic state and can be exchanged by the cation exchange resin. Then alkaloids can be alkalized with ammonia and refluxed with organic solvent.

3. Experimental Procedure

3.1 Pretreatment of Ion Exchange Resin

Add 70 g resin of polystyrene sulfonic acid type (3% of the cross-linking degree) into the beaker, add 200 ml distilled water (80℃) and swell for 30 minutes, pour out the distilled water and add 300 ml 2 mol/L hydrochloric acid, stir it thoroughly and stand a while for half an hour (static transformation), load it in the resin column (2 cm×100 cm), and make all the acid solution pass through the resin column (dynamic transformation). Outflow velocity of liquid should be appropriate. Finally, rinse to neutral with distilled water for use. Notice: Keep the liquid level above the resin bed in the process of packing column to the washing.

3.2 Extraction and Purification of Total Alkaloids

Weigh about 200 g of the root powder of *Sophora flavescens*, add about 260 ml 0.5% hydrochloric acid to keep wet, stir evenly, stand a while for 20 min and pack into the percolator. Then add some 0.5% hydrochloric acid until it flows from the exit, and there is no bubble in cylinder.

Connect the percolator to resin column, calculate the percolation velocity, and then begin to percolate and ion exchange at appropriate flow rate. Check the pH value and alkaloid reaction of the percolation fluid and exchange fluid at the beginning of the experiment and every hour during the course of the experiment, and discuss the reason for change. Stop the experiment when the extraction finishes completely or the resin is completely saturated.

Wash the resin to neutral with distilled water after stopping the percolation, pour out the water layer, add the resin into the enamel dish, pave it and dry in the air. Weigh the dried resin and put it into the beaker, add 14% ammonia to keep humid (the resin swells fully and has no excessive water), cover it and stand for 20 minutes. Then add it into Soxhlet extractor, use 300 ml 95% ethanol to extract alkaloids for approximately 6 hours, and pay attention to check whether the alkaloids have been extracted completely in the process. Recycle the resin after stopping the experiment; add the extract into a 500 ml Erlenmeyer flask for preservation.

3.3 Obtainment of Crude Oxymatrine

Recover and concentrate ethanol in the extract at atmospheric pressure to a small volume (about 6 ml), add 70~80 ml chloroform to dissolve it, shift it to a separatory funnel, stand for layering, separate the chloroform layer and preserve oily substance. Dry the chloroform solution with anhydrous sodium sulfate for 1 to 2 hours (oscillate during the course of drying), and recover chloroform to dry. The residue is recrystallized with acetone, get the precipitation of yellow-white solid, and stand a while. Collect the precipitate by pump filtration, wash with a little acetone, get crude oxymatrine, put it into desiccator, and then preserve mother liquor. The crude is recrystallized with acetone for several times, which can get refined oxymatrine.

3.4 Separation of Oxymatrine

(1) Identification of crude product (exploration of separation conditions):

Methods: Silica gel HF_{254}-CMC alkaline thin layer.

Adhesive: 0.5% CMC solution-4% NaOH (9:1) (5 cm×15 cm, 4 pieces each person)

Developer:

①chloroform-methanol (4:1).

②chloroform-methanol-hydroxide ammonium (5:0.6:0.3 lower layer).

③chloroform-methanol-hydroxide ammonium (10 ml:1.2 ml:2 drops).

④benzene-acetone-ethyl acetate-ammonium hydroxide (2:3:4:0.2).

(2) Separation of oxymatrine.

①Preparative thin layer chromatography:

Glass plate: 20 cm×20 cm.

Silicon HF_{254}: 20 g.

Adhesive: the same with the former (identification of crude product), dosage is 60 ml or so.

Sample: 300 mg oxymatrine crude product.

Developer: customize, dosage is 250 ml/4 person.

Color reaction: customize.

Elution: Scrap the oxymatrine ribbon, add it into the elution column, elute with mixed solvent of chloroform-methanol (7 : 3) until the elution has no alkaloid, and recover the solvent. Dissolve the residue in acetone, filter it, recover acetone to small volume, and stand a while. Filter and collect the crystal after complete crystallization, and dry it.

②Flash column chromatography:

Column dimensions: 2 cm × 50 cm.

Adsorbent: flash column silica gel 35 g passing 230~400 mesh.

Pressure: 0.3~0.5 kg/cm^2.

Sample: 120 mg refined oxymatrine dissolved in 1 ml chloroform, pack column by wet column method.

Eluent: chloroform-methanol-ammonium hydroxide (5 : 0.6 : 0.3) (fully oscillate, stand a while, use lower layer).

Elution: Collect a portion of 5 ml which is identified by alkaline silica gel thin layer, combine the portions with a single color point, recover the solvent, and get the purified oxymatrine.

3.5 Structural Identification of Oxymatrine

(1) Purity testing: Check by TLC, with optional conditions.

(2) Determination of the m.p.

(3) Determination of the product IR and the MS, ^{1}H-NMR spectrum.

4. Notice

(1) Flavescens meal should pass 10 mesh sieve, which won't make it too thick or too thin.

(2) Resin should be fully expanded with water before use, otherwise it has low exchange efficiency and poor reproducibility.

(3) The residual developing agent on TLC plate should volatilize in air before spraying the chromogenic reagent of modified potassium iodide.

5. Experimental Supplies and Arrangement of Class Hour

Experimental supplies: Soxhlet extractor, percolator, cation exchange resin, 500 ml beaker, 100 ml beaker, 10 ml beaker, 10 ml test tube, test tube rack, pallet scales, measuring cylinder, triangular funnel, Buchner funnel, water bath, 10 cm × 20 cm thin layer board, 10 cm × 20 cm thin layer chromatography tank, capillary for dropping sample, ultraviolet lamp, glass rods, bone spoon, adsorbent cotton, reagent spray bottle, small air compressor, chromatographic column (φ1.5 cm), flavescens meal, filter paper, pH test strips, hydrochloric acid, acetone, improved bismuth potassium iodide reagent, the thin layer with silica gel H, 0.5% CMC-Na, 4% sodium hydrate, reference substance of methanol, matrine and oxymatrine. Developer of matrine: toluene-ethyl acetate-methanol-water (2∶4∶2∶1, store at 10℃ and take the upper solution). Developer of oxymatrine: chloroform-methanol-concentrated ammonia solution (5∶0.6∶0.3, store at 10℃ and take the lower solution), NaCl, anhydrous sodium sulfate.

Arrangement of class hour: to be completed within 12 class hours.

6. Questions

(1) What is the principle of acidic water extraction and ion exchange purification in alkaloids?

(2) How to check: ①whether the sample contains the alkaloid in percolation liquid? ②whether alkaloids are exchanged in resin? ③whether ion exchange resin is saturated?

(3) Please sketch out the principle and characteristics of Soxhlet extractor.

(4) What is the flash column chromatography? What are their advantages and disadvantages?

(5) What are the characteristics of the preparative thin layer chromatography?

(6) Please sketch out the procedure of extraction, separation and identification of alkaloids and analyze the spectrum datum of oxymatrine.

New Words and Phrases

oxymatrine [ɒk'sɪmətrɪn]　*n.* 氧化苦参碱

sophora flavescen　苦参

legume ['legjuːm]　*n.* 豆科植物,豆类蔬菜

disinsection [ˌdɪsɪn'sekʃən]　*n.* 昆虫扑灭;除虫

diuresis [ˌdaɪjʊə'riːsɪs]　*n.* 多尿,利尿

dysentery ['dɪsənˌteriː]　*n.* 痢疾;脏毒

urticaria [ˌɜːtə'kɛərɪə]　*n.* 风疹;隐疹;荨麻疹

eczema ['eksəmə]　*n.* 湿疹

tracheitis [ˌtreɪkɪ'aɪtɪs]　*n.* 气管炎

antiarrhythmic [ˌæntɪə'rɪθmɪk]　*adj.* 抗心律失常的,抗心律不齐的

anti-aging ['æntɪ'eɪdʒɪŋ]　*n.* 抗衰老

sophoridine　槐定,槐定碱

sophocarpine [səʊfə'kɑːpiːn]　*n.* 槐果碱

matrine ['mætʃiːn]　*n.* 苦参碱

polystyrene [ˌpɒlɪ'staɪəriːn]　*n.* 聚苯乙烯

sulfonic [sʌl'fɒnɪk]　*adj.* 磺酸基的

hydroxide [haɪ'drɒksaɪd]　*n.* 氢氧化物

ammonium [ə'məʊnjəm]　*n.* 铵

customize ['kʌstəˌmaɪz]　*vt.* 定制,定做

bismuth ['bɪzməθ]　*n.* 铋

potassium [pə'tæsiːəm]　*n.* 钾

Experiment 2 Extraction, Separation and Identification of Berberine from Phellodendron Bark

Cortex phellodendron comes from the dry bark of *Phellodendron chinense* Schneid (see fig. 4-21). Berberine belongs to quaternary ammonium alkaloids, which is yellow needle crystal, soluble in water, and has larger solubility in hot water and ethanol. But it is difficult to be soluble in acetone, chloroform or benzene, and its salt has smaller solubility in water, such as berberine hydrochloride that is insoluble in cold water (1 : 500) but soluble in hot water. Berberine and its salts have good antibacterial effect that is used for the treatment of dysentery and general inflammation in clinical practice.

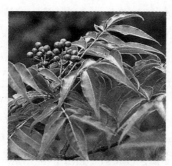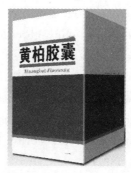

Fig. 4-21 **Plant and preparation of *Phellodendron Chinense* Schneid**

Berberine

Berberine mainly exists in coptis, phellodendron, barberry and other Chinese herbs. The content range of Berberine is from 1.4% to 4% (higher content in Cortex Phellodendron Chinese). It is yellow crystal, containing 5.5 molecules of crystal water, m. p. 145℃. It is slowly soluble in cold water (1 : 20), slightly soluble in cold ethanol (1 : 100), easily soluble in hot water and ethanol, slightly soluble or insoluble in benzene, chloroform and acetone. Its nitrate is hardly soluble in water, its hydrochloride is slightly soluble in cold water (1 : 500), but more easily soluble in boiling water, and its sulfate and citrate have high solubility in water (1 : 30). Berberine is a yellow crystal and containing bimolecular crystal water. It is decomposed at 220℃, changed into brownish red berberis, and melt completely at 285℃.

1. Experimental Purpose

(1) Master the general principle and method of extraction, separation and identification of berberine from phellodendron bark.

(2) Be familiar with the application of percolation and column chromatography in the

active ingredient of Chinese herbal medicine.

2. Experimental Principle

Berberine is a quaternary ammonium base whose free type has high solubility in water, but its hydrochloride has low solubility in water. Using the solubility and its characteristic of containing mucoid substances, we can first precipitate mucoid substance with lime milk, extract berberine with alkaline water, and add the hydrochloric acid to change it into precipitation of berberine hydrochloride.

3. Experimental Procedure

3.1 Extraction

Install the percolator whose bottom is covered with gauze, fix it on an iron stand with iron circle and iron clamp, and tighten the screw clamp at the lower latex pipe.

Weigh 50 g meal (decoction pieces should be properly smashed), put it in a beaker, add lime milk and stir evenly (the meal should be kept humid without excessive liquid). Load the percolator while pressing tightly with a glass rod, smooth it to keep the meal even, cover a round filter paper at the top of meal surface, then add some small stones on the filter paper, and pour into 500 ml saturated limewater slowly along the percolator wall and try to keep the liquid colorless above the meal. Percolate after soaking for 2 hours, control the flow rate to 5 ml/min, collect 500 ml percolation liquid, add the salt whose volume is 7% volume of percolation fluid (W/V), stir and stand overnight, and get precipitation and filter it (do not shake the precipitate before filtering; first use a dropper to adsorb the most supernatant). Wash the precipitation with distilled water to neutral, dry at 80℃, and get crude berberine hydrochloride.

3.2 Refinement

(1) Add some crude product (about 60~80 ml, gradually add the boiling water) into the boiling water and dissolve it in a water bath, filter it while hot. Heat the filtrate in a water bath to clarification, add concentrated hydrochloric acid and adjust pH to 2~3, stir and keep cooling, filter it with filter paper, wash the precipitate with distilled water to neutral, dry at 80℃, and get berberine hydrochloride crystal.

(2) Column chromatography.

Adsorbent: neutral alumina.

Eluent: 95% ethanol.

Sample solution: Take a little berberine hydrochloride crystal and dissolve in 95% ethanol.

Dry column method (packed dosage is 2/3 length of the column), add the sample, elute with 95% ethanol to colorless and concentrate in a water bath (do not use the stove) to a small volume (about 10 ml), and stand a while for crystallization.

3.3 Identification

(1) General identification of alkaloids. Take a little refined berberine, dissolve it in acidic water, divide the solution into four portions, and drop the following reagents respectively:

①Bismuth potassium iodide reagent (Dragendorff reagent), observe the color of the precipitation.

②Mercuric potassium iodide reagent (Mager reagent), observe the color of the precipitation.

③Iodine-potassium iodide reagent (Wagner reagent), observe the color of the precipitation.

④Silicotungstic acid reagent (Bertand reagent), observe the color of the precipitation.

(2) Special identification of berberine.

①Take a little berberine hydrochloride, add a little bleach (or sodium hypochlorite), and the color becomes cherry red.

②Take a little berberine hydrochloride, add 2 ml dilute sulfuric acid to dissolve it, add 1 or 2 drops of concentrated nitric acid, and the color becomes cherry red.

③Take about 0.05 g berberine hydrochloride and dissolve it in 5 ml hot water, add 2 ml 10% NaOH solution, and the color becomes orange. Cool the solution, add about 0.5 ml acetone, stand a while, get yellow crystal of acetone berberine.

④Take a little berberine hydrochloride and dissolve it in 2 ml water, then add a little zinc powder, and gradually drop concentrated sulfuric acid, shake it, drop concentrated sulfuric acid every 10 min and observe whether the yellow fades at last.

4. Notice

(1) Cortex Phellodendron Chinese with higher content of berberine should be used as experimental material.

(2) The purpose of adding sodium chloride is that it will change berberine into berberine hydrochloride whose salting-out effect reduces its solubility in water. The dosage should not be too low, otherwise salting-out effect will be not good and the yield will be too low.

(3) Berberine hydrochloride is almost insoluble in cold water and cooling the solution causes precipitation of the crystal, difficult filtration, and low yield.

5. Experimental Supplies and Arrangement of Class Hour

Experimental supplies: percolation tube, water bath, vacuum pump, thermometer, small chromatographic column, oven, beakers, plastic head dropper, filtration devices, glass rod. Cortex Phellodendron Chinese, lime, neutral alumina, 95% ethanol, acetone, hydrochloric acid, salt, bleaching powder, bismuth nitrate, iodine, potassium iodide, mercuric chloride, acetic acid, sodium hydroxide, silicotungstic acid, distilled water, calcium hydroxide or calcium oxide (add water in a bucket or pot to prepare the lime milk, stand a while and produce for saturated limewater), gauze, filter paper, roll paper, latex tube, pH test paper.

Arrangement of class hour: to be completed within 6 class hours.

6. Questions

(1) How to determine the purity of berberine?

(2) How to identify the chemical structure of berberine?

(3) How to extract and isolate berberine hydrochloride from phellodendron? What is

the principle? Why do we add the lime milk?

(4) When choosing alumina and silicon gel as the adsorbent in order to identify berberine hydrochloride by thin layer chromatography (TLC), what difference do the adsorbents and developers make?

New Words and Phrases

    berberine [ˈbɜːbəriːn]   *n.* 黄连素,小檗碱
    quaternary [kwəˈtɜːnəri]   *n.* 四,四个一组
    phellodendron [ˌfeləˈdendrən]   *n.* 黄柏
    barberry [ˈbɑːbəri]   *n.* 小檗属植物;小檗属植物的浆果
    cortex [ˈkɔː(r)teks]   *n.* 树皮;果皮
    latex [ˈleɪteks]   *n.* 胶乳,橡浆
    bismuth potassium tartrate   酒石酸钾铋
    iodine [ˈaɪəˌdaɪn]   *n.* 碘
    mercuric [mɜːˈkjʊərɪk]   *adj.* 水银的,含水银的
    silicotungstic acid   硅钨酸
    bleach [bliːtʃ]   *vt. & vi.* 漂白;使褪色
                          n. 漂白剂;漂白
    drop [drɒp]   *vt.* 滴;使降低
    salting-out   *n.* 盐析
    bucket [ˈbʌkɪt]   *n.* 水桶;一桶(的量)

Experiment 3   Extraction and Infrared Analysis of Caffeine in Tea

Caffeine is a kind of alkaloid which exists in plants such as tea, coffee (see fig. 4-22), and cocoa. For example, tea contains 1%～5% caffeine, also contains tannic acid, pigment, and cellulose etc.

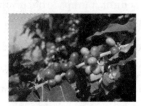 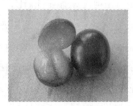 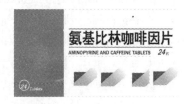

Fig. 4-22   **Plant and preparation of coffee cherry**

Caffeine is a kind of weak basic compound, which is soluble in chloroform, propanol, ethanol and hot water, and hardly dissolve in ether and benzene (cold). Melting point of its pure product is 235～236℃. Caffeine containing crystal water is usually colorless needle-like crystal, but it will lose crystal water at 100℃ and begin to sublimate. It is significantly sublimated at 120℃ and rapidly sublimated at 178℃. This nature can be used to purify caffeine. The structure of caffeine is as follows:

Chapter 4 Extraction and Separation of Various Compositions

Caffeine

Caffeine (1,3,7-trimethyl-2,6-dioxypurine) is a mild stimulant which has the effect of heart stimulating, central nervous stimulating and diuresis. Industrial caffeine is mainly obtained by synthetic. It is the component of Compound Aspirin (Aspirin, Phenacetin, and Caffeine).

1. Experimental Purpose

(1) Master the principle and application of Soxhlet extractor.

(2) Master the principle and operation of sublimation.

(3) Understand the principle and operation of Fourier transform infrared spectrometer.

(4) Be familiar with the infrared preparation method of solid materials—KBr pellets.

(5) Learn the method of qualitative structure identification by IR.

2. Experimental Principle

The extraction method of caffeine contains alkali extraction and Soxhlet extraction. In this experiment, take ethanol as extraction solvent, use Soxhlet extractor to extract caffeine, and then concentrate and sublimate it to get the caffeine containing crystal water.

3. Experimental Procedure

3.1 Experimental Process

Tea fragments $\xrightarrow{\text{reflux extract}}$ Extraction solute $\xrightarrow{\text{distillation}}$ Crude extract $\xrightarrow{\text{evaporate for drying}}$ $\xrightarrow[\text{(2) collect}]{\text{(1) sublimate}}$ Caffeine

3.2 Extraction of Caffeine

Weigh 5 g dried tea leaves, add it into a filter paper cylinder, press it lightly, plug a piece of cotton wool in the filter paper cylinder, put it in a Soxhlet extractor, add 60~80 ml 95% ethanol into a round bottom flask, heat to boiling, extract continuously for 2 h, and stop heating when the condensate goes into the flask because of siphonage.

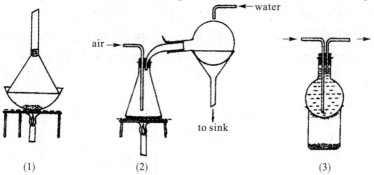

Fig. 4-23 Sublimation device of caffeine

Convert the instrument into a distillation unit (see fig. 4-23), and recover most of the ethanol. Dump the residual liquid (about 10~15 ml) into a evaporating dish, wash the flask with a little ethanol, pour the washing liquid into the evaporating dish, and evaporate it to almost dry. Add 4 g lime powder, stir evenly, heat with a electric jacket (100~120 V), evaporate it to dry and remove all the water. After cooling, wipe off the powder on the edge of evaporating dish in order to avoid pollution.

Cover the evaporating dish with a round filter paper which has many small holes, take an appropriate glass funnel to cover it, and plug a piece of cotton wool to its funnel neck loosely.

Heat the evaporating dish with an electric jacket carefully, and slowly increase the temperature in order to make caffeine sublimate. Caffeine passing through the filter paper holes encounters the inner wall of the glass funnel and becomes solid attached to the inner wall of the glass funnel and filter paper. When white needle-like crystals appear, stop heating, cool it to 100℃ or so, open the funnel and filter paper, and scrape carefully the caffeine attached to the filter paper and funnel wall with a knife into a glass dish. Stir the residue in the evaporating dish, put away the filter paper and funnel, and sublimate once again with higher temperature. At this point, the temperature should not be too high, otherwise a lot of smoke comes from the evaporating dish, which leads to pollution and loss of the product. Combine the collected caffeine, and measure its melting point.

3.3 Identification of Caffeine

(1) Precipitation reaction: Put half of caffeine crystal in a small test tube, add 4 ml water, and heat slightly to make the solid soluble. Put the solution in two test tubes, add 1~2 drops of 5% tannic acid solution in one tube, and record the phenomenon. Add 1~2 drops of hydrochloric acid (or 10% sulfuric acid), then add 1~2 drops of iodine-potassium iodide reagent in another tube, and record the phenomenon.

(2) Oxidation reaction: Add 8~10 drops of 30% H_2O_2 in the rest caffeine on the glass dish, evaporate in a water bath, and record the residue color. Add a drop of concentrated ammonia in the residue, observe and record the change of the color.

(3) Other identification method: Caffeine can be identified by measuring the melting point and determining the spectrometry. In addition, you can comfirm it further by the preparation of caffeine salicylate derivatives. As a kind of alkali, it can react with salicylic acid to produce salicylic acid salt that has the melting point of 137℃. Its chemical reaction process is as follows:

Preparation of caffeine salicylate derivatives: Add 50 mg caffeine, 30 mg salicylic acid and 2.5 ml toluene in a test tube, heat in a water bath and shake it for solubility, then add about 1.5 ml petroleum ether (60~90℃), and cool it in an ice bath for crystallization. If there is no crystal precipitation, rub the tube wall with a glass rod or blade. Use a glass funnel to filter it, collect the product, and measure the melting point. The melting point of pure salt is 137℃.

(4) Determination of infrared absorption spectrum: Solid sample can be prepared by tablet and paste methods. Mix the sample with KBr powder, press it into transparent sheet with about 1 mm thickness, which is called tablet method; grind the sample to fine powder, then stir with liquid paraffin or carbon tetrachloride to paste, and then smear the paste on a KBr wafer.

①Turn on the instrument, open the computer and enter the OMNIC window.

②Pellet method: Take 1~2 mg dry sample into the agate mortar, add about 100 mg potassium bromide powders, and grind evenly. As shown in the fig. 4-24, put lampstand, bed die, bottom die, sample paper and the die body in right order, and then add the sample with KBr powder carefully into the hole of the center specimen paper, press the die body into the die body, and gently rotate to make the potassium bromide powder spread evenly. Put the entire die on the work bench plate of the tablet machine (see fig. 4-24 and fig. 4-25), rotate the handwheel of pressure screw to press the die tightly, rotate oil discharge valve to the bottom in a clockwise direction, then press slowly the handlebar, and observe the piezometer. When it reaches the pressure, stop pressure, stand a while for 2~3 min, and rotate oil discharge valve to the bottom in a anti-clockwise direction. Relieve the pressure to make the piezometer back to "0", unscrew the handwheel of pressure screw, remove the die, and get a transparent tablet fixed in the sample paper hole. Put the sample paper carefully in the middle of the magnetic sample holder for determination of the sample drawing in the next step.

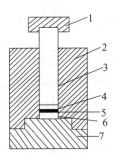

1. pressing lever cap 2. die body
3. pressing lever 4. head die 5. sample paper 6. bed die 7. lampstand

Fig. 4-24 Die structure

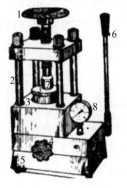

1. handwheel of pressure screw 2. stress bolt
3. workbench plate 4. oil discharge valve 5. machine base 6. handlebar 7. die 8. piezometer

Fig. 4-25 Tablet machine

③Draw the map of IR spectra and retrieve the standard library. The whole process includes the following procedures: Set the collection parameters; collect background datum; collect sample drawing; give baseline correction to the obtained sample spectra; retrieve the standard library; print the spectrum.

④After collecting sample drawing, remove the sample holder from the sample chamber, use the cotton soaked in ethanol to clean the used mortar, tweezers, scrapers and dies, and dry in the infrared drying lamp to prepare for next sample.

4. Notice

(1) Adding quicklime has the effect of neutralization which can remove the tannic acid and other acidic substances. Quicklime must be ground.

(2) When the ethanol is evaporated to dry, the solid easily spills out of the dish, so we must be careful to prevent fire.

(3) Before sublimation, remove the water completely, otherwise water will appear inside the funnel during the course of sublimation. When encountering this case, wipe away water inside the funnel with the filter paper quickly and roast for a moment, and then go on sublimation. If the flask contains some water before extracting caffeine, it will produce some smog that pollutes the container and sample during the course of sublimation.

(4) In the sublimation process we must strictly control the heating temperature because too high temperature will lead to charring of the drying materials and filter paper and bring out some colored materials, which can affect quality of the product. Indirectly heat with small fire during the course of sublimation because too high temperature makes the product become yellow. The thermometer should be placed at the right position so that it can accurately reflect the sublimating temperature. If there is no sand bath, you can also use the simple air bath to sublimate, namely make bottom of the evaporating dish slightly away from the asbestosed wire gauze while heating, and hang a thermometer beside the heat source to indicate the sublimation temperature.

(5) If there is no Soxhlet extractor, we can replace it by reflux extracting device. However, it usually costs more solvent and has lower extraction effect than Soxhlet extractor.

(6) In the process of preparing the sample, sample dosage must be appropriate because excessive sample will obtain too thick tablets which has bad transmittance, and get strong peaks beyond the detection range; less sample will get too thin tablets which get bad signal-noise ratio.

(7) IR spectra should be carried out in a dry environment because transmission parts of the infrared spectrometer are made of potassium bromide or other substances which are soluble in water, and are easily damaged in a humid environment. In addition, water can adsorb infrared light and produce strong adsorption peak which interferes with spectra of the sample.

5. Experimental Supplies and Arrangement of Class Hour

Experimental supplies: tea, 95% ethanol, lime, 60 ml Soxhlet extractor, evaporating dish, glass funnel, Claisen distilling head, receiving tube, 50 ml conical flask, straight condenser; infrared spectrometer, infrared drying lamps, stainless steel tweezers, the sample scraper, agate, sample paper, dies, tablet machine, the magnetic sample holder, cotton wool soaked in ethanol and so on.

Arrangement of class hour: to be completed within 9 class hours.

6. Questions

(1) What color is the precipitation of the reaction between caffeine and tannic acid?

(2) What color is the precipitation of the reaction between caffeine and iodine-potassium iodide reagent?

(3) How does IR spectrum come about? What important structural information does it supply?

(4) Why does methyl stretching vibration appear at high frequency region?

(5) Does it get the exact structure of unknown material only by infrared spectral analysis? Why?

(6) Does sample containing water be directly used to measure infrared spectrum? Why?

New Words and Phrases

caffeine [kæˈfiːn]   *n.* 咖啡因
cocoa [ˈkəʊkəʊ]   *n.* 可可；可可饮料
sublimate [ˈsʌblɪmət]   *n.* 升华物
                         vt. （使某物质）升华；使净化
sublimation [ˌsʌblɪˈmeɪʃən]   *n.* 升华，升华物
propanol [ˈprəʊpənəʊl]   *n.* 丙醇
phenacetin [fɪˈnæsɪtɪn]   *n.* 乙酰对氨苯乙醚，非那西汀（一种解热镇痛剂）
siphonage [ˈsaɪfənɪdʒ]   *n.* 虹吸（作用）
salicylate [sæˈlɪsɪleɪt]   *n.* 水杨酸盐
salicylic [ˌsælɪˈsɪlɪk]   *adj.* 水杨酸的
derivative [dɪˈrɪvətɪv]   *n.* 衍生物，派生物
pellet [ˈpelɪt]   *n.* 小球；小子弹
                 v. 将……制成丸状；把……弄成小球形
paraffin [ˈpærəfɪn]   *n.* 硬石蜡；石蜡
                       vt. 用石蜡处理；涂石蜡于……
tetrachloride [ˌtetrəˈklɔːraɪd]   *n.* 四氯化物
wafer [ˈweɪfə]   *n.* 圆片，晶片
lampstand [ˈlæmpstænd]   *n.* 灯柱；三脚架
handwheel [ˈhændwiːl]   *n.* 手轮，驾驶盘
piezometer [ˌpaɪəˈzɒmɪtə]   *n.* 压力计，压强计

retrieve [rɪˈtriːv] vt. 取回；恢复；检索
head die   模头
bed die   底模
handlebar [ˈhændlbɑː(r)] n. 手把
die n. 钢型，硬模；骰子
quicklime [ˈkwɪklaɪm] n. 生石灰
signal-noise ratio   信号噪音比
tweezer [ˈtwiːzə] n. 镊子，钳子
agate [ˈæɡɪt] n. 玛瑙；玛瑙制（或装有玛瑙的）工具
scraper [ˈskreɪpə] n. 刮刀
potassium chlorate   氯酸钾
hydrogen peroxide   过氧化氢

Experiment 4 Systematic Separation of Corydalis's Alkaloids

Corydalis tuber comes from dried tuber of *Corydalis yanhusuo* W. T. Wang of Papaveraceae (see fig. 4-26), which is mainly produced in Hebei, Shandong, Jiangsu and Zhejiang. It has the effect of invigorating the circulation of the blood, regulating the flow of *qi*, alleviating pain, easing the pain of chest and hypochondria, gastric cavity, gonorrhea or dismantle, blood stasis of post partum, traumatic injury and so on. Its main chemical components are alkaloids (including 0.65% tertiary amine, about 0.3% quaternary ammonium). 20 kinds of alkaloids are separated currently.

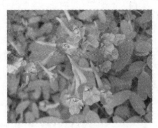
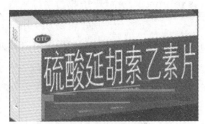

Fig. 4-26 Plant and preparation of corydalis tuber

1. Experimental Purpose

(1) Understand the principle and application of systematic separation of alkaloids.
(2) Master the concrete operating sequences of systematic separation of alkaloids.

2. Experimental Principle

Except water soluble alkaloids, most alkaloids are soluble in organic solvent and insoluble in water, whereas alkaloid salts are soluble in ethanol or water and hardly soluble in organic solvents. Therefore, alkaloid salts cannot be extracted from water solution with ether, so we should add the alkali to trigger alkalization and make alkaloids free. Thus we can extract the alkaloids because free alkaloids are soluble in organic solvents. Commonly used alkaloid extraction solvents are ether and chloroform. Alkaloids can be divided into four types, and physical and chemical properties of alkaloids are connected with their structures. According to their different properties, they can be separated (see fig. 4-27).

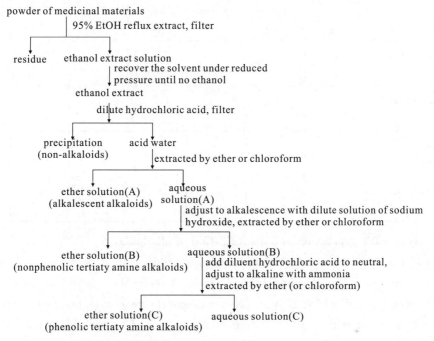

Fig. 4-27 Flow chart of systematic separation in corydalis alkaloids

(1) Alkalecent alkaloid: Because of its extremely weak alkaline, it reacts with acid to yield an unstable salt, which is easy transfered from the neutral or acidic aqueous solution to organic solvent. So it may appear in ether solution A.

(2) Non-phenolic tertiary amine alkaloid: It generally has strong alkaline. Alkalizing its salt makes the alkaloid free, which makes it dissolve in organic solvent. So it is in ether solution B.

(3) Phenolic tertiary amine alkaloid: It reacts with caustic soda (NaOH, KOH or Ca(OH)$_2$) to yield the sodium salt, potassium salt or calcium salt, which makes it soluble in water and insoluble in organic solvent. After acidizing, adding alkali (use ammonia or sodium carbonate) can free the alkaloid which is soluble in organic solvent. So it is in the ether solution C.

(4) Water soluble alkaloid: It contains quaternary ammonium alkaloid, nitrogen oxide, etc. They are soluble in water and insoluble in organic solvents and retain in the final aqueous solution.

3. Experimental Procedure

3.1 Preliminary test

Identify chemical composition according to corresponding experimental method, fill the results in tab. 4-4.

Tab. 4-4 Results of alkaloid precipitation reaction

solution \ sample reagent	preliminary solution	ether solution (A)	aqueous solution (A)	ether solution (B)	aqueous solution (B)	ether solution (C)	aqueous solution (C)
mercuric potassium iodide solution							
bismuth potassium iodide solution							
iodine-potassium iodide solution							
silicotungstic acid solution							

3.2 Systematic separation and identification of alkaloids

Take 10 g corydalis powder, add 15 ml 95% ethanol, reflux for 30 min in water bath, and transfer the extract to a round bottom flask. The residue should be extracted once more by the former method for 10 min. Then combine the two extracts, concentrate it until it has no alcohol taste with a rotary evaporator. Add 30 ml 5% hydrochloric acid, stir it to dissolve, filter it after cooling, and get clear aqueous solution. Add 15 ml 5% hydrochloric acid into the residue, operate once again according to the former method, and combine the two aqueous solution.

(1) Separation of alkalescent alkaloids: Take 8 ml ethyl ether to extract the former acid water solution, take 4 ml solution of ether layer, extract with dilute acid water again, take the solution of acid water layer to react with four alkaloid reagents respectively, and decide whether to extract or not according to the production of precipitation. When precipitation reaction shows negative at last, get ether solution (A).

(2) Separation of non-phenolic tertiary amine alkaloid: Take 2 ml aqueous solution (A), divide it into four portions for precipitation reaction. When precipitation appears obviously, take the rest of aqueous solution (A) and adjust pH$\geqslant$10 with 2 mol/L NaOH. Extract with 8 ml ethyl ether, operate again by the former method, and get ether solution (B).

(3) Separation of phenolic tertiary amine alkaloid: Take 2 ml aqueous solution (B) for acidification until pH$<$3, divide it into four portions for precipitation reaction. When precipitation appears obviously, add 2% hydrochloric acid in the rest aqueous solution (B) for neutralization, then add 5% ammonia and adjust pH to 9 or so, repeat the former operation, and get ether solution (C).

(4) Identification of aqueous alkaloid: Take 2 ml aqueous solution (C) to acidize it with 2% hydrochloric acid until pH$<$3, divide it into four portions for precipitation reaction. If precipitation appears, it indicates that the aqueous solution contains

hydrosoluble alkaloid.

3.3 Experimental Record Format

After organic layer and water layer react with alkaloid reagent under various pH conditions, "−" represents the negative reaction, "+", "+ +" and "+ + +" represent respectively the intensity positive reaction. Record them in tab. 4-4, and infer the type of alkaloids.

4. Experimental Supplies and Arrangement of Class Hour

Experimental supplies: corydalis, 95% ethanol, hydrochloric acid, ether, sodium hydroxide, ammonia, bismuth potassium iodide solution, mercuric potassium iodide solution, iodine-potassium iodide solution, silicotungstic acid solution, pH test paper, rotary evaporator, round bottom flask, dropper, test tube, reflux extraction device, separating funnel, beaker.

Arrangement of class hour: to be completed within 6 class hours.

5. Questions

(1) In the alkaloid precipitation reaction, when checking whether the alkaloid extraction is complete, can we use the ether layer to examine directly? Why?

(2) When the following four components are separated by systematic separation method, which part do they exist in? Ether solution A, B, C, or aqueous solution A, B, C?

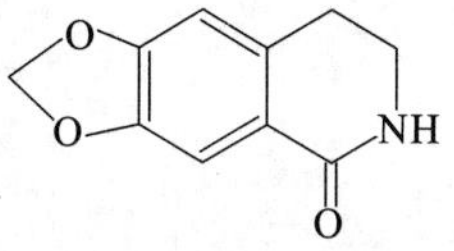

① Noroxyhydrastinine

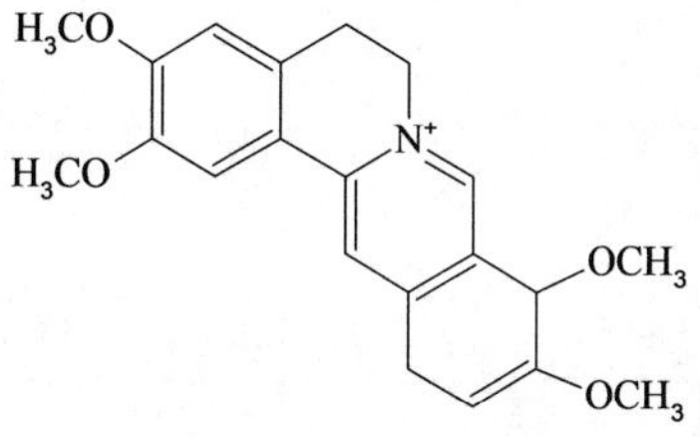

② Dehydrocorydaline

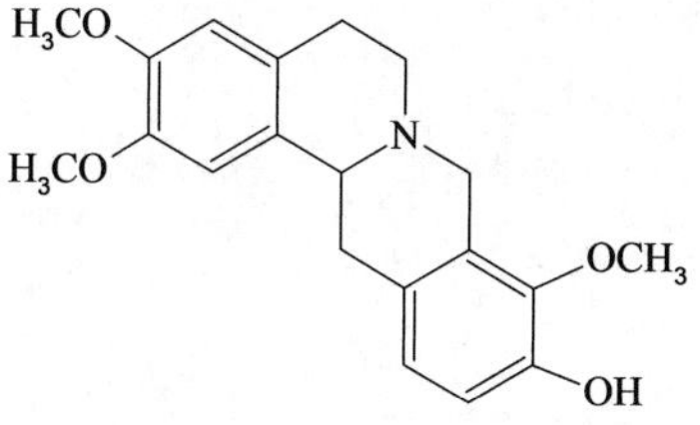

③ Corypalmine

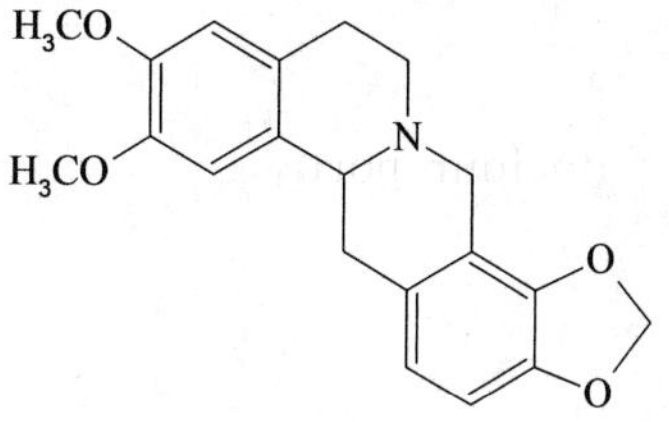

④ Tetrahydrocoptisine

New Words and Phrases

corydalis [kəˈrɪdəlɪs]   *n.* 紫堇属,延胡索
hypochondrium [ˌhaɪpəʊˈkɒndrɪəm]   *n.* 忧郁症,疑病症
gastriccavity [ˌgæstrɪkˈkævɪtɪ]   *n.* 脘,胃脘
amenorrhea [eɪˌmenəˈriːə]   *n.* 无月经(因生病或怀孕);停经
dysmenorrhea [ˌdɪsmenəˈriːə]   *n.* 月经困难,痛经;经行腹痛

post-partum 产后
traumatic [trɔːˈmætɪk] adj. 外伤的，损伤的
alkalescent [ˌælkəˈlesənt] adj. 弱碱性的，碱性的
phenolic [fɪˈnɒlɪk] adj. 苯酚的
tertiary [ˈtɜːʃiˌeriː] adj. 第三的；叔的
amine [ˈæmiːn] n. 胺
basicity [bəˈsɪsɪtɪ] n. 碱度，碱性度
mercuric [mɜːˈkjʊərɪk] adj. 水银的，含水银的
iodide [ˈaɪədaɪd] n. 碘化物
silicotungstic acid 硅钨酸
potassium [pəˈtæsiːəm] n. 钾
dehydrocorydaline [diːhaɪdrəʊkəˈraɪdəlaɪn] n. 去氢紫堇碱
corypalmine [kɒraɪˈpɑːmaɪn] n. 延胡索单酚碱
tetrahydrocoptisine [tetrəaɪdrəʊkɒpˈtaɪsaɪn] n. 四氢黄连碱
stasis [ˈsteɪsɪs] n. 停滞，静止

Chapter 5
Preliminary Test of Chemical Compositions

Section 1 Systematic Preliminary Tests on Chemical Composition of Natural Medicine

There are many kinds of chemical components in natural products, so that we must first understand what kind of chemical compositions they are, such as akaloids, saponins, flavones, etc. The preliminary judge can be done by systematic or single preliminary test, which gives color or precipitation reaction. If the extract has the darker color, it is essential to separate the extract by the thin layer chromatography (TLC) or paper chromatography(PC) before doing preliminary tests, because it may influence the accuracy of color reaction.

1. Experimental Purpose

Master the method of preliminary extraction and separation of natural products and know the operation and identification of color reaction in test tubes, precipitation reaction, PC and TLC.

2. Experimental Principle

The systematic test on the chemical composition of natural medicine by test tubes, PC and TLC give a preliminary judge for the chemical components.

3. Experimental Procedure

On the basis of the different solubility of chemical compositions, three kinds of solvents can be chosen for extraction and identification.

3.1 Water Extract

Take 5 g the crude powder of Chinese herbal medicine, heat it for 1h at 50~60℃ in a water bath, filter it, and do preliminary tests as table 5-1.

Tab. 5-1 Preliminary tests of water extract

chemical compositions	reagent	result
saccharides	* 1. phenol-formaldehyde condensation reaction	
	* 2. Fehling reagent	
organic acid	△ 1. pH test paper	
	△ 2. bromocresol green reagent	
phenols	△ 1% $FeCl_3$	
tannin	△ 1. 1% $FeCl_3$	
	* 2. gelatin reagent	

Continued

chemical compositions	reagent	result
amino acid	△ ninhydrin reagent	
protein	* biuret reaction	
glycoside or polysaccharide	* 1. phenol-formaldehyde condensation reaction	
	* 2. add 6 mol/L HCl to the sample, heat it for several minutes, cool it and produce floc precipitation	
	* 3. add Fehling reagent to observe if the precipitation of Cu_2O increases apparently	
saponin	* foam test	
akaloid	* 1. bismuth potassium iodide reagent	
	* 2. silicotungstic acid reagent	

Remarks: * indicates tube test, △ indicates the test on PC or Silica gel-CMC-Na thin layer plate, similarly hereinafter.

3.2 Ethanol Extract

Take 10 g the crude powder of Chinese herbal medicine, add 5~12 times of 80% ethanol to reflux for 1h in a water bath, filter it, and take 2 ml filtrate for test as table 5-2. Recover the ethanol completely, concentrate it to ointment, and divide it into two parts. Add 2% HCl to one part and shake vigorously, filter it, use the filtrate for test as table 5-3, take a little ethanol to dissolve the filter cake and use the filtrate for test as table 5-4; add a little ethyl acetate to dissolve another part, put the solution in a separating funnel, add appropriate 5% NaOH solution, shake it, which can make phenolic substance and organic acid move into the low layer of NaOH solution. Rinse the upper layer of ethyl acetate solution with water to neutral, take 2~3 ml ethyl acetate solution and evaporate it to dryness in a water bath, and use 1~2 ml ethanol to dissolve it for test as table 5-5.

Tab. 5-2 Preliminary test 1 of ethanol extract

chemical compositions	phenols	tannin	organic acid
reagent	△ 1% $FeCl_3$	△ 1% $FeCl_3$	△ bromocresol green reagent
result			

Tab. 5-3 Preliminary test 2 of ethanol extract

chemical compositions	reagent
akaloids	* 1. bismuth potassium iodide reagent * 2. silicotungstic acid reagent * 3. gallic acid reagent * 4. picric acid reagent
result	

Tab. 5-4 Preliminary test 3 of ethanol extract

chemical compositions	flavonoid	anthraquinone
reagent	△1. 1% AlCl₃ reagent * 2. HCl-Mg reaction	△1. 10% KOH reagent △2. 0.5% Mg(Ac)₂ reagent △3. fumigate with ammonia
result		

Tab. 5-5 Preliminary test 4 of ethanol extract

chemical compositions	coumarin and terpene lactone	cardiac glycoside
reagent	* 1. open-loop and closed-loop reaction △2. 4-aminoantipyrine-potassium ferricyanide color reaction △3. hydroxylamine reaction	△1. Kedde reagent △2. acetocaustin reagent * 3. picric acid reagent
result		

3.3 Petroleum Ether Extract

Take 1 g the crude powder of Chinese herbal medicine, add 10 ml petroleum ether (b. p. 60~90℃), stand a while for 2~3 h, filter it, move the filtrate to a glass-surface vessel for evaporation, take the residue for test as table 5-6.

Tab. 5-6 Preliminary test of petroleum ether extract

chemical compositions	steroids or triterpenes	volatile oil and axunge
reagent	* 1. Liebermann-Burchard reaction △2. 25% phospho-molybdic aicd solution	drop the petroleum ether extract on a filter paper, observe if it has the grease mark which can evaporate while heating.
result		

Identification of cyanogenic glycoside: Take 0.2 g the crude powder of Chinese herbal medicine, put it to a tube, add 3~5 ml 5% sulphuric acid, shake it evenly, place a filter paper strip soaked in sodium picrate solution, plug the tube (don't let the filter paper touch the solution), put the tube into a boiling bath, and heat it for more than ten minutes. If red color appears on the filter paper, it indicates the existence of cyanogenic glycoside.

In addition to color and precipitation reaction, chromatography with the above identification method can also be used for preliminary tests on Chinese herbal medicine, which not only reduces the disturbance among the different chemical components, but also improves the accuracy of the identification according to the characteristics of polarity and solubility (infer according to developing solvent or Rf value).

As is shown in tab. 5-7, preliminary test conditions for different chemical compositions are shown roughly. The proportion of developing solvent should be adjusted according to the specific object.

Tab. 5-7 Preliminary test conditions for different chemical compositions

chemical compositions	type of chromatography	developing conditions	color reagent
phenols	silica gel-TLC	chloroform-acetone (8:2)	1% ferric chloride ethanol solution
organic acid	silica gel-TLC	chloroform-acetone-methanol-acetic acid (7:2:1.5:0.5)	bromocresol green
amino acid	PC	n-butyl alcohol-acetic acid-water (4:1:5, upper layer)	ninhydrin
alkaloid	silica gel-TLC	chloroform-methanol (9:1), fumigate with ammonia	bismuth potassium iodide solution
cardiac glycoside	PC talcum powder-TLC (take formamide as the stationary phase)	chloroform-acetone-methanol-formamide (8:2:0.5:0.5)	xanthydrol
steroids or triterpenes	silica gel-TLC	chloroform-acetone (8:2)	sulphuric acid-acetic anhydride or 5% sulphuric acid-ethanol
anthraquinone	silica gel-TLC	cyclohexane-acetic ether (7:3)	fumigate with ammonia
volatile oil	silica gel-TLC	petroleum ether-acetic ether (85:15)	vanillin-sulphuric acid
coumarin	silica gel-TLC	n-butyl alcohol-acetic acid-water (4:1:1)	spray 5% KOH-methanol, observe the fluorescence
flavonoid glycosides and aglycone	PC	acetic acid-water (15:85), n-butyl alcohol-acetic acid-water (4:1:1)	aluminium muriate
saccharides	PC	n-butyl alcohol-acetic acid-water (4:1:1), acetic ether-pyridine-water (2:1:2)	aniline-phthalic acid

Section 2   Identification Method of the Chemical Composition of Natural Medicine

1. Alkaloid

Sample preparation: Add 2% hydrochloric acid (or 1% acetic acid) to water or ethanol extract of medicinal materials, shift it to a tube, add 1~2 drops of alkaloid precipitation reagents, observe and record the phenomenon such as precipitation, turbidity, crystal and color. The test is also done as follows: water or ethanol extract is dropped on a thin layer plate with a capillary tube, and then add the following precipitation reagent and observe the result compared with the blank sample.

1.1 Precipitation Reagent

(1) Bismuth iodide (Dragendorff) reagent: nacarat or yellow precipitate.

(2) Mercuric potassium iodide (Mayer) reagent: white or light yellow precipitate; black spot appears after heating if it is done on a thin layer plate.

(3) Picric acid (Hager) reagent: yellow crystalline precipitate (add the reagent after

adjusting the pH value to neutral).

1.2 Example of Recording Contents

Samples:

Result and phenomenon:

Analysis of thin layer chromatography:

1.3 Example of Silica gel-CMC-Na TLC

Sample: extract of coptis chinensis and corydalis tuber; standards of palmatine, berberine, jateorhizine and tetrahydropalmatine.

Developer: chloroform-methanol (3 : 1), thin layer plate should be pre-saturated for 5 min in a development tank with ammonia water.

Chromogenic reaction: Observe the fluorescence under UV lamp, and then observe the color after spraying the solution of modified bismuth potassium iodide.

Remarks: choose chloroform as the developer if we use the thin layer plate prepared by neutral or alkaline alumina.

Record: the spectrum of TLC.

2. Phenols and Tannin (identify the water or ethanol extract)

(1) 1% iron trichloride water or ethanol solution reagent: The color becomes blue, green or bluish violet (the test can also be performed on the filter paper).

(2) Ferric chloride-potassium ferricyanide reagent: Take 1% iron trichloride water solution and 1% potassium ferricyanide water solution and mix them together in equal volume before using. Drop the sample solution on the filter paper, then drop the chromogenic reagent, and the blue spot appears apparently. The background becomes blue after it is exposed to the air for a long time.

(3) gelatin reagent: Take 0.5% gelatin water solution and 10% sodium chloride water solution and mix them in equal volume. The precipitate is formed after dropping the reagent, which indicates the existence of tannin.

3. Organic acid (identify the water or ethanol extract)

(1) Inspection of pH test paper: It is acidic.

(2) Bromcresol green reagent: Drop the sample solution on the filter paper, then drop 1% bromcresol green 70% ethanol solution, and then yellow spot appears under the blue background. If the phenomenon is not apparent, spray the ammonia water on it and expose it to the hydrochloric acid vapour.

4. Amino acid, Protein and Glycoside (identify the water extract below 60℃)

(1) Ninhydrin reagent: 0.2% ninhydrin ethanol solution. Drop the sample solution on the filter paper, drop the chromogenic reagent, then heat it in an oven at 110℃ for 2 min, and the purple or blue spot appears if the sample contains amino acid or peptide. In rare cases the yellow spot appears.

(2) Biuret reaction reagent: Take 1% copper sulfate water solution and 40% sodium

hydroxide water solution and mix them together in equal volume, add 1~2 drops of the chromogenic reagent to 1 ml the sample water extract, shake and cool it, and the color turns purple if the sample contains protein.

5. Glycosides, Saccharides and Glucoside (identify the water or ethanol extract)

(1) Aldol condensation reaction (Molisch reagent): 10% α-naphthyl hydroxide ethanol solution, concentrated sulfuric acid. Shift the extract to a tube, add 1~2 drops of chromogenic reagent, shake it and tilt the tube, and add several drops of sulfuric acid along the tube's wall. Purple circular substance produced in the interface of two solutions indicates the existence of reducing sugar.

(2) Fehling reagent.

Solution I: Take 69.3 g cupric sulfate crystal and dissolve in 1000 ml water.

Solution II: Take 349 g potassium sodium tartrate and 100 g sodium hydrate and dissolve in 1000 ml water.

Solution I and II should be mixed together before using. If the following solution produce turbidity, it should be filtered. Mix them in equal volume before using.

Add an equivalent amount of Fehling reagent to water extract of the sample, shake and heat it for 2~3 min in a boiling bath. Red copper oxid precipitate produced in the solution indicates the existence of reducing sugar.

If the sample has no reducing sugar, it can be acidified by 6 mol/L HCl and boiled for several minutes to 0.5h. The production of floc indicates the existence of glycosides or oligosaccharide. Besides, add sodium carbonate to alkalize the extract, then add equivalent Fehling's solution, shake and heat it for 2~3 min in a boiling bath. Red copper oxid precipitate produced in solution indicates the existence of reducing sugar which has been hydrolyzed from glycosides or saccharides. The content of precipitation has apparently increased than before.

(3) Ammoniacal silver nitrate reagent (Tollens reagent).

Preparation: Add 2 ml 5% silver nitrate water solution in a tube, add a drop of 10% sodium hydrate solution, then drop 20% ammonia water solution, and shake it until silver oxide precipitate has completely dissolved (It is not advisable to add the ammonia too much because it can affect the results). The chromogenic reagent should be prepared before using because it is probably arouses hydrolyzed and produces a high explosive precipitate.

Operation: Drop the extract on the filter paper, drop the freshly prepared chromogenic reagent, heat it for 5~10 min at 100℃. It indicates the existence of aldehyde group of reducing sugar if the solution turns puce.

(4) Aminobenzene-phthalate reagent.

Preparation: Take 0.93 g aminobenzene and 1.66 g phthalate and dissolve in 100 ml n-butanol saturated by water.

Operation: Drop the extract on the filter paper, drop the chromogenic reagent, heat it at 105 ℃ for 10 min. Cherry red or brown spot appears if the extract has reducing sugar. General speaking, red spot indicates the existence of aldopentose and 2-ketohexose acid, yet brown spot indicates the existence of aldohexose and 5-ketohexose acid.

(5)(Basic) lead acetate water solution: Add lead acetate water solution to the extract, and it probably indicates the existence of organic acid, mucoid substance, tannin, protein and glycoside if the precipitate appears in the solution. Filter it, add the basic lead acetate water saturated solution, and it probably indicates the existence of glycoside if the precipitate appears.

(6) Iodine solution or potassium iodide-iodine solution (Wagner reagent).

Preparation of 5% iodine chloroform solution: Take 1 g iodine and 10 g potassium iodide and dissolve in 50 ml water, heat it, add 2 ml acetic acid, and dilute it to the volume of 100 ml with water.

Operation: Take 1 ml concentrated water solution of the extract, add five times ethanol, and then the precipitate appears. Filter it, and rinse it with a little hot ethanol. Take the precipitate and dissolve in 3 ml water, add a little iodine solution or Wagner reagent, and observe the different color reactions. For example, the brown spot indicates the existence of dextrin, and blue-black spot indicates the existence of lichen saccharide.

(7) Saponins.

①Foam test: Take 2 ml the water extract from *Discorea nipponica* Makino to a tube, shake it for 1 min. It indicates the existence of saponins if the foam doesn't disappear after 10 minutes. Then take two tubes and add respectively 1 ml the water extract from *Discorea nipponica* Makino, add 2 ml 0.1 mol/L sodium hydrate solution to a tube, add 2 ml 0.1 mol/L hydrochloric acid solution, shake it violently for 1 min, observe the foam produced in the two tubes. It indicates the existence of triterpenoid saponin if the height of foam is similar, and it indicates the existence of steroidal saponin if the height of foam in alkali liquor tube is higher than that in acid liquor tube.

②Hemolysis test: Take two tubes, add 0.5 ml distilled water to one tube, add 0.5 ml water extract from *Discorea nipponica* Makino to another tube, add 0.5 ml 0.8% sodium chloride solution to each tube respectively, shake evenly and then add 1 ml 2% erythrocyte suspension, shake evenly and observe the hemolysis.

Judge the test results according to the following conditions:

Complete dissolution—transparent scarlet solution, no red precipitate in the bottom of the tubes.

Insolubilization—transparent scarlet solution, large amounts of erythrocyte in the bottom of the tubes, shaking the tube produces the precipitate.

(8) Sapogenin: Take sapogenin extracted from the yam and do the following tests.

①3%~10% phospho-molybdic acid ethanol solution: Drop the mother liquid after recrystallized by ethanol on a filter paper or thin layer plate, drop the phospho-molybdic acid reagent, heat it quickly, and the color becomes blue compared with the blank.

②Trichloroacetic acid reagent (Rosen-Heimer reaction): Take a little diosgenin crystal to a dry tube, add the equal amount of trichloroacetic acid, heat for several minutes at 60~70℃ in a water bath. It indicates the existence of steroidal saponin if the solution color turns from red to purple, and indicates the existence of triterpenoid saponin if the solution color turns from red to purple at 100℃.

③Sulphuric acid-anhydride acetic acid reagent (Liedermann-Burchard reaction): Take a little diosgenin crystal to a white porcelain plate, add 2~3 drops of sulphuric acid-anhydride acetic acid reagent, the color changes as the following order: red→purple→blue, and turns to dirty green finally.

④Sulphuric acid reagent: Take a little diosgenin crystal to a white porcelain plate, add 2 drops of sulphuric acid reagent, and the solution color turns from purple to dirty green.

Thin layer chromatography (TLC):

Thin layer plate: Silica gel CMC-Na plate.

Sample: crude product of diosgenin, mother liquid recrystallized by ethanol, refined diosgenin ethanol solution.

Reference substance: standard diosgenin ethanol solution.

Developer: petroleum ether-acetic ether (7:3).

Chromogenic reagent: Spray 5% phospho-molybdic ethanol solution on the thin layer plate, heat it, and blue spot appears.

6. Flavonoids

(1) Hydrochloric acid-powdered magnesium reaction: Take 1 mg rutin or quercetin to a tube, add 2 ml 50% ethanol, heat it in a water bath, add 2 drops of hydrochloric acid, add 50 mg powdered magnesium, and the solution color turns from yellow to red.

(2) Fumigation with ammonia: Drop the extract of flavonoids on a filter paper, fumigate it with ammonia, observe the color under a fluorescent lamp, and bright yellow spot appears.

(3) 1% Aluminium muriate ethanol solution: Drop the extract of flavonoids on a filter paper, drop the chromogenic reagent, and yellow spot or bright yellow fluorescence spot appears under a UV lamp.

(4) Potassium (sodium) borohydride reaction: Take 5 drops of hesperidin to 50% ethanol and dissolve it, add a grain of potassium borohydride, then add a little hydrochloric acid. It indicates the existence of flavanones if the solution color turns from red to purple.

(5) Magnesium acetate reaction: Weigh several milligram of rutin and rutin and dissolve in 50% ethanol solution, take a little solution to a tube or filter paper, add 1% magnesium acetate methanol solution. Yellow fluorescence appears if flavones exist, and cerulean fluorescence appears if flavanones exist.

(6) Concentrated sulfuric acid reaction: Weigh several milligram of rutin on a white perforated porcelain plate, drop a little concentrated sulfuric acid, and the color becomes

orange; dilute it with much water, and then the solution color turns to pale yellow and yellow rutin precipitate appears.

(7) Zirconium dichloride-citric acid reaction: Weigh 0.1 mg quercetin and baicalein respectively and put in two tubes, add a little methanol and heat it in a water bath for dissolution, add 3~4 drops of 2% zirconium dichloride methanol solution, and bright yellow appears if C_3—OH of flavones exists. Then add 3~4 drops of 2% citric acid methanol solution, yellow fades if only C_5—OH of flavones exists, yet yellow doesn't fade if C_3—OH of flavones exists.

(8) Iron trichloride reaction: Take the extract of flavonoids on a filter paper, then drop a little 1% iron trichloride ethanol solution, and observe the color.

7. Coumarins

(1) Fluorescence: Ash bark water solution produces blue fluorescence in the sunlight or under a UV lamp, and produce yellow fluorescence after adding the ammonia.

(2) 1% Iron trichloride water solution: Add several drops of 1% iron trichloride water solution to ash bark water solution, the color becomes blue-green and turns to dirty red after adding the ammonia.

(3) Hydroxamic acid iron reaction (hydroxylamine reaction): Take 1 ml 1% coumarin methanol solution to a tube, add 0.5 ml newly prepared 1 mol/L hydroxylamine hydrochloride methanol solution, alkalize it by adding 0.5 ml 2 mol/L caustic potash methanol solution, heat it in a water bath and cool it. Add 1~2 drops of 1% iron trichloride, acidify it by adding a little 5% hydrochloric acid. It indicates the existence of coumarins, inner ester group or esters if the solution color becomes aubergine.

(4) Gibb's reaction.

Conditions: The test is positive if the structure of coumarin has at least one phenolic hydroxyl group with no para orientation. Blue substance is produced because of condensation reaction between the Gibb's reagent and para-orientating hydrogen of phenolic hydroxyl group.

Reagent A: 0.5% 2,6-dichloroquinone-4-chlorimide ethanol solution; Reagent B: boric acid-potassium chloride-sodium hydrate buffer solution (pH=9.4). Drop respectively 7,8-dihydroxycoumarin and 7-hydroxycoumarin ethanol solution on a filter paper with a capillary tube, blow and dry it, drop the solution A with a capillary tube, dry it in the air, then drop the solution B. The color turns from mazarine to blue on the filter paper.

(5) 4-aminoantipyrine-potassium ferricyanide (Emerson reaction).

Reagent Ⅰ: 2% 4-aminoantipyrine ethanol solution; Reagent Ⅱ: 8% potassium ferricyanide water solution; or 0.9% 4-aminoantipyrine and 5.4% potassium ferricyanide water solution.

Method: Drop the extract on a filter paper, spray the solution Ⅰ on it, then spray the solution Ⅱ on it, the color becomes red; or continue to fumigate it in a sealing cylinder which is filled with 25% ammonium hydroxide solution, the color turns from orange red to crimson.

(6) Closed-loop and open-loop reaction of esters: Take 1 ml the ethanol extract, add 2 ml 1% sodium hydrate, heat it for 3~4 min in a boiling water bath, the solution becomes limpid because of open-loop reaction. Then acidify it with 2% hydrochloric acid, the precipitate or turbidity appears because of the closed-loop reaction.

8. Cardiac glycosides

8.1 Identification of cardiac glycoside

Type A cardiac glycoside can react with active methylene reagent in alkaline solution, and produce a color reaction.

(1) Sodium nitroferricyanide-sodium hydrate reagent (Legal reagent).

Application: It usually applied for identification of unsaturated lactone, methyl ketone or active methylene of cardiac glycoside. Red or purple spot appears.

Preparation of spraying reagent: Take 1 g sodium nitroferricyanide and dissolve in 100 ml mixed solution of 2 mol/L sodium hydrate-ethanol (1 : 1).

(2) 3,5-dinitrobenzoic acid (Kedde reagent).

Application: It is applied for identification of type A cardiac glycoside or α, β-unsaturated lactone. Aubergine spot appears if cardiac glycosides exist.

Preparation of spraying reagent: Take 1 g 3,5-dinitrobenzoic acid and dissolve in 50 ml methanol, and then add 50 ml 1 mol/L potassium hydrate solution.

(3) Baljet reaction: Drop total glycosides ethanol solution extracted from *Digitalis lanata* Ehrh. on a silica gel plate, add one drop of prepared newly alkaline picric acid solution (equivalent mixed solution of picric acid ethanol and 5% sodium hydrate water solution). The color becomes range or orange red (the color can be seen 15 min later because of low reaction speed).

(4) Toluene-sodium-sulfonchloramid-trichloroacetic acid.

Preparation of spraying reagent. Solution I: prepare newly 3% toluene-sodium-sulfonch-loramid water solution; solution II: 25% trichloroacetic acid ethanol solution (available within one day). Take 10 ml solution I and 40 ml solution II and mix them together before use, heat it for 7 min at 110℃, and blue or yellow fluorescence appears under a UV lamp.

8.2 Chromogenic reaction of 2,6-deoxysugar

(1) Keller-Killani reaction: Take 1 mg total glycosides extracted from *Digitalis lanata* Ehrh. and dissolve in 1 ml glacial acetic acid, add a drop of 2% iron trichloride water solution, shift it to a tube, add 0.5 ml concentrated sulphuric acid along the tube wall, observe the color of the interface and the acetic acid layer, the color of acetic acid layer becomes blue if 2,6-deoxysugar exists.

(2) Xanthydrol reaction: Drop total glycosides ethanol solution extracted from

Digitalis lanata Ehrh. on a silica gel plate, add a drop of xanthydrol, heat it for 3 min with hair drier, and the color becomes red.

9. Volatile oil

Preparation of vanillic aldehyde-concentrated sulphuric acid reagent: Take 0.5 g vanillic aldehyde and dissolve in 100 ml mixed solution of concentrated sulphuric acid-95% ethanol (4:1), spray it on thin layer plate, heat it at 105℃, different colors appear in different volatile oils.

Experiment Preliminary Test, Extraction and Design of Separation process of Chemical Components from Herba Clinopodii

Herba clinopodii comes from dry aerial part of *Clinopodium polycephalum* (Vaniot) C. Y. Wu et Hsuan or *C. chinensis* (Benth.) D. Kuntze in the Labiatae family (see fig. 5-1) as a kind of special medicinal material in Anhui Province of China, which has the effect of hemostasis for uterine bleeding, hematuria, epistaxis, traumatic hemorrhage, hysteromyoma hemorrhage etc. Herba Clinopodii has complex chemical compounds, and saponins and flavones are its main components. Its clinical application includes Herba Clinopodii tablet, capsule and granule etc.

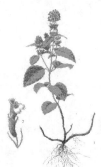
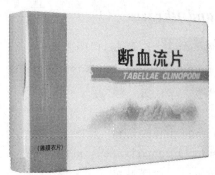

Fig. 5-1 Plant and preparation of Herba Clinopodii

1. Experimental Purpose

(1) Grasp the preliminary test design of Herba clinopodii's chemical compounds.

(2) Be familiar with the design method of extraction and separation process of chemical components from Herba clinopodii.

(3) Understand the commonly used apparatuses, equipments, reagents and drugs during course of extraction and separation process of chemical components from Herba clinopodii.

2. Experimental Procedure

(1) Design different methods of preliminary test to identify the chemical compounds in Herba Clinopodii.

(2) Look up some information and design the process of extracting and separating the

saponins and flavones.

(3) Look up some information and design the separation process of clinodiside A and didymin.

(4) Select a optimal extraction and separation process of saponins and flavones.

3. Notice

(1) Each group of students finish the experimental design, reagent preparation and experimental operation indenpendently. Their process shouldn't repeat with other groups.

(2) Record the advantages and disadvantages of extraction and separation process design according to the yield and discuss the reason.

(3) According to the experiment, students should master the method of consulting literature material, experimental design, reagent preparation, experimental operation and writing a design report, and obtain certain scientific research ability.

4. Questions

Calculate the yield of saponins and flavones according to experimental data, and discuss how to optimize the extraction process on the basis of existing conditions and improve the extraction yield.

New Words and Phrases

gelatin [ˈdʒelətɪn]   *n*. 凝胶,白明胶

ninhydrin [nɪnˈhaɪdrɪn]   *n*. (水合)茚三酮

biuret [bjəˈret]   *n*. 缩二脲

floc [flɒk]   *n*. 絮状物

coeruleum [kəʊˈruːlɪəm]   *n*. 蓝色

bromocresolis [bˈrɒmkriːsɒlɪs]   *n*. 溴甲酚

chrysolepic acid   *n*. 苦味酸

ferricyanide [ˌferɪˈsaɪənaɪd]   *n*. 铁氰化物

acetocaustin [æsɪtəˈkɔːstɪn]   *n*. 三氯乙酸

molybdophosphoric acid   *n*. 磷钼酸

cyanogenic [ˌsaɪənəʊˈdʒenɪk]   *adj*. 生氰的

picrate [ˈpɪkreɪt]   *n*. 苦味酸盐

sulphuric [sʌlˈfjʊərɪk]   *adj*. 硫黄的

formamide [fɒˈmæmaɪd]   *n*. 甲酰胺

triterpene [traɪˈtɜːpiːn]   *n*. 三萜烯

cyclohexane [ˌsaɪklə(ʊ)ˈheksein]   *n*. 环己烷

ammonia [əˈməʊnɪə]   *n*. 氨

aluminium [æl(j)ʊˈmɪnɪəm]   *adj*. 铝的

muriate [ˈmjʊərɪət]   *n*. 氯化物

aniline [ˈænɪliːn]   *n*. 苯胺

phthalic [ˈθælɪk] adj. 邻苯二甲酸的
phthalate [ˈ(f)θæleɪt] n. 邻苯二甲酸酯；邻苯二甲酸盐
picric [ˈpɪkrɪk] adj. 苦味酸的
palmatine [ˈpælməti:n] n. 巴马亭；非洲防己碱
jateorhizine [dʒeɪˈtɔːhaizin] n. 药根碱
tetrahydropalmatine [tetrəaɪdrəʊˈpælmɪti:n] n. 四氢帕马丁，延胡索乙素
ferricyanide [ˌferɪˈsaɪənaɪd] n. 铁氰化物
naphthyl [ˈnæfθɪl] n. 萘基
tilt [tɪlt] vi. 倾斜；翘起
alkalize [ˈælkəlaɪz] vt. 使成碱性；使碱化
nitrate [ˈnaɪtreɪt] n. 硝酸盐
aldehyde [ˈældɪhaɪd] n. 醛；乙醛
aminobenzene [əˌmɪnəʊˈbenzin] n. 氨基苯；苯胺
aldopentose [ˈældəpentəʊs] n. 戊醛糖
ketohexose [ˌki:təʊˈheksəʊs] n. 己酮糖
mucoid [ˈmju:kɔɪd] n. 类黏蛋白；类黏液
            adj. 类黏蛋白的；黏液状的
dextrin [ˈdekstrɪn] n. 糊精；葡聚糖
anhydride [ænˈhaɪdraɪd] n. 酸酐；脱水物
muriate [ˈmjʊərɪət] n. 氯化物
borohydride [ˌbɔːrəʊˈhaɪdraɪd] n. 硼氢化物
cerulean [sɪˈru:lɪən] adj. 蔚蓝的，天蓝色的
quercetin [ˈkwɜːsɪtɪn] n. 槲皮素
baicalein [ˈbeɪkælɪn] n. 黄芩素，黄芩苷元
zirconium [zɜːˈkəʊnɪəm] n. 锆
dichloride [daɪˈklɔːraɪd] n. 二氯化合物
citric [ˈsɪtrɪk] adj. 柠檬的
caustic [ˈkɔːstɪk] adj. 腐蚀性的；苛性的
potash [ˈpɒtæʃ] n. 碳酸钾；苛性钾
aubergine [ˈəʊbəʒi:n] n. 茄子；紫红色
mazarine [ˌmæzəˈri:n] n. 深蓝色
aminoantipyrine [æmɪˈnəʊæntɪpaɪərɪn] n. 氨基比林
magnesium [mægˈni:zɪəm] n. 镁